Noninvasive Ventilation. The Essentials

Series Editor
Antonio M. Esquinas, Hospital Morales Meseguer, Murcia, Spain

Nowadays, Noninvasive Ventilation (NIV) is widely accepted in medical practice. This Series, titled "Noninvasive Ventilation: Clinical and Practice," is a culmination of extensive prior publications on the topic. It aims to define current clinical developments in NIV technologies, including equipment and ventilator modes, and provide practical recommendations primarily in Critical Care (CC), Pulmonary, Emergency, and Sleep Medicine.

Building on previous publications, a group of experienced Editors and top international contributors aim to present new books that take a multidisciplinary approach and provide a comprehensive overview of Non-invasive Ventilation. The main goals of this Series are as follows:

- Establish a scientific reference for NIV clinical practice, covering pathophysiology, clinical indications, and evidence-based concepts
- Present significant advances in CC, pneumology, anesthesiology, sleep medicine, pediatrics, and healthcare organization in acute and chronic respiratory failure
- Analyze technological advancements and complementary procedures associated with NIV, such as aerosol therapy, humidification, and airway clearance, crucial for effective NIV techniques.
- Serve as a valuable teaching reference for healthcare professionals, including residents, consultants, and allied healthcare professionals, as well as undergraduate and postgraduate students and fellowship participants.

The Series will produce focused thematic volumes, led by internationally recognized guest editors, providing comprehensive coverage of specific areas of NIV advancement in CC, emergency medicine, pulmonary, and sleep medicine.

Omar Alibrahim
Umberto Vincenzi • Nabil A. Shallik
Editors

Biphasic Cuirass Noninvasive Ventilation

Science and Clinical Practice

Springer

Editors
Omar Alibrahim
Pediatric Critical Care Medicine
Duke University Hospital
Durham, NC, USA

Umberto Vincenzi
Pneumology and Intensive Respiratory Care Unit
Ospedali Riuniti di Foggia
Foggia, Italy

Nabil A. Shallik
Department of Anesthesiology
Weill Cornell Medicine - Qatar
Doha, Qatar

ISSN 2948-2747 ISSN 2948-2755 (electronic)
Noninvasive Ventilation. The Essentials
ISBN 978-3-032-20932-0 ISBN 978-3-032-20933-7 (eBook)
https://doi.org/10.1007/978-3-032-20933-7

This Springer imprint is published by the registered company Springer Nature Switzerland AG
The registered company address is: Gewerbestrasse 11, 6330 Cham, Switzerland

This textbook exists because of the dedication, skill, and perseverance of countless individuals who care for patients with respiratory failure across ICUs worldwide.

To the respiratory therapists, whose expertise forms the foundation of safe and effective negative pressure ventilation—we are indebted to your vigilance, technical mastery, and unwavering advocacy for patient comfort and dignity.

To the ICU nurses, who remain the constant presence at the bedside, balancing precision and compassion, adjusting therapies minute by minute, and ensuring that complex respiratory support strategies are carried out with extraordinary consistency and care—thank you.

To our critical care physicians, advanced practice providers, fellows, and trainees, whose curiosity and commitment continue to advance the science and practice of NPV—your contributions shape the future of this field.

To the biomedical engineers, innovators, and industry partners who work tirelessly to improve technology, safety, and usability—this book reflects your impact as well.

Our deepest gratitude extends beyond professional roles or institutional walls. We especially acknowledge healthcare workers serving in conflict zones and areas of humanitarian crisis—physicians, nurses, respiratory therapists, paramedics, and volunteers—who continue to deliver care amid bombardment, displacement, shortages, and unimaginable danger. Many have lost their lives over the past several years while trying to save the wounded and critically ill, often children. Their courage represents the highest ideals of our profession. Their sacrifices remind us that medicine is not only a scientific endeavor but also a profoundly moral one.

This book is dedicated to all who serve, teach, innovate, and stand at the bedside—often quietly and anonymously—to improve the lives of patients who depend on us.

Omar Alibrahim, Umberto Vincenzi, and Nabil A. Shallik

About the Book

In the history of respiratory support, negative pressure ventilation has long occupied a unique place—once a lifesaving mainstay, later overshadowed by positive pressure technologies, and now re-emerging with renewed relevance. This textbook arrives at a critical moment, filling an important gap by offering the first comprehensive and contemporary exploration of noninvasive negative pressure ventilation across pediatric and adult critical care.

What distinguishes this work is not only its scientific rigor but also its grounding in the lived realities of bedside care. Negative pressure ventilation, more than many therapies, requires collaboration: respiratory therapists adjusting pressures and seals, nurses monitoring comfort and positioning, physicians interpreting physiology and response, engineers refining interfaces and devices. This book honors that collective expertise and provides a roadmap for clinicians seeking to apply NPV with precision and purpose.

But its significance extends beyond technology and clinical algorithms. This text carries a profound acknowledgment of the global community of healthcare workers whose commitment to caring for the critically ill persists even under the most dangerous circumstances. Numerous clinicians in war zones and humanitarian disasters have lost their lives while treating injured and critically ill patients—often working in makeshift ICUs, basements, field hospitals, or facilities under active siege. Their bravery is not abstract; it is a daily act of service carried out amid risk, scarcity, and fear, motivated solely by the belief that every human life deserves care.

In highlighting these individuals, the editors remind us that critical care is both a science and a calling. It demands technical excellence, but also resilience, courage, and unwavering humanity. This book stands as a testament to that dual identity.

For trainees, it offers clarity.

For seasoned clinicians, it offers depth and renewed perspective.

For the field, it establishes an essential foundation on which future research and practice can be built.

It is a privilege to introduce this remarkable contribution to the respiratory and critical care communities.

Omar Alibrahim
Umberto Vincenzi
Nabil A. Shallik

Contents

Historical and Epidemiological Applications of Noninvasive Negative Ventilation

1

Giancarlo Garuti and John Robert Bach

1.1 Introduction

Negative pressure pulmonary ventilation is based on the idea that applying pressure to the chest, lower than atmospheric pressure, can cause air to flow into the lungs. This is done by creating a pressure gradient that leads to the expansion of the lungs and the reduction of intrapleural pressure. During inspiration, the increase in lung volume leads to a decrease in alveolar pressure, causing air to enter from the outside. Under normal conditions, intrathoracic negative pressure is formed by the contraction of the inspiratory muscles, such as the diaphragm and intercostals. This type of ventilation is essential to understand the operation of devices such as the cuirass ventilator, and for clinical application in different conditions of respiratory failure [1].

The main difference between negative pressure and positive pressure ventilation is that in negative pressure ventilation, the diaphragm is active, and expiration is usually passive, induced by the low pressure inside the chamber. In positive pressure ventilation, negative pressure is imposed on the chest and abdomen, and then positive pressure is imposed on the airway, usually with a valve between the endotracheal tube and the external ambient. If there is partial obstruction of the

G. Garuti (✉)
Pneumology Unit, Santa Maria Bianca Hospital, AUSL Modena, Mirandola, Italy
e-mail: g.garuti@ausl.mo.it

J. R. Bach
Department of Physical Medicine and Rehabilitation, Rutgers University – New Jersey Medical School, Newark, NJ, USA
e-mail: bachjr@njms.rutgers.edu

O. Alibrahim et al. (eds.), *Biphasic Cuirass Noninvasive Ventilation*, Noninvasive Ventilation. The Essentials, https://doi.org/10.1007/978-3-032-20933-7_1

upper airway, mechanical means such as continuous negative pressure are used. CNEP is possible but does not directly assist ventilation any more than CPAP does. These methods are generally used in infants and small children. Negative pressure ventilation (NPV) has very rarely been used for small children. Negative pressure ventilation refers to the mechanical respiration of patients with the chest enclosed in a rigid chamber or cuirass covered with airtight clothing and connected to an apparatus that lowers the air pressure inside the chamber. The resulting negative pressure around the chest expands the lungs by distension of the chest wall, rather like an iron lung.

1.2 History of Pulmonary Ventilation

Since ancient times, writings and references have appeared that intimately correlate ventilation with resuscitation. The history of lung ventilation has ancient roots, with attempts to use positive pressure to aid breathing dating back at least to ancient Egypt. The Bible records that the prophet Elisha resurrected the son of a Shunammite woman by applying mouth-to-mouth resuscitation (2 Kings 4:34-35) [2]. Galen was the first to apply mechanical pulmonary insufflation [3]. Andrea Vesalio, founder of modern anatomy, in his treatise "De humani corporis fabrica", published in 1543, described the artificial ventilation obtained by inserting a cannula into the trachea of animals. In 1667 Robert Hook conducted an experiment based on Galen's theories. He was able to demonstrate how closely connected the respiratory and circulatory systems are, conducting experiments on dogs for which he had provided a hole that connected the lungs with the external environment [4]. In 1732, Thossac succeeded in reviving a Scottish miner through mouth-to-mouth ventilation. From then on, this type of ventilation was widely used both in England and throughout Europe. In 1774, following the discovery of oxygen by Priestly and Whillelm, Lavoisier was able to demonstrate the use and function of ventilation for oxygenation of the blood [5]. In the mid-nineteenth century, several attempts were made to initiate ventilation in clinical practice, initially on animals. In 1908, the New York Times reported the use of the first mechanical ventilator made by Prof. George Poe on asphyxiated animals [6].

Instead, the history of negative pressure pulmonary ventilation has its roots in the nineteenth century, with pioneers such as John Dalziel, Theodor Billroth, and Ferdinand Sauerbach. In 1838, John Dalziel in Scotland first began the application of negative pressure ventilation by enclosing the body in a sealed box and creating negative atmospheric pressure around it using a bellows in the treatment of a patient who had suffered respiratory paralysis as a result of polio: The patient was placed inside a box leaving only the head outside [7]. The negative pressure that was generated inside the metal structure allowed the lungs to expand and therefore, the patient to "breathe". Initially, operation was by manually operating a pump system, which was replaced by an electrical system in 1927 [8].

1.2.1 The Iron Lung

The essential concept of a negative pressure ventilator was developed by Woillez in 1876, but it was impractical since the negative pressure was generated by manually operated bellows. In 1904, Sauerbruch introduced a technique to overcome this problem, which he called the "negative pressure" ventilation method [9]. With this technique, the lungs were kept expanded by placing the patient's body inside a chamber where the pressure was cyclically lowered below atmospheric, while his head remained outside, allowing the patient to breathe air in a normal atmospheric pressure environment.

From this period onward, various ideas about negative pressure ventilation have developed.

One of the first attempts was Thunberg's "*Barospirator Tank*": this was also a tank style ventilator. Dr. T. Thunberg produced it in 1920 in Scandinavia [10]. The entire patient was placed in the tank and the pressure changed rhythmically into positive and negative due to the presence of a connection with a cylinder. The later versions had been scaled up to room size to accommodate medical staff inside it. The results of treatment with the "Barospirator" were scarce.

Another negative pressure device was Dr. Eisenmenger's *Biomotor Cuirass* that appeared in the second half of the 20 s. In 1927, Eisenmenger registered in the United States, a motorized version of his cuirass "Dr Eisenmenger's Biomotor" [11]. The power unit was a half-horse power fan motor. The shell of the "Biomotor" cuirass had a soft rubber sack that was pushed onto the abdomen during exhalation by positive pressure. A systematic use of this device appeared from 1935.

In 1926, in Germany, Wilhelm Schwake patented a "*pneumatic chamber*". This device was portable but negative pressure was provided by large bellows operated by the erect patient: this machine was not useful for very ill patients.

In 1928, an engineer, Philip Drinker, a pediatrician, Charles F. McKhann, and physiologist, Louis A. Shaw, at Harvard Medical School, announced the development of America's first mechanical tank ventilator [12].

The first "*iron lung*" was a cylinder sealed at one end (Fig. 1.1a). The other end had a flat lid to which a rubber collar was attached. Head and neck protruded through the collar and rested on an adjustable support attached to the outside of the tanktag. The patient was lying on a frame covered by a mattress. This ran on rails welded to the sides of the tank. The tank was hermetically sealed between the cylinder with the locks for commercial refrigerators. Into the sides of the cylinder had been placed portholes for the observation of patients and for nursing care. Other small sealed holes were designed to insert medical instruments such as pressure gauges (a simple water pressure gauge measured internal pressure, which in turn was regulated by a variable leak on top of the cylinder), blood pressure cuffs, stethoscopes, etc. The pumps were manufactured by the Electric Blower Company of Boston [13]. The pumps ran continuously and the positive and negative pressure was fed into the tanks via a valve system. In the following years, several new versions were produced: the *Collins Drinker tank*, the *Emerson iron lung* [14], the *Henderson tank*,

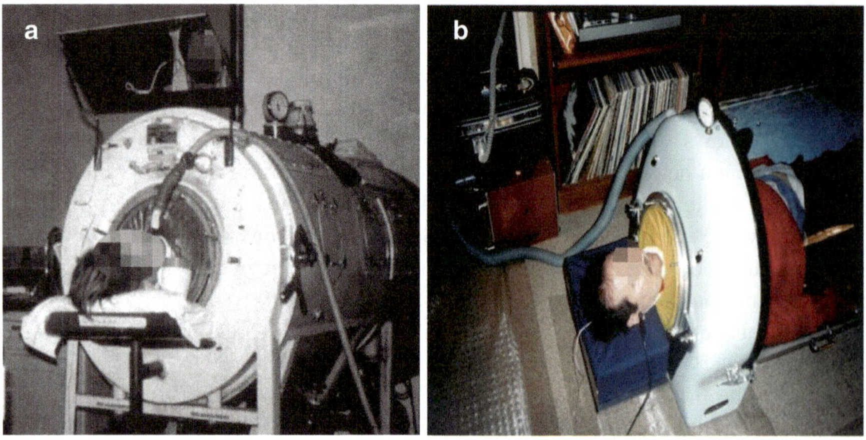

Fig. 1.1 (**a**) Example of Iron lung user supplementing negative pressure with mouthpiece positive pressure ventilatory support, 1b Example of Portalung, a 110 (**b**) tank respirator operative by negative pressure ventilator

and the Both Cabinet Respirator (Fig. 1.1b). Drinker showed his respirator in the UK in 1931. Siebe Gorman began production of the Drinker respirator in Britain in 1934. The main use of the respirator was for poliomyelitis patients.

Due to the massive polio epidemic in the United Kingdom in 1938, the only device available was the Drinker iron lung and the *Bragg-Paul "pulsator"* [15]. Sir William Bragg, the Nobel Prize-winning physicist, produced a pneumatic belt made of rubber football bladders that were tied around the abdomen and lower chest. The bladders were inflated by a small air pump. The abdomen was compressed and the chest was lowered. Robert W. Paul improved the belt by making it of hollow rubber hoses. The belt has been used successfully in many cases. Unfortunately, the rapid deterioration of the rubber created some problems.

In 1938, a Medical Research Council committee reviewed all respirator devices available and recommended models to be purchased and when and where they should be distributed. Prior to the first meeting of the Committee, Lord Nuffield declared that respirators would be provided free of charge, both cuirass and tank respirators, to any hospital in the Empire. His declaration changed the MRC Committee's mandate into decisions on the distribution of this generous offer. Many respirators (like the Both Cabinet Respirator) were difficult to store (for their size), so they were placed in regional centers and distributed as needed (as the Wingfield Morris Orthopaedic Hospital in Oxford for the Oxford area).

The development of the tank from 1929 was much faster than the cuirass (Fig. 1.2). The next commercially available cuirass after the *Biomotor* did not appear until 1930 when Sahlin, working at the Institute of Physiology in Lund, Sweden, developed a cuirass produced by the Stille—Werner family of Stockholm [16]. The cuirass had a shell made of a sheet metal with a rubber edge and bolted to an operating table on which the patient was treated. The power unit could

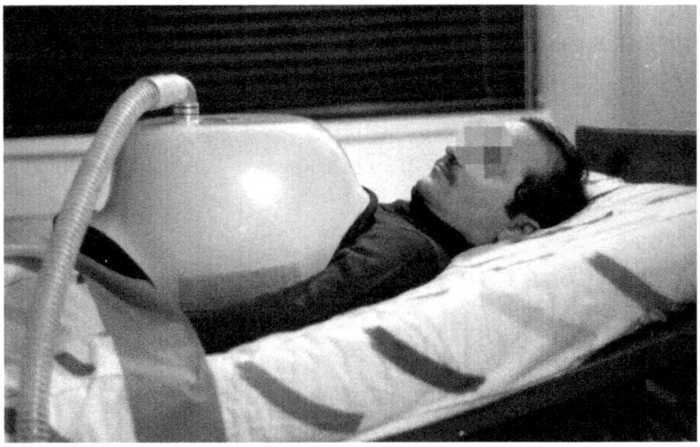

Fig. 1.2 Example of Cuirass Shell Ventilation used by patient with 0 ml of vital capacity for sleep for 11 years

provide both negative and positive pressure. A 21-year-old medical student with polio was kept alive for 7 months using the Sahlin cuirass, and it was reportedly used by 827 victims of polio, of which 127 survived. P. Peterson produced the *Pulsatorgurtel* [17], a portable cuirass unit for emergency resuscitation in places such as swimming pools. The energy source was a gas cylinder (with 95% oxygen and 5% carbon dioxide). Leather straps narrowed the lower chest and abdomen. To initiate the inhalation, the gas was directed through a valve that inflated the balloon and moved the metal plates apart, filling the cylinder. A spring in the piston returned the cuirass to the expiratory position and the balloon collapsed under the weight of the patient when the valve closed the gas supply. The exhaust gas passed through a Venturi valve to drag in the air and pass it to the head piece. This produced external respiratory support in an atmosphere with 70% oxygen in the air. This complex device had not popular use.

In 1937, at the beginning of a serious polio epidemic in the state of Victoria, Australia, there were only two tank respirators, but by the end of the year there were 200 in operation. Aubrey Burstall, Professor of Engineering at the University of Melbourne, produced the *Burstall Jacket* [18]. After the presentation (on January 27, 1938), a week later, this device went into clinical use at Melbourne Children's Hospital. This cuirass was made of a piece of aluminum hammered down to the shape of the chest and abdomen down to the waist. A rubber sponge vest one inch thick protected the patient from the shell. A tight seal was achieved with rubber sheet sleeves and collar. For energy source, the Drinker power unit was used, but due to its small volume, different liners could be run from a single power source.

The Burstall jacket was not a replacement for the tank respirator, but a cheaper and more portable device for patients in the convalescence phase of the disease. The device had the advantages as price, portability, ease for treating patients in splints in regular hospital beds, and ease of sterilization of the unit. The disadvantages were the time to dress the patients with the jacket (this was normally 7 min and could be 10–12 min if the patient was in an ordinary bed) and to get an airtight seal.

Burstall sent a sample jacket to Dr. Andrew Topping of London County Council (LCC). On the basis of this was developed another kind of cuirass jacket, the LCC cuirass [19]. This was made in two bolted halves together with wing nuts: the arm holes and in the airtight seal were modified, for easier application and greater freedom for the patient. The appliance had its own 1/8 hp. electrical power supply unit. This operated a small suction bellows at a fixed speed of 20 rpm with a maximum negative pressure of 25 cmH_2O. The negative pressure was controlled by a variable leak valve on the jacket. There was a manual mechanism if the power unit failed.

1.2.2 The Cuirasses

During World War II, the development of these respirators halted and new models did not appear until the late 1940s. The years 1948–1950 saw several new American cuirasses with the following examples:

1. *Blanchard's Portable Plastic Respirator*
   This was developed by Bergene Inc. of Los Angeles. It was a type of jacket made of plastic using an electric drive [20].
2. *The Chestspirator*
   The Chestspirator was a portable chest respirator (Fabrikators Inc. of Boston, Massachusetts): it was probably the first thoracoabdominal cuirass that covered the front surface of the body from the collar bones to the pubis [21].
3. *The Fairchild–Huxley chest respirator*
   The Fairchild–Huxley chest respirator (Fairchild Camera and Instrument Corporation, New York) was made in three shell sizes and two types (thoracic only and thoraco-abdominal) and had an alarm system to warn of power failure and excessive leakage [22].
4. *The Monaghan Portable Respirator*
   This device, developed by the Monaghan Company Inc. of Denver, continued to be used until the end of the 1980s. It originally had a set of six plastic thoraco-abdominal shells that had pneumatic rubber seals [23].

The polio epidemic in Copenhagen in 1952 would radically change the treatment of respiratory paralysis: until this time, anesthesiologists had used manual ventilation with the bag during anesthesia both during respiratory depression and electively in anesthesia-curaro applications. Dr. Lassen demonstrated that intermittent positive pressure (IPPV), that he learned from Professor Andre Cournand in New York City in 1946 when delivering medications via intermittent positive pressure breathing to COPD patients, could be applied via tracheostomy tubes for artificial respiration. He described how, over a 19-week period toward the end of 1952, the Blegdam hospital in Copenhagen had 2722 admissions for acute polio, 866 of them paralytic, and 316 required respiratory assistance [24]. At the beginning of the epidemic, the hospital had a tank ventilator and six cuirasses but, at one time, 70 patients needed assistance at the same time. After the first month, Dr. Lassen, in collaboration with his anesthesiologist colleague Dr. B. Ibsen, surgically placed tracheostomy tubes and had 400 medical and dental students apply intermittent manual positive pressure ventilation (IPPV) via the tubes for paralytic patients.

The Blegdam hospital had treated 76 polio victims between 1934 and 1944 in cuirasses with a mortality rate of 80%. In 1952, during the first month of the Danish epidemic, the 80% mortality rate markedly decreased to 40% by using tracheostomy IPPV. The results were confirmed during the much smaller outbreak in Stockholm the following year.

Lassen's work essentially ended the use of negative pressure as a treatment method for acute respiratory failure [25]. It was natural, however, that its popularity declined more slowly in the United States, where he had been so successful. In fact, with the advent of the Cof-flator, mechanical insufflation-exsufflation (MIE) device by Dr. Alvin Barach of Columbia University in New York City in 1953, the U.S. death rate from paralytic polio decreased to 20% because much, if not most of the mortality in both the U.S. and in Europe was due to inability to effectively clear airway secretions [26]. Barach, Beck, and Bickerman published numerous publications demonstrating the effectiveness of MIE to prevent pneumonia post-thoraco abdominal surgery, to eliminate atelectasis for postpolio survivors, and in conjunction with methods of noninvasive ventilatory support but MIE was not reportedly used via a tracheostomy or translaryngeal tube until Bach et al. reported this in 1990 [27].

In 1955, Pask made observations on the optimal use of the cuirass ventilator through three statements: (1) it had to be built comfortable enough for continuous use for long periods, (2) it had to be made capable of producing really adequate ventilation in all patients, (3) it had to be modified in such a way as to be able to entice the patient to sleep in the supine position.

E. J. Tunnicliffe produced his jacket in 1955 in an attempt to overcome some of these issues. The jacket was made from a blend of cotton and nylon [28]. The straps sealed it to its arms, neck, and through its buttocks, and it was kept away from its chest by a plastic shell. The original powerplant was based on a Rootes type air pump. The manufacturers said that more than twice the tidal volume could be achieved with the same negative pressure compared to a normal cuirass. This fact was demonstrated by Spalding and Opie when they compared the jacket with armor and intermittent breathing at positive pressure in cases suffering from chronic respiratory insufficiency from paralytic polio and myasthenia gravis [29]. After this period of research for efficient devices, in the following years, machines were designed whose purpose was greater portability and above all use in chronic respiratory failure.

1.2.3 Pneumobelt, Ventilation Belt, or Intermittent Abdominal Pressure Ventilator (IAPV)

Rhythmic abdominal compression can provide artificial respiration as has been known for some time. The device, first described by Adamson and Stern, consisted of a large flat bladder embedded in a belt [30] (Fig. 1.3). Inflating the bladder produces exhalation. Inhalation is produced by the elastic recoil of compressed abdominal tissues and organs and redescent of the diaphragm. The force applied to the

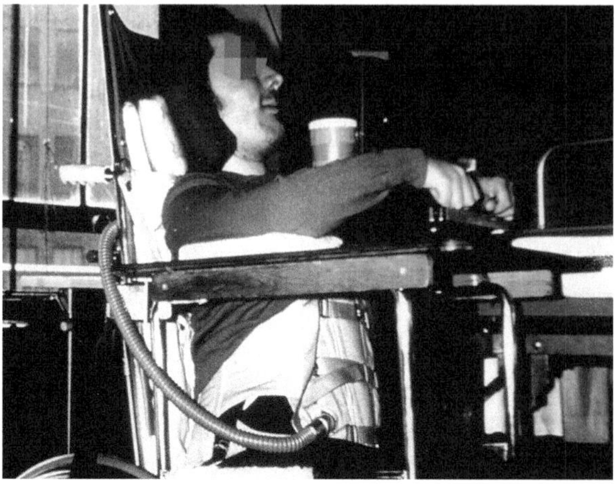

Fig. 1.3 Example of intermittent abdominal pressure ventilation (IAPV) used by patient with Duchenne muscular dystrophy for daytime ventilatory support

abdomen pushes the diaphragm toward the head to expel air from the lungs before removal of the force causes the elastic recoil of compressed tissues to draw air into the lungs. If the subject is standing or sitting, gravity assists inspiration. If the subject is lying down, it is the elastic recoil of the compressed tissues and organs that provides inspiration but the device is rarely useful under 30° from the horizontal. The pressure cycle is synchronized with a patient's breathing to provide respiratory assistance or even full support. Adequate ventilation of all subjects was achieved with less than 50 cm of H_2O applied to the abdomen with subjects in a sitting position. Ventilation increases progressively as the subjects' trunks are lifted from the lying position to the sitting position and, likewise, as abdominal pressure increased. The respirator has proved to be a valid complement to other respiratory aids in allowing rehabilitation activities without hypoxia. For some activities, it is the respirator of choice since it is almost impossible for anyone to tell that the user is using a respirator.

A similar device has been described by Miller et al. [31]. In a study of 15 patients, a bladder pressure of less than 50 cmH_2O produced a normal tidal volume and they strongly recommended wider acceptance for the high tetraplegic population. Bach et al. reported transitioning over 50 daytime chest cuirass users to ventilation belts in 1991 [32]. This device is back on the market with the Dima Italia company in Italy, and Dano Carbone's group in Colorado that makes 3 sizes of IAPV.

1. *The Rocking Bed*: This device is similar to the IAPV in moving the diaphragm and using gravity to ventilate the lungs. The concept originated with Eve in 1932, who postulated that abdominal contents would raise the diaphragm when the head and thorax were tilted downward and that inspiration would occur when the head and thorax were tilted upward. Besides being an effective ventilator, interestingly it may be useful for constipation and has been used for intimate sexual relations by married couples since the frequency and amplitude of the rocking can be adjusted during use [33].

2. *The Exovent* is a newly developed armor-like ventilator in response to COVID (coronavirus disease). Exovent is larger than a cuirass but smaller than an iron lung ventilator. It has its own inner mattress. The patient lies on it and the cover is placed over the entire body and arms and equipped with neck support and hip seals [34].

The Hayek Oscillator is a versatile ventilator with a lightweight, flexible, and airtight chest envelope with a soft seal around the chest and abdomen. It rests on a backplate or flexible cushion. Its piston pump can provide negative pressure ventilatory support when negative pressures of 40–50 cmH_2O are cyclically cycled under the shell. It can also provide oscillation for high-frequency negative pressure in resonance with the mucociliary elevator to mobilize secretions. It usually oscillates at a frequency of 2 hertz. Above 2 hertz, it acts like a high-frequency ventilator and provides oxygen and ventilation by diffusion [35].

Over the last few years, the concept of negative pressure ventilation has remained unchanged but the products are evolving. Technological evolution has allowed us to produce lighter and more comfortable devices, with innovative solutions in terms of materials, technology (e.g. the introduction of the trigger to coordinate the patient's breathing with the machine), portability, transport, and comfort. Despite this, this method remains relegated as secondary ventilation and not very practical. Another limitation of negative pressure ventilation is that it usually causes obstructive apneas during sleep since the negative pressure expands the lungs but closes the upper airways. The solution is to combine this with continuous positive airway pressure (CPAP) or place a tracheotomy, however, switching to noninvasive positive pressure ventilation not only ventilates the lungs but keeps the airway open to do so.

Nevertheless, some clinicians still advocate the use of reservoir respirators in the acute phases of respiratory disease when there is no pharyngeal paralysis and secretions are minimal and in some cases of chronic paralysis in chronic hospital units. There are also some patients living at home depending on the use of the Armour Respirator for 25 years or more. One of the most interesting uses for negative pressure ventilation is to facilitate ostomy closure for ventilator unweanable people whose tracheostomy tubes have been removed in favor of continuous noninvasive ventilatory support. After decannulation, when continuous noninvasive ventilatory support (NVS) must been continued via nasal or oronasal interfaces, the NVS tends to blow out of the ostromy even when sealed using a pressure dressing. However, if they are decannulated to negative pressure ventilation rather than NVS, the negative pressure ventilation also facilitates ostomy closure (Fig. 1.4). Since negative pressure respirators are rarely seen in acute care hospitals, few physicians have knowledge of these devices.

Besides countering obstructive sleep apneas, challenges in adopting negative pressure lung ventilation include the need to ensure proper application and monitoring. In addition, the limited availability of specialized devices and high cost can be barriers to widespread implementation. Some limitations also concern tolerability by patients, who may experience discomfort or difficulty with prolonged use of the devices. It is essential to address these challenges to ensure proper and safe

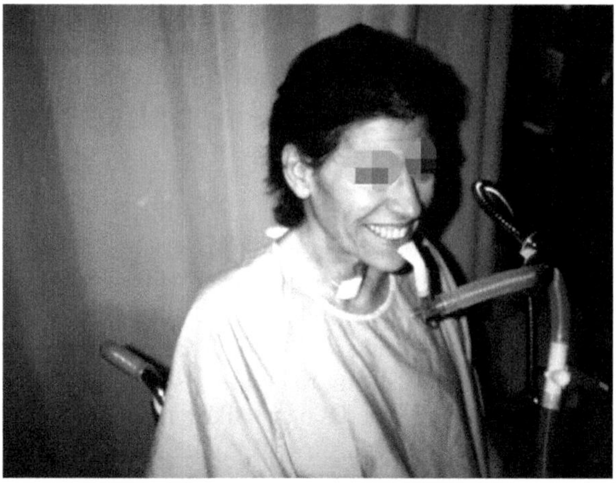

Fig. 1.4 52 year old woman with muscular dystrophy with no ventilator-free breathing ability, decannulated of her tracheostomy tube with her lungs ventilated for 16 h by Porta-Lung ventilator. This facilitated ostomy closure. The ostomy closed in 16 h when this usually takes 2 months or more when nasal ventilatory support is required after decannulation. (*All the photos appearing on this chapter were published with kind permission of Dr. HR Bach)

application of negative pressure pulmonary ventilation for patients who may benefit from it. Future prospects for negative pressure pulmonary ventilation will focus on integrating innovative technologies to improve treatment efficacy and safety. The development of lighter, quieter, and more portable devices can make this technique more accessible and comfortable for patients. The implementation of advanced sensors for users to trigger the devices can decrease the risk of obstructive apneas. Control algorithms may allow more accurate personalization of the therapy. In addition, research is moving more toward the creation of remote monitoring and telemedicine systems to enable more efficient management of patients using negative pressure pulmonary ventilation.

1.3 Conclusions

In conclusion, negative pressure pulmonary ventilation is configured as a technique with deep historical roots and solid physiological foundations, that has found important clinical applications in acute and chronic respiratory failure, both in adults and in children and in the elderly. Epidemiological evidence supports the efficacy of this ventilatory modality despite the challenges and limitations that may arise in practical implementation. However, future prospects with technological developments may open new frontiers and further improve clinical outcomes, supporting the value of negative pressure pulmonary ventilation in modern medical practice.

References

1. Levine S, Levy S, Henson D. Negative-pressure ventilation. Crit Care Clin. 1990;6(3):505–31.
2. Karpovich P. Adventures in artificial respiration. New York: Association Press; 1953.
3. Sternbach G, Varon J, Fromm R, et al. Galen and the origins of artificial ventilation, the arteries and the pulse. Resuscitation. 2001;49(2):119–22.
4. Fulton J. The history of physiology. Springfield: Charles C Thomas; 1930. p. 150–2.
5. Gottlieb Ls: A history of respiration. Springfield, Charles C Thomas, 1964, 52–54.
6. Garrison F. History of medicine. Philadelphia: Wb Saunders; 1929. p. 101–12.
7. As S. History of mechanical ventilation. From Vesalius to ventilator-induced lung injury. Am J Respir Crit Care Med. 2015;191(10):1106–15.
8. Woollam CM. The development of apparatus for intermittent negative pressure ventilation. Anaesthesia. 1976;31(5):537–42.
9. Sauerbuch F. Zur Pathologie der Offenen Pneumothorax Und die Grundlagen Seines Verfahren Zu Seiner Ausschaltung. Mitt Grentsgreb Med Chir. 1904, 13:299–306.
10. Drinker P. New apparatus for artificial respiration: The Barospirator of professor T. Thunberg. Journal Of Industrial Hygiene. 1928;10:7–11.
11. Eisenmenger R. Heart failure and its treatment with the biomotor. Wiener Medizinisch Wochenschrift. 1936;86:1129–40.
12. Drinker P. Prolonged Administration of Artificial Respiration. Lancet. 1931;1:1186–95.
13. Drinker P, Mckhann CF. The use of a new apparatus for the prolonged administration of artificial respiration. JAMA. 1929;92:1658–170.
14. Emerson JH. Exhibition at the Brussels World's Fair. 1958.
15. Paul RW. The Bragg-Paul pulsator. Proc R Soc Med. 1935;28:436–54.
16. Bergman R. Eight hundred cases of poliomyelitis treated in the Sahlin respirator. Acta Paediatr. 1948;36:470.
17. Peterson P. Der Pulsatorgurtel, Eine Tragbare, Selbsttbtige Vorrichtung Zur Kunstlichen Atmung Mit Sauerstoff-Kohlensbureadministration. Acta Med Scand. 1936;Suppl. 78:880–90.
18. Burstall F. New type of 'Jacket' respirator for The treatment of poliomyelitis. Br Med J. 1938;2:611–3.
19. Menzies F. Mechanical respirators. Med Off. 1938;60:231–5.
20. The Council on Physical Medicine. Acceptability report on the Blanchard portable plastic respirator. J Am Med Assoc. 1949;137:867.
21. The Council on Physical Medicine. Acceptability report on the chestspirator portable chest respirator. J Am Med Assoc. 1994;9(141):658.
22. The Council on Physical Medicine. Acceptability of the Fairchild Huxley cuirass respirator. J Am Med Assoc. 1950;143:1157.
23. The Council on Physical Medicine. The Monaghan portable respirator acceptance. J Am Med Assoc. 1949;139:1273.
24. Lassen HCA. Preliminary report on the 1952 epidemic of poliomyelitis in Copenhagen with special reference to the treatment of acute respiratory insufficiency. Lancet. 1953;1(6749):37–41.
25. D'avignon P, Sundell L, Werneman H. Treatment in cuirass and or positive pressure respirator; primary lethality, invalidity and physical fitness of respirator patients after one year. Acta Med Scand. 1956;316:107–10.
26. Barach AL, Beck GJ, Bickerman HA, Seanor HE, Smith W. Physical methods simulating mechanisms of the human cough. J Appl Physiol. 1952;5(2):85–91.
27. Bach JR, Zaniewski R, Lee H. Cardiac arrhythmias from a Malpositioned greenfield filter in a traumatic quadriplegic. Am J Phys Med Rehabil. 1990;69(5):251–3.
28. Pask EA. Maintenance of respiration in respiratory paralysis. Proce R Soc Med. 1955;48(3):239–44.
29. Spalding JM, Opiel L. Artificial respiration with the Tunnicliffe breathing jacket. Lancet. 1958;1(7021):613–5.

30. Adamson JP, Stern JD. Application of abdominal pressure for artificial respiration. JAMA. 1959;169(14):1613–7.
31. Miller HJ, Thomas E, Wilmot CB. Pneumobelt use among high quadriplegic population. Arch Phys Med Rehabil. 1988;69(5):369–72.
32. Bach JR, Alba AS. Intermittent abdominal pressure ventilator in a regimen of noninvasive ventilatory support. Chest. 1991;99(3):630–6.
33. Eve FC. Actuation of the inert diaphragm by a gravity method. Lancet. 1932;220(5697):995–7.
34. Exovent Development Group. Exovent: a study of a new negative-pressure ventilatory support device in healthy adults. Anesthesia. 2021;76(5):623–8.
35. Lerman SI. The Hayek oscillator. Anaesthesia. 1996;51(6):606.

Part I

Physiology

The Work of Breathing

2

Esteban Salas Rezola

2.1 Definitions of Work and Energy

The *work* done by a force on an object is the product of that force and the distance travelled, while *energy* is the capacity to do that work. The work required to move an object across a smooth surface will require less force than sliding it over a rough surface. This would translate into less energy needed to do that work.

$$W = F \times d\left(F \text{ is force,} d \text{ is distance}\right)$$

The work done by a mechanism can have a positive or negative value depending on whether the energy is transferred from the system or into the system. Once the work has been done, the energy is transformed according to the principle of conservation of energy, and efficiency is defined as the ratio of energy delivered to energy output expressed as a percentage with the difference being lost as heat.

There are many types of energy (kinetic, potential, electrical, etc.), including elastic energy defined as the energy stored in a deformed elastic material, such as a lung. The unit of energy is the joule (J) and one joule is the amount of energy required to generate a force of one newton over a distance of one meter (the calorie is another unit of energy and is equivalent to 4.2 joules).

The *power* delivered to that process refers to the rate at which that work is done (or energy is transferred). The unit of power is the Watt (W) which is equivalent a 1 J/s.

When discussing the work performed by a ventilator, we must imagine a piston pushing a plunger inside a cylinder. The pressure (P) generated will depend on the force (F) of the pump and the area (A) of the cylinder.

E. S. Rezola (✉)
Department of Anaesthesiology and Reanimation, Hospital General Universitario Dr. Balmis, Alicante, Spain

O. Alibrahim et al. (eds.), *Biphasic Cuirass Noninvasive Ventilation*, Noninvasive Ventilation. The Essentials, https://doi.org/10.1007/978-3-032-20933-7_2

$$P = F / A \text{ or } F = P \cdot A$$

It follows that:

$$W = P \cdot A \cdot d$$

If we know that volume (V) is equal to area per distance:

$$W = P \cdot V$$

If there is no change in airway resistance, an unforced inspiration that moves 450 ml of tidal volume generates 0.8 kPa of pressure and 0.36 J of work.

2.2 Work of Respiration

Work of breathing is defined as the energy required to overcome the elastic and resistive forces of the respiratory system during the ventilatory cycle, and depends mainly on lung and thoracic compliance, airway resistance, and an inertial component, due to changes in the lung parenchyma caused by volume acceleration. It is accepted that for respiratory rates below 1 Hz (60 breaths/min) the component due to the inertia of the system is negligible [1].

The physiological parameters that allow tissue deformation and its cost to be quantified are stress and strain [2]. Stress is the force required to deform a body. In this case, to inflate the lung, equivalent to the transpulmonary pressure. We understand the concept of strain as the amount of deformation, represented as a ratio with respect to the initial state. Some authors use residual functional capacity as the initial situation and others use the end-expiratory lung volume (EELV) [3].

2.2.1 Compliance and Hysteresis

An integrated understanding of lung compliance, hysteresis, and the application of BCV is essential for optimizing ventilatory work in negative pressure ventilation (NPV) settings. Adjusting the system parameters to the mechanical properties of the lung promotes more efficient, physiological, and potentially less harmful ventilation.

We define compliance (C) as the change in volume relative to the change in pressure. Its unit is liter per centimeter of water (L/cmH_2O).

$$C = \Delta V / \Delta P \left(\text{where } \Delta V \text{ is the change of volume and } \Delta P \text{ the change of pressure}\right).$$

Highly compliant lungs have reduced elasticity and therefore reduced expiratory capacity, requiring greater work from the expiratory muscles during exhalation. During BCV, we would need less negative pressure and more external positive pressure for active exhalation.

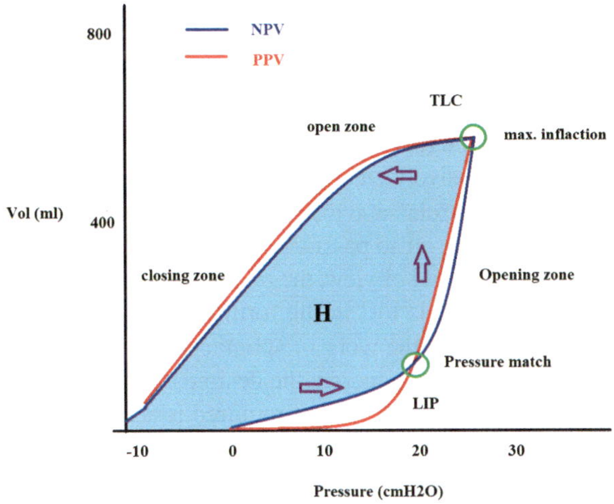

Fig. 2.1 Adapted from Sattari et al. [5]. Experimental comparison of hysteresis curves between a lung ventilated with PPV (red line) and NPV (blue line). The blue area is the hysteresis area (H). TLC: Total Lung Capacity. LIP: Lower Inflexion Point. Opening zone: first part of inspiration; the peripheral airways are opened exponentially. Open zone: second part of expiration, the peripheral airways remain open. Closing zone: third part of expiration; the peripheral airways close [6]

In lungs with low compliance, such as those with atelectasis, edema, pneumonia, or surfactant deficiency, extra work is needed to expand the lung. In this case, we would need greater negative pressure during BCV.

Pulmonary hysteresis is a phenomenon whereby, at the same transpulmonary pressure, there is greater volume during exhalation than during inhalation. This follows the principle that all elastic material does not return exactly to its original size. In a volume versus pressure graph, we obtain a hysteresis loop.

In isolated pig lungs (without the rib cage factor), Sattari et al. found notably dissimilar inflation paths between PPV and NPV hysteresis loops (Fig. 2.1). At the start of inspiration, the PPV curve produces a sudden rise when it reaches 20 cm H_2O, while with NPV there is a more gradual increase in volume, remaining above the PPV curve. Energy loss was significantly greater in PPV than in NPV. They also calculated the anisotropic index [4], a measure of tissue stretch distortion. NPV reduced surface strain concentrations, caused homogenous stretch contours [5].

2.2.2 Work Done during Spontaneous Breathing

It is the pleural membrane lining the inside of the rib cage that prevents lung collapse. During spontaneous breathing, the diaphragm descends 1–1.5 cm and the intercostal muscles move the rib cage outwards. This causes the pressure to become subatmospheric and air passively enters to equalize both pressures. During exhalation, the intercostal muscles relax and the forces of pulmonary elasticity and pulmonary surfactant tension cause air to passively exit the lungs.

From a purely physical point of view, the respiratory muscles are extremely inefficient. Up to 90% of energy is lost in the form of heat. The rest is distributed in mechanical energy to perform the work of spontaneous breathing and some potential energy in the lungs that will generate the desired elasticity.

Due to this 10% inefficiency, the power required is actually close to 900 mW. If a person's resting metabolic rate is 80–90 W, the power of respiration represents 1% of the body's total energy.

During exercise, both tidal volume and respiratory rate increase, and respiratory power can reach 25% of the total metabolic rate.

Under ideal conditions, NPV reduces the patient's respiratory work because it replaces part of the muscular effort required to generate negative intrathoracic pressure.

Respiratory work can be quantified by integrating pressure over inspired volume:

$$WR = \int P \cdot dV$$

where PPV is the pressure required to inflate the lungs. In NPV, this pressure is generated externally, so the net work performed by the patient's respiratory muscles can be reduced, depending on the degree of support provided (Fig. 2.2).

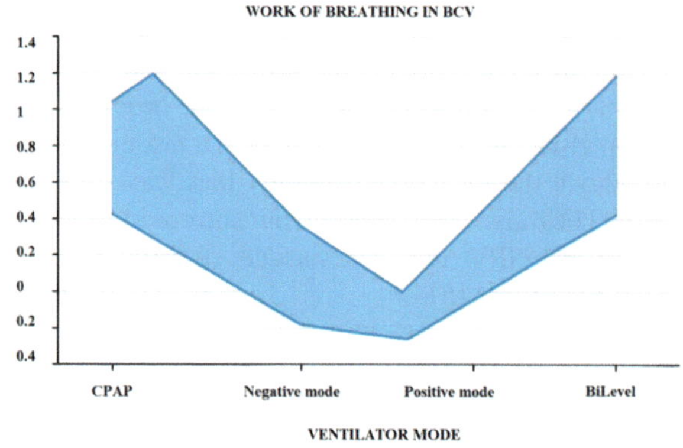

Fig. 2.2 Representation of respiratory work measured in J/L during ventilation in different ventilation modes

However, in practice, the effectiveness of NPV in reducing respiratory work depends on:

- *Synchronization* between the ventilator cycle and the patient's inspiratory effort. Patients who remain persistently asynchronous with control mode may get superior results on respiratory synchronized mode.
- *Integrity of the rib cage*: chest deformities or muscle weakness can hinder the transmission of negative pressure.
- *Cuirass tightness*: pressure leaks reduce effectiveness. Lines, tubes, and drains will work fine with BCV as long as the point of entry into the skin is not directly beneath the seal [7].

For all these reasons, we can establish some exclusion criteria for BCV:

- Burned skin or draining wounds under cuirass or seal area.
- Indwelling lines or tubes that are located under seal (within cuirass is acceptable).
- Patients weighing more than 180 kg.
- Patient's thoracic structure precludes establishment of good seal.
- Lack of viable airway either natural or artificial.
- Cardiopulmonary arrest.

2.2.3 Measurement of Respiratory Work During BCV

During positive pressure ventilation, measuring airway pressures is easier than when applying negative pressure through a chest wall with the cuirass. These are mainly the methods used:

- *Esophageal manometry*: indirect measurement of pleural pressure via esophageal pressure allows us to calculate transpulmonary pressure, which is a basic measurement in understanding and analyzing respiratory mechanics [8, 9].
- *Thoracic electrical impedance (TEI)* is a noninvasive, radiation-free method of diagnostics imaging, allowing for a bedside, real-time dynamic assessment of lung function [10].
- *External pressure–time curves*: recorded by the cuirass ventilator, useful for estimating assistance (Fig. 2.3).

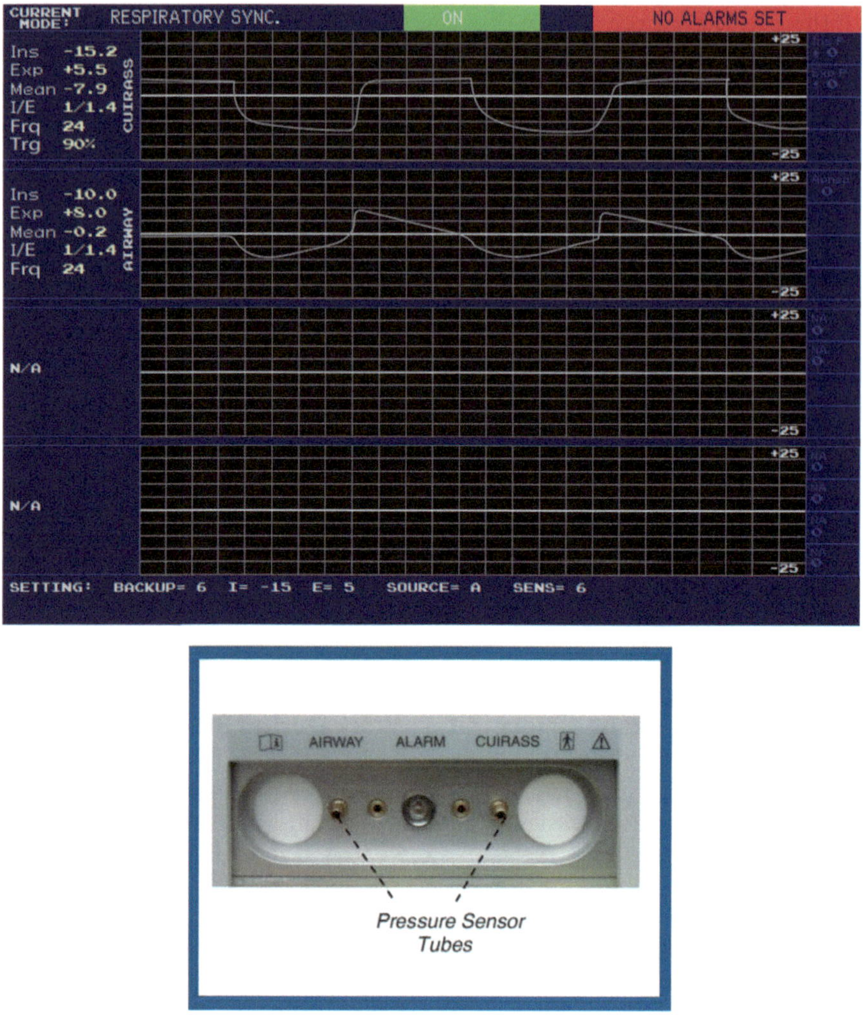

Fig. 2.3 Pressure sensors for airway sensing (connected to nasal cannula or T-piece) and for inspiratory/expiratory pressures sensing (connected to Hayek RTX ventilator). Above, we can see the screen display of the Hayek RTX ventilator showing the pressure curves in both the cuirass and the airway during inspiration (negative) and active exhalation (positive) in synchronized ventilation mode. All permissions and copyrights have been granted by United Hayek Industries

2.3 Conclusions

Knowledge of the basic physical and physiological concepts of the work of breathing is essential for understanding lung behavior in different clinical situations. The study of hysteresis curves, the relationship between volume and pressure, the comparison of inflection points, maximum insufflation, and lung opening and closing zones allows us to see certain differences in lung function between PPV and NPV.

Lung injury or damage caused by PPV in mechanical ventilation is a well-known phenomenon. Negative pressure ventilation responds to our search for certain modalities that reproduce a more physiological and less harmful type of ventilation. On the one hand, biphasic chest wall ventilation can help reduce the work of breathing, as it is a device that reduces inspiratory effort and has active exhalation modes; on the other hand, it could reduce energy loss by making each respiratory cycle more efficient. Under certain circumstances, it can even reduce pulmonary strain values.

The use of cuirass ventilation in neuromuscular diseases is well established. Due to all these advantages, a wide range of applications (it was not the aim of this chapter to discuss all of them) in the surgical field and in resuscitation and critical care units are opening up. Upper airway surgery and tracheal endoscopy are promising areas of research. Its use as an additional tool to conventional ventilation (it can be combined with invasive and noninvasive mechanical ventilation devices and even high-flow oxygenation therapies) allows for the creation of new protocols for weaning from mechanical ventilation, which is particularly relevant in critically ill patients with neuropathy, in whom the reduction of respiratory muscle mass increases the work and failure of such weaning. We even have data on the advantages of its use in postoperative cardiac surgery.

We must continue researching and persisting in our quest, which began over a century ago, to find the best tools to improve the quality of ventilation for our patients.

References

1. García-Prieto E, Amado-Rodríguez L, Albaiceta GM. Monitoring respiratory mechanics in ventilated patients. Intensive Care Med. 2012;38(1):49–55.
2. Chiumello D, Carlesso E, Cadringher P, Caironi P, Valenza F, Polli F, et al. Lung stress and strain during mechanical ventilation for acute respiratory distress syndrome. Am J Respir Crit Care Med. 2008;178(4):346–55.
3. Gonzalez-Lopez A, Garcia-Prieto E, Batalla-Solis E, Amado-Rodriguez L, Avello N, Blanch L, et al. Lung strain and biological response in mechanically ventilated patients. Intensive Care Med. 2012;38(2):240–7.
4. Mitzner W, Fallica J, Bishai J. Anisotropic nature of mouse lung parenchyma. Ann Biomed Eng. 2008;36(12):2111–20.
5. Sattari S, Mariano CA, Kuschner WG, Taheri H, Bates JHT, Eskandari M. Positive- and negative-pressure ventilation characterized by local and global pulmonary mechanics. Am J Respir Crit Care Med. 2023;207(5):577–86.
6. Schmitt DA, Gehr P, Bachofen M. Lung hysteresis: a morphological view. Histol Histopathol. 2004;19(1):159–66.
7. Hayek Medical. Application of the Hayek RTX guidelines [Internet]. Hayek Medical; [cited 2025 Sep 12]. Available from: https://hayekmedical.com/resources/.
8. Lanteri CJ, Petak F, Gurrin L, Sly PD. Influence of inertance on respiratory mechanics measurements in mechanically ventilated puppies. Pediatr Pulmonol. 1999;28(2):130–8.
9. Ortiz-Ruiz G, Dueñas-Castel C, Garay-Fernández M. Utility of oesophageal pressure measurement in mechanical ventilation: individualizing physiological variables. Acta Colomb Cuid Intensivo. 2022;22(3):200–8.
10. Maciejewski D, Putowski Z, Czok M, Krzych ŁJ. Electrical impedance tomography as a tool for monitoring mechanical ventilation: an introduction to the technique. Adv Med Sci. 2021;66(2):388–95.

The Hemodynamic Profile of Biphasic Cuirass Ventilation: Beyond Respiratory Support

3

Mostafa Elshazly and Heba Hesham

3.1 Introduction

The advent of mechanical ventilation revolutionized medicine, enabling the survival of patients with acute respiratory failure. The overwhelming majority of modern ventilators operate on the principle of positive-pressure ventilation (PPV), where gas is delivered into the lungs under positive pressure, forcing alveolar inflation. While life-saving, this nonphysiological approach fundamentally alters the physiological relationship between the heart and the lungs. The increase in intrathoracic pressure (ITP) inherent to PPV is known to cause a cascade of adverse hemodynamic effects, including decreased venous return, reduced cardiac output, and increased right ventricular (RV) afterload, which can be particularly deleterious in patients with pre-existing cardiovascular compromise [1, 2].

In the search for less invasive and more physiologically sound methods of respiratory support, there has been a resurgence of interest in negative-pressure ventilation (NPV). The iron lung is the most famous historical example, but modern technology has refined this concept into more practical and sophisticated forms. Biphasic Cuirass Ventilation (BCV) represents the pinnacle of this evolution. BCV utilizes a rigid shell, the cuirass, which covers the patient's thorax and abdomen (Fig. 3.1). A pump connected to the cuirass cyclically generates negative pressure to actively assist inspiration and a controlled positive pressure to actively assist expiration [3].

Unlike PPV, the negative inspiratory phase of BCV decreases ITP, thereby mimicking the mechanics of spontaneous breathing. This fundamental difference is the source of its unique and often favorable hemodynamic profile. BCV is not simply a tool to move air in and out of the lungs; it is a powerful modulator of cardiopulmonary hemodynamics. This chapter will delve into the physiological mechanisms

M. Elshazly (✉) · H. Hesham
Chest Department, Faculty of Medicine, Cairo University, Cairo, Egypt

O. Alibrahim et al. (eds.), *Biphasic Cuirass Noninvasive Ventilation*, Noninvasive Ventilation. The Essentials, https://doi.org/10.1007/978-3-032-20933-7_3

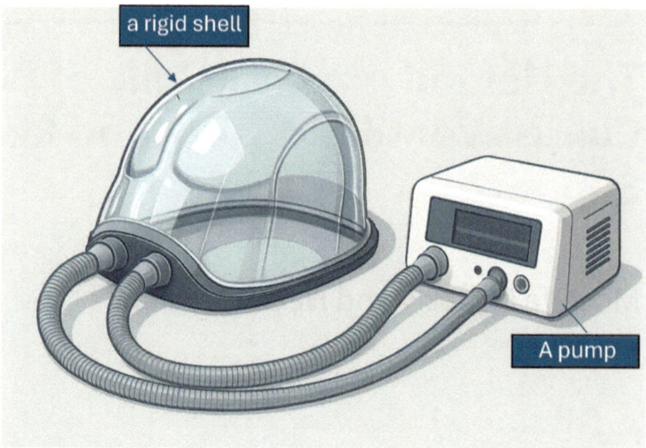

Fig. 3.1 Biphasic Cuirass Ventilation (BCV). BCV utilizes a rigid shell, the cuirass, which covers the patient's thorax and abdomen, a pump connected to the cuirass cyclically generates negative pressure to actively assist inspiration and a controlled positive pressure to actively assist expiration. (Courtesy of Mohamed Moawad)

underpinning the hemodynamic effects of BCV, contrast them with those of conventional PPV, and review the clinical evidence supporting its use as a genuine cardiopulmonary assist device.

3.2 Principles of Cardiopulmonary Interaction: The Role of Intrathoracic Pressure

To understand the effects of any mode of ventilation, one must first appreciate the heart and lungs as a single, integrated functional unit which lie within the thoracic cavity. Intrathoracic pressure (ITP) is the critical variable that links the function of these two systems. In a spontaneously breathing individual at rest, ITP becomes negative during inspiration (approximately −5 to −8 cmH_2O) and slightly positive during expiration. This negative inspiratory pressure is the driving force for both airflow into the lungs and venous blood flow back to the heart.

PPV reverses this dynamic. During a positive-pressure breath, ITP rises significantly, directly impacting several key hemodynamic parameters [4]:

Preload Venous return to the right atrium is determined by the pressure gradient between the mean systemic filling pressure and the right atrial pressure. By increasing ITP, PPV directly increases right atrial pressure, thus reducing this gradient and impeding venous return. This leads to decreased right ventricular end-diastolic volume (preload) and, subsequently, a fall in cardiac output via the Frank–Starling mechanism [5].

Right Ventricular (RV) Afterload The afterload of the RV is the resistance it must overcome to pump blood into the pulmonary circulation. PPV increases RV afterload by two mechanisms: (1) direct compression of pulmonary capillaries by high alveolar pressures (West zones 1 and 2), and (2) the potential for hyperinflation, which stretches and narrows alveolar vessels, increasing pulmonary vascular resistance (PVR) [1, 6].

Left Ventricular (LV) Afterload The effect of PPV on LV afterload is more complex. LV afterload is approximated by the LV transmural pressure during systole (Systolic Arterial Pressure - ITP). By increasing ITP, PPV decreases LV transmural pressure, thereby reducing LV afterload. This effect can be beneficial in patients with severe LV dysfunction, but it is often overshadowed by the profound reduction in preload [4, 7].

BCV, by generating a negative ITP during its inspiratory phase, fundamentally alters these interactions in a manner that is often hemodynamically advantageous.

3.3 The Hemodynamic Signature of Biphasic Cuirass Ventilation

The defining feature of BCV is its ability to lower ITP during inspiration. This simple yet profound difference from PPV is the primary driver of its distinct hemodynamic effects. The "biphasic" nature—coupling a negative inspiratory phase with a positive expiratory phase—further refines its clinical utility.

3.3.1 Augmentation of Preload and Venous Return

The most significant and well-documented hemodynamic effect of BCV is the augmentation of venous return [8]. During the negative pressure inspiratory phase, the cuirass expands the thoracic cage, causing a drop in pleural and, consequently, intrathoracic pressure. This lowers the pressure in the right atrium (Pra). According to the venous return equation (Venous Return = {mean systemic filling pressure − right atrial pressure} / Resistance to Venous Return), lowering right atrial pressure while mean systemic filling pressure remains constant increases the pressure gradient for blood flow from the systemic circulation back to the heart.

This mechanism effectively "pulls" venous blood into the thorax, increasing RV filling and preload. Several studies have directly demonstrated this effect. In a seminal study by Grasso et al. (2008), BCV was compared to PPV in patients with acute respiratory failure. The researchers found that switching from PPV to BCV resulted in a significant increase in the global end-diastolic volume index, a measure of cardiac preload, which was directly correlated with an increase in cardiac index [9]. Similarly, a study on patients with stable congestive heart failure showed that BCV increased stroke volume and cardiac output, an effect attributed primarily to enhanced diastolic filling [10].

This preload-enhancing effect positions BCV as a noninvasive cardiac assist device. In situations where cardiac output is limited by inadequate preload (e.g., hypovolemia, distributive shock, or right-sided heart failure), BCV can provide crucial hemodynamic support simultaneously with respiratory support, a combination not achievable with PPV.

3.3.2 Effects on Right Ventricular Afterload

The impact of BCV on RV afterload is more nuanced than its effect on preload. While lung inflation, regardless of the method, can increase PVR by stretching alveolar vessels, the concomitant decrease in ITP during BCV's inspiratory phase has a countervailing effect. Unlike PPV, especially with high levels of Positive End-Expiratory Pressure (PEEP), BCV avoids the direct alveolar compression and overdistension that dramatically elevates PVR [6].

Studies suggest that the net effect of BCV on PVR is generally neutral or slightly reduced compared to PPV. By avoiding high airway pressures and lung hyperinflation, BCV is less likely to precipitate acute RV failure in susceptible patients, such as those with acute respiratory distress syndrome (ARDS) or pulmonary embolism [11]. The active positive-pressure expiratory phase of BCV can also be beneficial in patients with dynamic hyperinflation (e.g., COPD), as it helps to fully empty the lungs, reducing the end-expiratory lung volume and thereby lowering the baseline PVR [12]. By unloading the RV, BCV can be a particularly attractive ventilation strategy for patients with cor pulmonale or RV dysfunction.

3.3.3 Effects on Left Ventricular Afterload

Theoretically, the negative ITP generated during BCV inspiration should increase LV afterload. As LV transmural pressure (LVTMP) is calculated as LVTMP = Systemic Arterial Pressure—ITP, a negative ITP would result in a higher transmural pressure, meaning the LV has to work harder to eject blood [7]. This is the physiological inverse of the afterload reduction seen with PPV.

However, in clinical practice, this theoretical increase in afterload is often clinically insignificant or is more than compensated for by the powerful preload-enhancing effects. According to the Frank–Starling law, a well-filled ventricle contracts more forcefully. The substantial increase in LV preload provided by BCV often leads to a greater stroke volume and cardiac output, despite the modest increase in afterload [9, 10].

Furthermore, for the afterload increase to be detrimental, the left ventricle must be failing and highly sensitive to afterload changes. In many clinical scenarios, the limiting factor is preload, not afterload. Moreover, the improved cardiac output and systemic blood pressure resulting from BCV can enhance coronary artery perfusion pressure, improving myocardial oxygen supply, which may further offset any increase in myocardial oxygen demand from the afterload effect [13].

3.3.4 Net Effect on Cardiac Output and Systemic Perfusion

The composite hemodynamic effect of BCV is a significant increase in cardiac output. The augmentation of venous return and preload is the dominant driver of this phenomenon. By increasing the volume of blood returned to the heart, BCV

Table 3.1 Comparative hemodynamic effects of PPV vs. BCV

Hemodynamic parameter	Positive-pressure ventilation (PPV)	Biphasic cuirass ventilation (BCV)
Intrathoracic pressure	Increased during inspiration	Decreased during inspiration
Venous return/ preload	Decreased (due to increased Pra)	Increased (due to decreased Pra)
RV afterload	Increased (due to alveolar compression and hyperinflation)	Neutral or decreased (avoids hyperinflation; active expiration helps)
LV afterload	Decreased (due to decreased LV transmural pressure)	Increased (due to increased LV transmural pressure)
Cardiac output	Often decreased, especially in preload-dependent states	Often increased, driven by preload augmentation
Primary mechanism	Pushing air into the lungs	Pulling the chest wall outwards

increases stroke volume, which, in turn, increases cardiac output (Cardiac Output = Stroke Volume × Heart Rate).

This has been consistently demonstrated across various clinical settings. In patients weaned from cardiopulmonary bypass after cardiac surgery, BCV was shown to increase the cardiac index by an average of 25% compared to PPV, facilitating a reduction in the need for inotropic support [14]. In a cohort of patients with cardiogenic shock, the use of BCV resulted in a marked improvement in cardiac index, mean arterial pressure, and mixed venous oxygen saturation (SvO_2), indicating improved systemic oxygen delivery [15]. A study by Foti et al. [16] directly compared the hemodynamic effects of BCV and PPV in septic patients, finding that BCV produced a significantly higher cardiac index and oxygen delivery (DO_2) without compromising gas exchange [16].

The contrast with PPV is stark (Table 3.1). While PPV is often necessary for oxygenation, it frequently comes at the cost of hemodynamic stability, requiring interventions like fluid boluses or vasopressor therapy. BCV offers the unique potential to support both respiration and circulation simultaneously.

3.4 Clinical Applications and Evidence

The unique hemodynamic profile of BCV makes it an attractive option in several clinical scenarios where the interplay between cardiac and pulmonary function is critical.

Cardiogenic Shock and Acute Decompensated Heart Failure: This is perhaps the most compelling application for BCV. In these patients, the heart's pumping function is severely impaired, and the hemodynamic compromise induced by PPV can be catastrophic. BCV acts as a "noninvasive ventricular assist device," augmenting preload, increasing cardiac output, and improving systemic perfusion, all while providing necessary respiratory support without the need for an invasive airway [15, 17]. This can serve as a bridge to recovery or to more definitive therapies like mechanical circulatory support or transplantation.

Weaning from Invasive Ventilation and Postextubation Support: Patients who are difficult to wean from PPV, particularly those with underlying cardiac dysfunction, often fail extubation due to the sudden hemodynamic shift. When PPV is removed, the ITP drops, venous return surges, and LV afterload increases, which can precipitate pulmonary edema in a compromised heart [18]. BCV can be used as a bridge during this process. It can be initiated prior to extubation to provide continued respiratory support while maintaining the augmented preload, preventing the abrupt hemodynamic collapse associated with weaning failure [19].

Postcardiac Surgery: The postoperative period following cardiac surgery is characterized by myocardial stunning and tenuous hemodynamics. PPV can exacerbate this instability. Studies have shown that using BCV in the immediate postoperative period can improve cardiac index, reduce the need for inotropes and vasopressors, and potentially facilitate earlier extubation [14].

Chronic Obstructive Pulmonary Disease (COPD): While the primary benefit discussed has been hemodynamic, the "biphasic" nature of BCV is crucial for COPD patients. These patients often suffer from dynamic hyperinflation and air trapping. The active positive-pressure expiratory phase of BCV can help stent open the airways during exhalation and actively assist in emptying the lungs, reducing the work of breathing and mitigating hyperinflation, which in turn can improve RV function [3, 12].

3.5 Limitations and Future Directions

Despite its significant physiological advantages, BCV is not without limitations. The proper fitting of the cuirass is essential for effective ventilation and to prevent air leaks or skin injury from pressure points. It may not be suitable for patients with recent thoracic or abdominal surgery, chest wall deformities, or significant ascites. In deeply obtunded patients, the negative pressure can cause passive collapse of the upper airway, necessitating careful monitoring or the use of a nasopharyngeal airway [20].

The primary barrier to widespread adoption has been a relative lack of large-scale, multicenter randomized controlled trials (RCTs). While the physiological data and smaller cohort studies are compelling, larger trials are needed to definitively establish its role in mainstream critical care algorithms and to compare its outcomes against modern PPV strategies and other noninvasive modalities like high-flow nasal cannula.

Future research should focus on refining cuirass design for better patient tolerance, integrating BCV with advanced hemodynamic monitoring systems for real-time feedback, and conducting robust RCTs in specific patient populations, such as those with cardiogenic shock or RV failure.

3.6 Conclusion

Biphasic Cuirass Ventilation represents a paradigm shift from conventional respiratory support. By leveraging negative pressure to create a more physiological breathing pattern, it does more than just ventilate the lungs—it actively supports the circulation. Its ability to decrease intrathoracic pressure, augment venous return, and increase cardiac output distinguishes it as a unique therapeutic tool. While PPV often forces clinicians to choose between oxygenating the patient and compromising their hemodynamics, BCV offers the potential to do both. As our understanding of cardiopulmonary interaction deepens, BCV is poised to find its place not as a replacement for PPV, but as a powerful, complementary therapy for critically ill patients in whom the heart–lung relationship is the key to recovery.

References

1. Pinsky MR. Cardiopulmonary interactions: the effects of positive-pressure ventilation on cardiac function. Respir Care. 2007;52(12):1851–63.
2. Jardin F, Farcot JC, Boisante L, Curien N, Margairaz A, Bourdarias JP. Influence of positive end-expiratory pressure on left ventricular performance. N Engl J Med. 1981;304(7):387–92.
3. Corrado A, Gorini M, Villella G, De Paola E. Biphasic cuirass ventilation in the treatment of ventilatory failure in patients with chronic obstructive pulmonary disease. Eur Respir J. 2002;20(5):1216–22.
4. Pinsky MR. The hemodynamic consequences of mechanical ventilation: an evolving story. Intensive Care Med. 1997;23(5):493–503.
5. Fessler HE, Brower RG, Wise RA, Permutt S. Effects of positive end-expiratory pressure on the canine venous return curve. Am Rev Respir Dis. 1992;146(1):4–10.
6. Vieillard-Baron A, Prin S, Augarde R, et al. Increasing argument for routine monitoring of TEE in patients with ARDS. Intensive Care Med. 2003;29(8):1371–7.
7. Scharf SM. Effects of continuous positive pressure breathing on cardiac output. Am Rev Respir Dis. 1991;144(3 Pt 1):538–50.
8. Anthonisen NR, Fleetham JA. Non-invasive mechanical ventilation. In: Fishman AP, editor. Pulmonary diseases and disorders. 3rd ed. New York: McGraw-Hill; 1998. p. 2565–74.
9. Grasso S, Terragni P, Birocco A, et al. Biphasic cuirass ventilation is a safe and effective tool for weaning from prolonged mechanical ventilation. Intensive Care Med. 2008;34(9):1588–96.
10. Skabkin O, Fomin A, Kiselev A, et al. Biphasic cuirass ventilation improves haemodynamics in patients with stable congestive heart failure. J Cardiovasc Med (Hagerstown). 2017;18(12):962–8.
11. L'Her E, Deye N, Lellouche F, et al. Physiologic effects of noninvasive ventilation during acute lung injury. Am J Respir Crit Care Med. 2005;172(9):1112–8.
12. Diaz O, Begin P, Torrealba B, Jover E, Lisboa C. Effects of noninvasive ventilation on lung hyperinflation in stable hypercapnic COPD. Eur Respir J. 2002;20(6):1490–8.
13. Pinsky MR. Heart-lung interactions. In: Tobin MJ, editor. Principles and practice of mechanical ventilation. 3rd ed. New York: McGraw-Hill; 2013. p. 865–95.
14. Borelli M, De Vita M, Anile A, et al. Biphasic cuirass ventilation in patients weaned from cardiopulmonary bypass. Crit Care Med. 2002;30(8):1753–8.
15. Koutoukas P, Koutsoukou A, Katsiari M, et al. Biphasic cuirass ventilation in the treatment of cardiogenic pulmonary edema. Intensive Care Med. 2005;31(11):1598–601.
16. Foti G, L'Her E, Ranieri VM, et al. Haemodynamic effects of non-invasive positive pressure ventilation in septic patients. Intensive Care Med. 2010;36(11):1854–60. (Note: This study

on NPPV provides context for BCV's contrasting effects, often cited in BCV literature for comparison)
17. Raymondos K, Stalder O, Rawal R, et al. Biphasic cuirass ventilation improves cardiac output in patients with low cardiac output state. Crit Care. 2009;13(Suppl 1):P455.
18. Lemaire F, Teboul JL, Cinotti L, et al. Acute left ventricular dysfunction during unsuccessful weaning from mechanical ventilation. Anesthesiology. 1988;69(2):171–9.
19. Ambrosino N, Vagheggini G. Non-invasive positive pressure ventilation in the acute care setting: where are we? Eur Respir J. 2008;31(4):874–86.
20. Goldstein RS, Molotiu N, Contreras M, Popkin J, helplessly S, Vellody K. Reversal of sleep-induced hypoventilation and chronic respiratory failure by nocturnal negative pressure ventilation in patients with restrictive ventilatory impairment. Am Rev Resp Dis. 1987;135:1049–55.

Part II

Equipment, Ventilatory Options

4 Equipment-Technology: Biphasic Cuirass Ventilator

Akiva Nachshon and Peter Vernon van Heerden

4.1 Introduction

The biphasic cuirass ventilator (BCV) is a device which is able to provide noninvasive mechanical ventilation (NIV) by means of pressure changes within a hollow shell (cuirass) closely applied to the anterior chest wall. The term cuirass is applied to this device because of the similarity of this hollow shell to a component of a medieval suit of armor—the piece of armor consisting of a breastplate and backplate fastened together. In turn, the word cuirass is derived from the French *cuirasse*, which came from the Latin word *corium* (leather). This chapter will deal with the equipment used to provide NIV using the BCV.

4.2 History

The BCV was derived from the initial concept of negative pressure ventilation applied using a body-enclosing apparatus. The first such apparatus was described in 1832 [1]. From this device was developed the first "tank" ventilators in 1928, where the entire body, except the head and neck, was placed within the negative pressure environment [2, 3]. Such tank ventilators came into their own (and gained widespread use) and provided effective supportive ventilatory care for patients during the polio epidemics of the 1950s. The history is discussed in greater detail in Chap. 1.

The original version of this chapter has been revised. Cross-references to other chapters on pages 34 and 36 have been updated accordingly.

A. Nachshon · P. V. van Heerden (✉)
Department of General Intensive Care, Hadassah University Hospital, Jerusalem, Israel

Department of Anesthesiology, Critical Care and Pain Medicine, Hadassah University Hospital, Jerusalem, Israel
e-mail: Akivan@Hadassah.org.il; Vernon@Hadassah.org.il

O. Alibrahim et al. (eds.), *Biphasic Cuirass Noninvasive Ventilation*, Noninvasive Ventilation. The Essentials, https://doi.org/10.1007/978-3-032-20933-7_4

Tank ventilators are very cumbersome, with the patient resting on a thin mattress within the device and the head protruding through a porthole at one end. There is a leather, rubber, or silicone seal around the neck and access to the patient is via additional portholes on the sides of the device (for monitoring devices or to carry out procedures). Negative pressure is generated by either a bellows within the ventilator structure or by external rotary pumps [4].

Various modes of ventilation can be provided by tank ventilators:

Continuous negative pressure (CNEP) ventilation—the patient breathes spontaneously, whilst the device maintains a subatmospheric pressure (SAP). This is somewhat equivalent to positive end-expiratory pressure (PEEP) in patients receiving positive pressure ventilation (PPV).

Cyclical *negative pressure ventilation* (NPV)—the tank ventilator provides SAP causing inspiration and then allows expiration to atmospheric pressure.

NPV and CNEP—this is a combination of the above two modes.

Negative and positive pressure ventilation (NPV/PPV)—the device provides sub-atmospheric pressure to cause inspiration as well as positive pressure during expiration (which may be useful in obstructive lung and chronic heart failure (CHF) conditions). This is also called biphasic ventilation.

The physiological effects of these modes of ventilation are further discussed in Chap. 5.

Cuirass ventilators superseded tank ventilators ("iron lungs") due to the bulkiness of the tank ventilators, as well as the restricted access to the patient being ventilated. The cuirass could provide the negative pressure (SAP) around the anterior chest wall and abdomen in order to inflate the lungs by applying negative pressure and allow the lungs to deflate passively during expiration. Addition of positive pressure within the cuirass could further aid expiration, thereby providing biphasic (negative and positive pressure) cuirass ventilation, BCV.

Although cuirass ventilation superseded negative pressure ventilation via tank ventilators, it was overshadowed by the rapid development of medications (e.g. muscle relaxants) and devices (e.g. endotracheal tubes, mechanical ventilators) that allowed IPPV to become the dominant mode of ventilation from the 1960s onwards. BCV was revived as a mode of ventilation in the 1990s, slowly developing until the utility of home ventilation using BCV was recognized in the early 2000s. Since cuirass ventilation is a negative pressure device it carries the advantages of being the most similar to natural physiological breathing: i.e. subatmospheric pressure in the pleural space during inspiration and atmospheric pressure at the end of expiration. IPPV of course has an inverse pressure signature to this.

Using a cuirass to apply the pressure changes to the chest wall and upper abdomen allowed for much greater mobility for the patient as well as access to the patient for carers, while maintaining the advantages of negative pressure ventilation (over invasive positive pressure ventilation (IPPV) via endotracheal tube or tracheostomy), namely:

Prevention of some of the complications of invasive ventilation (IPPV) such as impairment of the natural secretion clearance mechanisms and coughing in the presence of an endotracheal tube.

An option to effectively break up/loosen and remove secretions without the aid of a physiotherapist.

Patient autonomy. BCV allows patients the ability to eat, drink and talk while being ventilated, which allows patients to be an active participant in their treatment.

Patient comfort—there is no need for endotracheal intubation or tracheostomy.

BVC is available for both hospital and home care patients.

4.3 The Components of the Biphasic Cuirass Ventilator (BCV)

There are several manufacturers of biphasic cuirass ventilators in the world. The most prominent are listed in Table 4.1.

Regardless of the manufacturer the BCV has the following common components:

1. A *generator of airflow* which can be used to increase or decrease the pressure in the cuirass. Airflow can be generated using several devices such as.
   (a) A *diaphragm* which can be moved back and forth within a closed cylinder (somewhat like a large syringe), connected to the cuirass by a suitably sized tube. Unless the diaphragm and chamber are much larger than the cuirass volume this system may not be able to cope well with air leaks such as may occur between the cuirass and the chest wall. This setup also is not as responsive to rapid changes in patient effort due to the inertia of the movement of the diaphragm.
   (b) A *rotary pump*, such as was used in early tank ventilators, adapted for use with a cuirass. This device is more responsive to meeting changing patient demands and is more able to compensate for air leaks from the system as the

Table 4.1 Manufacturers of cuirass ventilators

Manufacturer	Address	Telephone number
Hayek Medical, A United Hayek Company	Unit 12 Northfields Prospect Business Centre Northfields, London SW18 1PE, UK	(+44) 844 415 7888
CareFusion Corp., A BD Company (US), Becton Dickson & Company	3750 Torrey View Ct, San Diego, CA 92130, USA	(+1) 858-617-2100
Medtronic International	Route du Molliau 31, Case Postale, CH-1131 Tolochenaz, Switzerland	(+41) 21 802 7000
Dräger Medical, Deutschland GmbH	Moislinger Allee 53-55, 23558 Lubeck, Germany	(+49) 0800 882 882 0
GE Health Care (UK)	Pollards Wood, Nightingales Lane Chalfont St Giles Buckinghamshire, HP8 4SP, UK	(+44) 01494 544 000
Respi USA	260 Geiger Rd, Number 31, Philadelphia PA 19115, USA	(+1) 877-428-1425

flows generated exceed those needed to generate the negative and positive pressures needed for patient ventilation.

(c) A *gas turbine*. This is a high-capacity airflow generator that is well able to cope with leaks from the system and is also able to meet patient requirements rapidly.

2. A *control system* which has inputs such as required pressure changes within the cuirass during the various phases of ventilation, patient effort required to trigger an assisted breath (e.g. pressure, flow or volume changes), electrocardiograph (ECG) signal and arterial oxygen saturation (SpO_2). These inputs are integrated by the controller to safely deliver the designated ventilator mode (spontaneous, intermittent or controlled—see Chaps. 5 and 7). The controller produces the outputs to control valves to vary the pressure within the cuirass in order to provide the desired mode of ventilation. The controller also has inbuilt and user-controlled alarm functions to enhance patient safety e.g. if physiological parameters (heart rate, SpO_2) deviate from preset limits, if the set ventilatory goals are not met or if unsafe pressures are being delivered. There is a screen (graphic user interface or GUI) showing both inputs and outputs (e.g. tidal volume, inspiratory and expiratory pressure, respiratory rate) as well as settings during functioning of the device. The controller also has a means of allowing user input, such as a keyboard or touch-screen, to adjust settings and set alarms.
3. The *cuirass shell*—this is a hard shell, suited to the patient size (for children and adults) applied to the anterior chest wall and upper abdomen. The edge of the cuirass is fitted with a soft rubber seal to reduce air leak and enhance patient comfort. It is secured via several broad straps which pass around the body. The cuirass is attached to the ventilator (containing the airflow generator and controller) via a wide-bore tube. In addition, there is a narrow bore pressure sensing tube which connects the cuirass to the ventilator. Negative pressure changes within the cuirass allow active inspiration due to downward and outward movement of the diaphragm and outward movement of the anterior chest wall. Expiration may be either passive (negative pressure within the cuirass returns to atmospheric pressure) or active (the pressure within the cuirass is above atmospheric pressure). These pressure changes are controlled by the controller opening and closing valves rapidly to allow air provided by the airflow generator to enter or leave the cuirass.
4. A power source—these devices commonly operate on mains power (120 V or 240 V), but many also have the ability to operate on 12 V or 24 V inputs such as from a car battery. Many devices also have an on-board battery, for portable use of the device.

An example of the components of a BCV system are shown in Fig. 4.1.

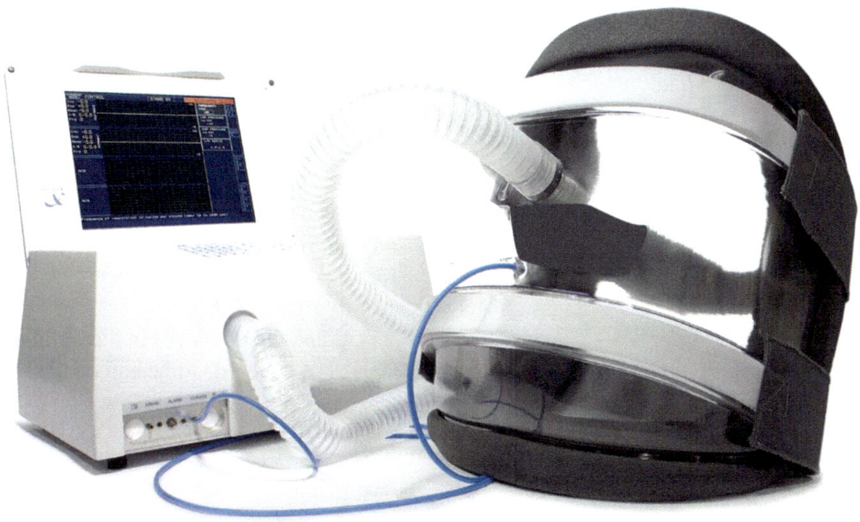

Fig. 4.1 A typical biphasic cuirass ventilation system

4.4 Conclusion

The components of a BCV system are not complex and allow for safe and comfortable non-invasive ventilation in both the hospital and the home.

References

1. Dalziel J. On sleep and an apparatus for promoting artificial respiration. Br Assoc Adv Sci. 1838;2:127–34.
2. Drinker P, Shaw LA. An apparatus for the prolonged administration of artificial respiration: I. A design for adults and children. J Clin Invest. 1929;7(2):229–47. https://doi.org/10.1172/JCI100226. PMID: 16693859; PMCID: PMC434785
3. Shaw LA, Drinker P. An apparatus for the prolonged administration of artificial respiration: II. A Design for Small Children and Infants with an appliance for the Administration of Oxygen and Carbon Dioxide. J Clin Invest. 1929;8(1):33–46. https://doi.org/10.1172/JCI100253. PMID: 16693884; PMCID: PMC424606
4. Corrado A, Gorini M, Villella G, De Paola E. Negative pressure ventilation in the treatment of acute respiratory failure: an old noninvasive technique reconsidered. Eur Respir J. 1996;9(7):1531–44. https://doi.org/10.1183/09031936.96.09071531.

5 Biphasic Cuirass Ventilation: Ventilatory Mode Options

Catarina Hilário

Biphasic Cuirass Ventilation (BCV) has evolved over the years and currently offers a wide range of ventilatory modes, enabling the application of many ventilation patterns typically achieved with positive pressure devices. Furthermore, it can deliver respiratory rates ranging from normal breathing to high-frequency oscillation, as well as provide expiratory assistance through forced expiration [1].

The biphasic function effectively allows for control of the inspiration-to-expiration (I:E) ratio, which refers to the proportion of time allocated to inspiration, during which air is pumped out of the cuirass to create negative pressure in the thorax, and expiration, during which air is pumped into the cuirass to generate positive pressure in the thorax [2, 3].

Most other ventilation methods, particularly those employing positive pressure, rely on the passive recoil of the patient's thorax, which inherently limits the achievable respiratory rate. In contrast, BCV enables the attainment of higher tidal volumes and increased respiratory rates overall [2, 3].

Moreover, BCV facilitates a ventilation pattern that closely mimics physiological breathing, through a noninvasive and efficient method, while minimizing associated risks such as infections and barotrauma [3].

This chapter will provide a detailed analysis of the ventilatory modes available in BCV.

C. Hilário (✉)
Pulmonology Department, Centro Hospitalar de Trás-os-Montes e Alto Douro, Vila Real, Portugal

O. Alibrahim et al. (eds.), *Biphasic Cuirass Noninvasive Ventilation*, Noninvasive Ventilation. The Essentials, https://doi.org/10.1007/978-3-032-20933-7_5

5.1 Modes of Cuirass Ventilation

5.1.1 Continuous Negative Pressure Mode

In this ventilatory mode, the cuirass applies continuous negative pressure to the thorax, producing sustained chest wall expansion. This facilitates passive air entry into the lungs while allowing the patient to maintain spontaneous breathing [1].

In contrast to the controlled biphasic mode, no active positive pressure is generated during exhalation, meaning expiration occurs passively. Although not a biphasic mode per se, continuous negative pressure ventilation is available on biphasic ventilation systems and is often selected as the initial mode.

This mode is functionally analogous to continuous positive airway pressure (CPAP), with the distinction that sustained negative pressure is applied throughout the respiratory cycle. There is no active control of expiration; air is expelled through the natural elastic recoil of the thoracic cage [1].

Continuous negative pressure ventilation offers several physiological benefits, including improved oxygenation through the prevention of alveolar collapse, enhanced alveolar capillary perfusion, and dilation of small airways. Additional advantages arise from the noninvasive nature of cuirass ventilation, such as reduced risk of barotrauma and greater patient comfort due to its closer approximation to natural breathing [1, 2].

This mode is particularly useful for promoting alveolar recruitment and improving ventilation-perfusion matching in patients with pulmonary atelectasis or respiratory infections leading to acute respiratory failure. It may also provide mild respiratory support in early-stage neuromuscular diseases where upper airway integrity is preserved. Furthermore, it is a safe and well-tolerated option following cardiac surgery or in selected patients who are intolerant to positive pressure ventilation [1, 4–6].

At initiation, the level of negative pressure must be carefully determined. This is always a subatmospheric value and varies with patient age. In adults, support typically begins at −8 cmH_2O and may be increased up to −15 cmH_2O in most cases of acute respiratory failure, or to more extreme levels (e.g., below −20 cmH_2O) when maximal alveolar recruitment is required. In pediatric patients, lower initial pressures are recommended: −6 to −10 cmH_2O in children, and −4 to −8 cmH_2O in infants [2, 6]. The negative pressure may be progressively adjusted based on clinical response.

5.1.2 Controlled Biphasic Mode

This mode allows precise control of the two phases of the respiratory cycle, inspiration and expiration, by alternately applying negative and positive pressure to the chest. During inspiration, the diaphragm moves downwards and the intercostal muscles and ribs move outwards, creating a negative pressure that expands the chest, allowing air to enter the lungs. Conversely, during exhalation, the creation of positive pressure compresses the chest, making it easier for air to escape [1, 2].

To do this, the clinician sets several ventilatory parameters, namely pressures, the inspiration/expiration ratio and the respiratory rate, in order to achieve a certain tidal volume or desired respiratory rate [2, 3].

When starting this mode, a negative and positive pressure should be set for application during inspiration (I) and expiration (E), respectively, maintaining an I:E ratio of approximately 3:1. The difference between the inspiratory and expiratory pressures determines the chest wall excursion and therefore the total volume. The ventilator's frequency is regulated slightly above the patient's respiratory rate, but should not exceed 60 cycles per minute. In controlled mode, pressures are delivered at a set rate and cannot be synchronized with the patient's efforts [6].

This mode is therefore often used in patients with acute respiratory failure secondary to lower respiratory tract infections who do not respond favorably to continuous negative pressure mode. By allowing stable ventilation, it can be indicated as the initial mode in critically ill patients with reduced lung compliance and unable to maintain a constant breathing pattern, offering support equivalent to invasive mechanical ventilation in some conditions, precise control of gas exchange and reduction of respiratory work, especially important in patients with muscle weakness [6]. Furthermore, unlike conventional positive pressure ventilation, it does not compromise venous return, maintaining cardiac output [3].

Thus, patients with acute and chronic respiratory failure, and more particularly neuromuscular patients with ventilatory compromise and patients with chronic obstructive pulmonary disease, can benefit from this ventilatory mode, especially by improving hemodynamic parameters and gas exchange [8, 9]. In addition, studies have demonstrated its usefulness in the postoperative context of heart surgery and in patients who are difficult to wean from ventilation, as well as in situations where conventional non-invasive mechanical ventilation is poorly tolerated or contraindicated [3, 4, 7].

This modality is currently available for hospital and home use, with portable devices that are easy to handle.

5.1.3 Respiratory Synchronized Mode

Synchronized ventilation offers optimized interaction between the ventilator and the patient's spontaneous breathing. In this mode, the ventilator detects the patient's spontaneous respiratory efforts, usually through pressure or flow sensors located in the cuirass, and coordinates the application of pressure, creating an assisted cycle according to the patient's demand.

Similar to the controlled mode, the ventilator applies negative pressure on inspiration, which allows the tidal volume to be increased, and then a positive pressure to facilitate airflow and prevent alveolar collapse. The main difference compared to the controlled mode is that, in this case, the ventilator does not impose a fixed rhythm, but assists the cycles triggered by the patient, avoiding ventilatory asynchrony. The ventilator automatically adjusts synchronization in real time, even in the presence of variations in the breathing pattern [2, 5].

Thus, synchronized mode improves ventilatory efficiency and reduces respiratory work, while maintaining spontaneous control of breathing by the patient. Compared to the controlled mode, it provides the patient with greater autonomy by allowing the preservation of the sensation of respiratory control, while also carrying a lower risk of patient–ventilator asynchrony.

Once again, this mode can also be useful for neuromuscular patients with residual respiratory effort and patients with chronic obstructive pathology who have signs of hypoventilation, with hypercapnia and respiratory muscle fatigue. It can also be useful as ventilatory support during weaning from invasive ventilation, allowing the patient to trigger cycles and gradually train the respiratory muscles without overloading them, while maintaining ventilatory support [2, 6].

The basic principles for setting inspiratory and expiratory pressure are similar to those applied in the controlled mode.

5.1.4 High Frequency Chest Wall Oscillation Mode (HFCWO)

High-Frequency Chest Wall Oscillation (HFCWO) consists of two main components: a vest that is fitted around the patient's thorax and an air pulse generator that delivers high-frequency oscillations to the chest wall through alternating cycles of inflation and deflation. The frequency of the oscillations can reach 1200 oscillations per minute (5–20 Hz) and the pressure applied can be adjusted according to each patient's therapeutic needs [10].

In addition, setting ventilation parameters in HFCWO mode must also take into account the patient's age group due to the anatomical and developmental differences at these different stages of life. Adults, owing to their larger chest diameter, greater lung volumes, and increased elastic resistance, typically require higher negative pressures (−20 to −40 cmH_2O) combined with lower oscillatory frequencies (600–800 cycles per minute) to ensure adequate ventilatory efficiency during therapy. In contrast, pediatric patients, especially infants, present with a more compliant thoracic cage, smaller airways, and reduced lung volumes. Consequently, lower negative pressures are necessary to reduce the risk of barotrauma (children: −15 to −30 cmH_2O; infants: −5 to −20 cmH_2O), while higher frequencies are generally more effective (children: 700–1000 cpm; infants: 800–1200 cpm). At the same time, adults have greater tolerance and a greater physiological reserve, so they can usually tolerate longer sessions. These physiological distinctions are essential considerations when individualizing ventilation parameters according to patient age and thoracopulmonary mechanics [2, 6].

High-frequency vibrations generate pressure changes that stimulate the ciliary beat, change the viscosity of the mucus, making it less thick, detach the mucus from the airway walls and consequently mobilize mucous secretions from the peripheral airways to the central airways, facilitating the exteriorization of secretions, clearing the airways and thus optimizing the effectiveness of ventilation [11]. Thus, although primarily used to mobilize secretions, HFCWO is integrated into BCV to improve overall respiratory function.

Scientific evidence has shown that HFCWO can improve lung function and oxygenation, decrease the frequency of respiratory exacerbations and hospitalizations, and increase the quality of life of patients with chronic respiratory diseases [11].

Thus, HFCWO is especially indicated in patients with difficulty mobilizing bronchial secretions, including patients with cystic fibrosis, bronchiectasis unrelated to cystic fibrosis, chronic obstructive pulmonary disease, and pulmonary complications of neuromuscular diseases. In addition, it can also be beneficial in patients with atelectasis or recurrent respiratory infections due to secretion impaction [11]. This therapy is usually well tolerated and can be self-administered, promoting greater patient autonomy in the management of their illness.

5.1.5 Cough Assist Mode

The Cough Assist mode in BCV provides additional support for secretion clearance, which is particularly important for patients with respiratory muscle weakness and reduced ability to generate an effective cough. In this mode, a sudden increase in negative pressure is applied during inspiration, followed by a rapid shift to positive pressure during expiration. This creates a high expiratory flow that mimics a natural cough, thereby facilitating the mobilization and clearance of secretions. The cough assist mode is integrated into the same device that delivers both ventilation and high-frequency oscillation, using the cuirass as a single interface. This eliminates the need to switch equipment or interfaces [2, 3].

Similar to HFCWO, the parameters in cough assist must be adjusted to the patient's age group. These parameters include inspiratory and expiratory pressures, the duration of each phase and the number of cycles per session. Synchronization with the patient's respiratory effort can be done manually or automatically, depending on the device model. In this mode, coughing is stimulated for 12–60 cycles/min, using variable inspiratory and expiratory pressures, with a high I:E ratio, usually 4:1 to 6:1. The patient can be encouraged to coordinate their efforts with those of the device. The assisted cough should be performed for approximately 2 min. Typical secretion clearance sessions range from 30 to 60 min [2, 6].

Thus, this mode can be indicated in all pathologies that compromise an effective cough, namely neuromuscular diseases, high spinal cord injuries with compromised expiratory muscle function and airway diseases, among other chronic pulmonary conditions characterized by the accumulation of secretions that are difficult to mobilize.

In these patients, assisted cough is essential to improve secretion elimination, thus reducing the risk of respiratory infections and the need for aspiration by more invasive methods, with a gain in improved oxygenation and alveolar ventilation. Compared to conventional methods from other interfaces, such as a face or mouth mask, BCV-assisted coughing can provide greater comfort and quality of life for the patient, allowing them to carry out other activities during therapy, such as talking and eating.

5.1.6 Cardiac Synchronized Mode

In this mode, it is possible to synchronize the ventilation cycle with the cardiac cycle. To do this, the patient must have electrocardiographic monitoring.

Several studies have already reported the benefits of using this mode in pediatric patients, before and after cardiac surgery for congenital malformations, namely by increasing cardiac output [12, 13].

An additional useful indication for BCV synchronized with the ECG is in the radiology department during magnetic resonance imaging. In highly sensitive magnetic resonance imaging of the heart and chest, synchronizing the ventilatory cycle with the heartbeat improves image quality and more accurately detects the presence of structural disease, particularly in the coronary arteries [1].

In conclusion, BCV stands out as a complete and multifunctional noninvasive approach that offers multiple ventilatory modes that can be tailored to the needs of patients with varying degrees of respiratory impairment. It includes ventilatory and secretion mobilization modes, which can be performed simultaneously and from a single device.

References

1. Linton DM. Cuirass ventilation: a review and update. Crit Care Resusc. 2005;7(1):22–8. Available from: https://www.sciencedirect.com/science/article/pii/S1441277223015661.
2. Hayek Medical. Application of the Hayek RTX. Hayek Medical. Available from: https://www.hayekmedical.com. Accessed May 2025.
3. EBME. Biphasic Cuirass Ventilation. Available from: https://www.ebme.co.uk/articles/clinical-engineering/biphasic-cuirass-ventilation. Accessed May 2025.
4. McBride WT, Ranaldi G, Dougherty MJ, et al. The haemodynamic and respiratory effects of continuous negative and control-mode cuirass ventilation in recently extubated cardiac surgery patients: part 2. J Cardiothorac Vasc Anesth. 2012;26(5):873–7. https://doi.org/10.1053/j.jvca.2012.05.021.
5. Onweni C, Rashid S, Goswami R, et al. Cuirass ventilation: an alternative home-based modality for chronic respiratory failure. Home Health Care Manag Pract. 2019;32(1):40–4. https://doi.org/10.1177/1084822319875111.
6. DeRusso M, Miller AG, Caccamise M, Alibrahim O. Negative-pressure ventilation in the paediatric ICU. Respir Care. 2024;69(3):354–65. https://doi.org/10.4187/respcare.11193.
7. Kristensen MS, Hesselfeldt R, Schmidt JF. Modern cuirass ventilation for airway surgery: unlimited access to the larynx and trachea in anaesthetised patients. Br J Anaesth. 2023;131:e106–9. https://doi.org/10.1016/j.bja.2023.07.010.
8. Jackson M, Kinnear W, King M, Hockley S, Shneerson J. The effects of five years of nocturnal cuirass-assisted ventilation in chest wall disease. Eur Respir J. 1993;6(5):630–5.
9. Sato Y, Saeki N, Asakura T, Aoshiba K, Kotani T. Effects of extrathoracic mechanical ventilation on pulmonary hypertension secondary to lung disease. J Anesth. 2016;30(4):663–70. https://doi.org/10.1007/s00540-016-2172-7.
10. McIlwaine MP, Alarie N, Davidson GF, et al. Long-term multicentre randomised controlled study of high-frequency chest wall oscillation versus positive expiratory pressure mask in cystic fibrosis. Thorax. 2013;68:746–51.

11. Marin A, Chiaradia VC, Dobre M, et al. High-frequency chest wall oscillation devices: an umbrella review and bibliometric analysis. Comput Biol Med. 2024;182:109135. https://doi.org/10.1016/j.compbiomed.2024.109135.
12. Shekerdemian LS, Bush A, Shore DF, Lincoln C, Redington AN. Cardiopulmonary interactions after Fontan operations: augmentation of cardiac output using negative pressure ventilation. Circulation. 1997;96(11):3934–42. https://doi.org/10.1161/01.cir.96.11.3934.
13. Shekerdemian LS, Shore DF, Lincoln C, Bush A, Redington AN. Negative-pressure ventilation improves cardiac output after right heart surgery. Circulation. 1996;94(9 Suppl): II:49–II55.

Ventilatory Aspects and Waveforms in Different Modes of Negative Mechanical Ventilation Monitoring and Setting

6

Umberto Vincenzi and Antonio M. Esquinas

6.1 Introduction

Although the first attempts to apply extrathoracic negative pressure were made in the nineteenth century, it can be said that only in 1929 did true negative mechanical ventilation begin with the application of forces acting outside the thorax using electric motors. In fact, in that year, Philip Drinker and Louis Agassiz Shaw [1], based on studies of human physiology, presented the first lung ventilator controlled by an electric motor, called *"iron lung"* (IL). This machine was based on the application of air pressures inside a hermetically sealed box which acted, alternately, on the patient's chest, placed entirely inside it with the exclusion of the head. The degree of the positive and negative pressures and their frequency resulted in a mobilization of the air present inside the chest with a consequent increased pulmonary ventilation. This type of mechanical ventilation, however unique at the time, was subsequently named *"negative pressure ventilation"* (NPV) and, in more recent years, *"biphasic cuirass ventilation"* (BCV) as it supports the patient's ventilatory action in both inspiratory and expiratory phases. NPV was very successful, remaining in continued use until the development and spread of *"positive pressure ventilation"* (PPV).

Over the years, however, various modifications were made to this type of ventilators.

Among these we recall, in 1969, the possibility of modulating the duration of inspiration and expiration, in order to establish varied I:E ratios and the introduction

U. Vincenzi (✉)
Pneumology and Intensive Respiratory Care Unit, Ospedali Riuniti di Foggia, Foggia, Italy

A. M. Esquinas
Intensive Care Unit Hospital Morales, Meseguer, Murcia, Spain

O. Alibrahim et al. (eds.), *Biphasic Cuirass Noninvasive Ventilation*, Noninvasive Ventilation. The Essentials, https://doi.org/10.1007/978-3-032-20933-7_6

of *"pauses"*, in the moments of inversion of the ventilatory cycle in order to allow greater persistence, in the box, of the pressure level reached [2].

In the 90s, the advent of electronics introduced the possibility of recognizing the triggering of the patient's inspiratory act by means of thermal sensors or flow sensors applied near the nostrils. This innovation made it possible to add the *"assisted"* mode to the *"controlled"* type of ventilation, which had been used until that time, with greater adherence on the part of the patient to the lung ventilator.

Soon, to the normal extrathoracic mechanical ventilation (NPV) carried out with the iron-lung, other devices acting on the patient's chest were added, i.e. cuirass-shaped prostheses, which supplied negative and positive pressures, or the use of the so-called *"poncho-wrap"* which supplied only negative pressures. The advantages of these devices, compared to the iron-lung, were: less weight, easy portability, and better handling while in use. The disadvantage, which resulted from the smaller area of pressure intervention on the patient's body, was a relative lower therapeutic efficacy. In fact, the decrease of the direct action of pressures on the patient's abdomen produced a lower effect on the mobilization of the diaphragm. For some years now, a lung ventilator has also been in use which has additional characteristics to those of a common extrathoracic ventilator. This is the Hayek ventilator, which, in addition to standard extrathoracic ventilation, with alternating negative and positive pressure (BCV), can deliver high-frequency oscillatory waves to the chest wall, causing so-called *"high-frequency chest wall oscillation"* (HFCWO). It also has a *"Cardiac Synchronized—Biphasic Cuirass Ventilation"* (CS-BCV) that allows the ventilatory cycle to be synchronized with cardiac activity detected by an ECG.

More recent applications of NPV have been the simultaneous combination of two modes of ventilation, such as extrathoracic NPV and *"positive pressure ventilation"* (PPV) delivered into the upper airways.

A first scientific work, concerning the treatment of a patient affected by ARDS, was published in 2015, as a "case report", by Raymondos et al [3]. On that occasion, given the worsening of a subject affected by ARDS, already tracheostomized and ventilated in *"Pressure-Support + PEEP"*, an extrathoracic negative pressure ventilation (CENPV) was also added. This was done by introducing the patient into a self-built container, with transparent and mobile hermetic walls in which the CENPV was dispensed. The box ventilator, which delivered a negative pressure of -33 cmH_2O on inspiration and $-$ 15 cmH_2O on expiration, was combined with the positive pressure ventilator. This combination of the two machines allowed complete recovery from ARDS with prolonged benefit of her life.

A second scientific work, published in 2021 by Vincenzi [4], based on the electronic connection and the perfect synchronization between the two ventilators, highlighted how the *"positive + negative synchronized ventilation"* (PNSV) or extrathoracic negative pressure ventilation using cuirass + positive pressure ventilation in pressure support mode, was very effective in treating patients with severe respiratory failure.

In this case, mechanical ventilation with the two machines was applied both in a completely noninvasive mode, i.e. with the combination of a NPV with a PPV with a face mask (Fig. 6.1a), and in a mixed mode (noninvasive + invasive) in which, to

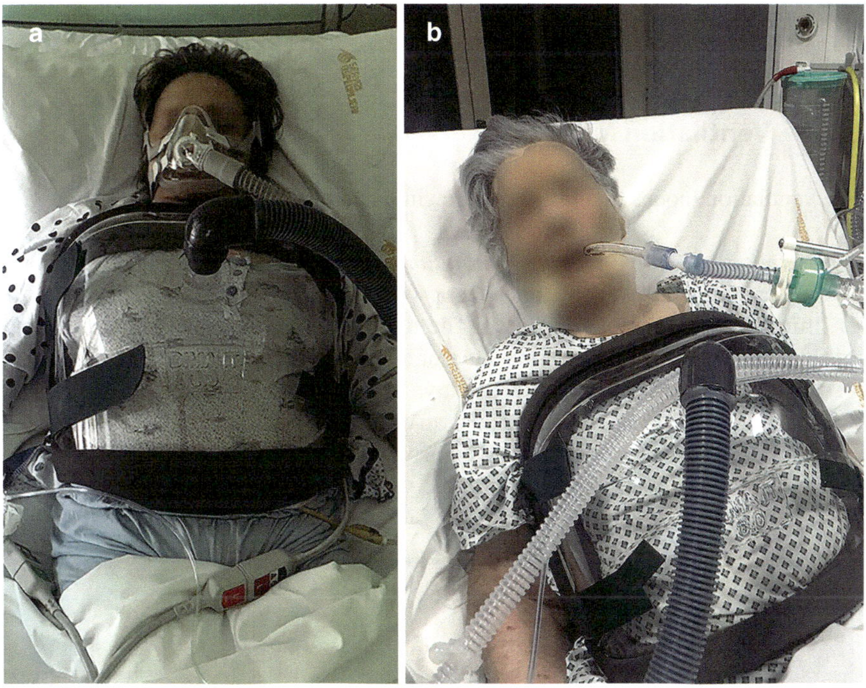

Fig. 6.1 In this figure, the application of "positive + negative synchronized ventilation" (PNSV) is noted. In image (**a**) the ventilation mode is completely noninvasive: NPV is combined with PPV using an oronasal mask. In image (**b**) the mode is "mixed" because NPV, which is noninvasive, is combined with PPV using invasive orotracheal intubation

the NPV, a positive pressure ventilation was added by means of a tracheal intubation (Fig. 6.1b). In both cases the patients were not sedated and could directly control the start, depth, and frequency of the entire ventilatory cycle with the exception of only the pressures preset on the machines by the operating doctor. Although the application of PNSV was administered for only 1 h on elderly patients with severe respiratory failure, the clinical and blood gas analysis benefits were immediate and very evident. The patients, despite being subjected to a treatment that doubled the transpulmonary pressure, not only immediately adapted to the new type of mechanical ventilation, but did not show any intolerance or side effects. Presumably, the fact that both pressures were of opposite value to each other, caused the alveolar pressure to zero during the entire inspiratory act, significantly lowering the ventilatory stress.

A latest evolution of negative pressure ventilators, presented in the COVID period, is the *"Exovent"*. Developed by the University of Warwick, Marshall Aerospace & Defense Group, and other collaborators, *"Exovent"* is a breathing support device that uses negative pressure ventilation. It resembles the old iron-lung, but, unlike the latter, it is shorter (it extends from the neck to the patient's hips), it is constructed of lighter materials, and it is more powerful. Furthermore, the patient, who has his legs free, can have a semi-seated position and can turn comfortably on his side.

6.2 Ventilation Modes

The ventilation modes that may be used with an extrathoracic ventilator are:

1. *Intermittent negative pressure ventilation* (called NPV) (Fig. 6.2a). In this case, the machine creates a subatmospheric (negative) pressure which results in the lifting of the chest and abdomen. The first determines an expansion of the rib cage, the second a lifting of the anterior abdominal part with the lowering of the diaphragm. Both determine a negative intrathoracic pressure with a suction mechanism of the air from the upper airways, in other words, they determine an inspiratory act. In the case of the "controlled" mode, the doctor sets the times of the ventilatory cycle, the I/E ratio, the ventilatory frequency, the extent of the

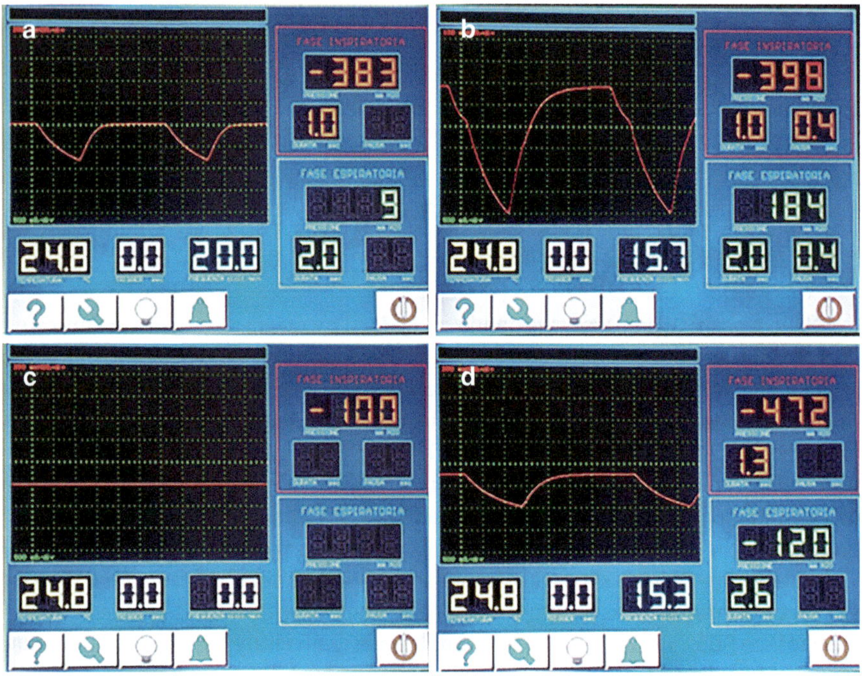

Fig. 6.2 Top left (**a**) shows the trend of the pressure curve during ventilation with negative pressure only. At the top right (**b**) the curve of negative pressure ventilation alternating with positive pressure can be observed. Bottom left (**c**), the curve indicates a constant negative pressure. In practice, this is not a true ventilatory modality and the patient, although facilitated in inhaling, is free to breathe autonomously. Bottom right (**d**) shows the ventilation curve at two levels of negative pressure where the end of inspiration corresponds to the maximum negative pressure and the end of expiration to the lowest negative pressure level

negative pressure, eventual pauses when the ventilatory cycle is reversed. In the case of the "assisted" mode, the doctor sets the entity of the negative pressure, while the patient determines the beginning of the inspiratory act, its duration and the moment to switch to the expiratory act. At the end of the inspiration, the machine interrupts the negative pressure and the expiratory act takes place passively due to the simple pulmonary elastic recoil up to the Functional Residual Capacity (FRC) position. If the ventilator uses a *"cuirass"* or a *"ponchowrap,"* the effect of the negative pressure on the patient's body is reduced, since part of the abdomen is not affected by the action created by the ventilator and the diaphragm has a smaller excursion.

2. *Negative and positive pressure ventilation* (also called: *"Biphasic Cuirass Ventilation"* or simply: NPV) (Fig. 6.2b). In this mode the ventilator adds, to the inspiratory phase, a positive pressure in the expiratory phase up to the equilibrium position (FRC). This force helps the elastic recoil of the chest and shortens expiratory times as both forces act in the same direction. However, a positive pressure in the expiratory phase may run the risk of causing air trapping phenomena with possible barotrauma phenomena, especially in patients with increased thoracic time constants (TC), such as in COPD. Even with this type of ventilation, the "controlled" or "assisted" mode may be used, depending on the clinical characteristics of the patient and his or her ability to interact with the ventilator. Positive pressure cannot be applied in "ponchowrap" ventilators that do not have a rigid external thoraco-abdominal support such as that of the "cuirass ventilator" or the IL.
3. *Extrathoracic continuous negative pressure ventilation* (CNPV) (Fig. 6.2c). In this mode, a continuous subatmospheric pressure is created which, by bringing the FRC value to a higher level, reduces the inspiratory effort, facilitates the expansion of the chest and, therefore, the inspiration itself.

   Just like a continuous positive pressure, delivered inside the airways such as CPAP, both raise the FRC level, but this modality cannot be considered a true mechanical ventilation in which the cyclical trend of a respiratory act can be recognized, characterized by an inspiration and an expiration, but only a support to the spontaneous ventilation of the patient.
4. *Ventilation with two levels of negative pressure* in which a negative end-expiratory pressure is added to a normal negative pressure ventilation (NPV-NEEP) (Fig. 6.2d). In practice, the ventilator implements the ventilatory cycle alternating it between two levels of negative extrathoracic pressure similar to what occurs with positive pressure ventilation to which a PEEP has been added (IMV + PEEP). To facilitate the onset of inspiration, a relatively low negative pressure is applied which raises the end-expiratory level (FRC), while the entire inspiratory act is consequent to the application of a higher negative pressure up to preset values. The expiratory act occurs by simple thoracopulmonary elastic recoil or also supported by extrathoracic positive pressure acting up to the pre-established FRC value.

One particular ventilatory modality is the *"high-frequency chest wall oscillation"* (HFCWO) of the Hayek ventilator. In this case, the positive and negative pressures are delivered at a high frequency, so much so as to cause the chest wall to oscillate.

Both the magnitude and frequency of the oscillation can be adjusted. Oscillation frequencies above 2 Hz can improve gas exchange in adults with ARF [5] or increase pulmonary blood flow in children undergoing cardiac surgery [6]. The *"high-frequency chest wall oscillation"* differs from the *"high-frequency chest wall compression"* (HFCWC) which causes a direct rhythmic compression of the chest wall, thus relying on its natural elastic rebound to return to the starting point. But, while HFCWC can lead to pulmonary atelectasis, HFCWO, based on the pendulum action of 2 forces applied in sequence on the chest, by means of rapid compression and then expansion movements, produces an oscillatory movement of its surface, does not create atelectasis and favors the mobilization of secretions present within the airways. A graphical representation of the ventilation mode of the Hayek ventilator is shown in Fig. 6.3.

"Cardiac Synchronized—Biphasic Cuirass Ventilation" (CS-BCV). This is a ventilation mode of the Hayek device that synchronizes the inspiratory and expiratory phases with the cardiac cycle. This type of ventilation has resulted in increased cardiac output and easier hospital discharge in pediatric patients undergoing cardiac surgery. The same mode, applied during cardiac magnetic resonance imaging (RM), has allowed for better definition of cardiac structures. Specifically, during coronary angiography, synchronizing the image acquisition phase with cardiac diastole and

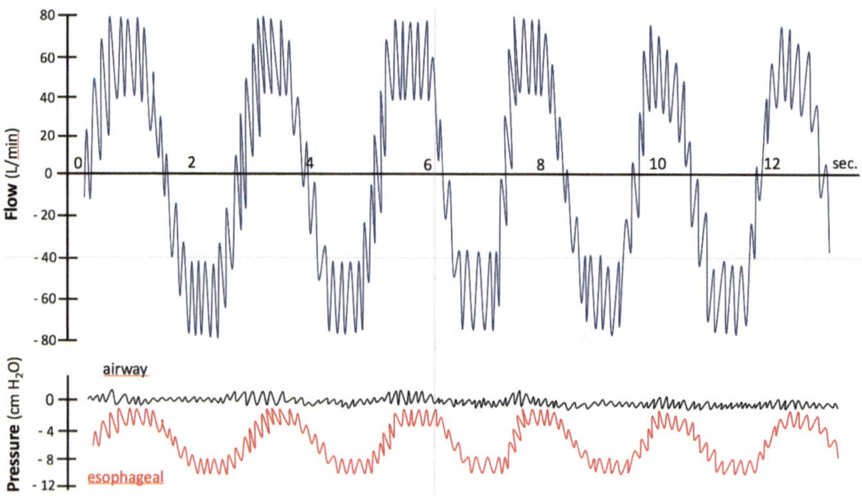

Fig. 6.3 Graphical reconstruction of the HFCWO showing both flow and pressure over time. The x-axis is measured in seconds. At the top, in blue, you can see how high-frequency thoracic oscillations, with rapid flow variations, affect the normale inspiratory (negative) and expiratory (positive) curves, The lower section shows the respective pressures, in cm. H2O, detected within the airways (in black) and esophagus (in red)

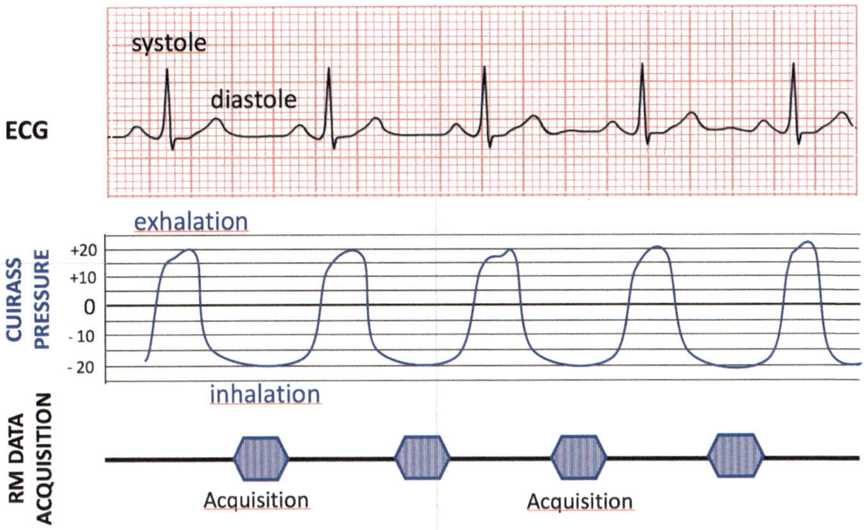

Fig. 6.4 Schematic representation of the RM acquisition mode during coronary angiography. The ventilator, synchronized with the ECG, is adjusted to have a short expiratory phase, coinciding with cardiac systole, and a long inspiratory phase, coinciding with diastole. Acquiring RM data during the diastolic phase allows for clearer and more legible data, as cardiac and respiratory movements are minimal

the inspiratory phase has resulted in shorter acquisition times and improved RM image quality (Fig. 6.4).

6.3 Monitoring

It is important to separate the monitoring of the functions of the negative pressure ventilator from the monitoring of the patient subjected to this ventilation method.

6.3.1 Ventilator Monitoring

As far as ventilator monitoring is concerned, modern equipment makes it possible to control the ventilatory frequency of the ventilator, the inspiration and expiration times, the temperature and the trend of the volume and pressure curves within the air space surrounding the patient. In the case of a large capacity ventilator, such as the iron-lung, in which the entire patient, with the exception of the head, enters the machine cabinet, the air volume will be decidedly higher and the volume and pressure variations will affect the whole body of the patient and, in particular, the chest and abdomen. Therefore, the variations in pressure and volume will determine the expansion and/or compression of these parts of the human body, with the indirect lowering or lifting of the diaphragm as well and relative mobilization of air in the airways and in the lung parenchyma.

On the other hand, in the case of ventilators with a lower volumetric capacity, in which the whole chest and only part of the abdomen will be involved, such as in the case of the cuirass or of the ponchowrap, the volume and pressure variations will mainly concern the chest, with less involvement of the diaphragm. Both in the first and in the second case, the trend of the pressure and volume curves in the air that will surround the patient will make it possible the monitoring of the ventilator.

Furthermore, modern ventilators also have a flow sensor with trigger function which, by means of a small probe placed near the upper airways, can detect the start of voluntary inspiration of the patient and initiate the inspiratory act of the ventilator, determining, thus, an "assisted" type of ventilation. However, there are no sensors that can determine the start of the expiratory act.

6.3.2 Patient Monitoring

The monitoring of the patient and in particular what happens, from a functional and metabolic respiratory point of view, inside the human body subjected to noninvasive extrathoracic mechanical ventilation, can be evaluated with various equipment.

Furthermore, monitoring can be defined as of first level or of second level. In the first case, the monitoring is of the noninvasive type, while in the second case, the monitoring is of the invasive type.

6.3.3 Noninvasive Patient Monitoring (1st Level)

The first monitoring of the patient is through observation and clinical evaluation by the health professionals. Added to this are the simplest noninvasive monitoring methods such as assessment of patient oxygenation by pulse oximetry (O_2 Sat), assessment of respiratory metabolic picture by arterial blood gas analysis (EGA), PaO_2/FiO_2 ratio, continuous ECG monitoring and body temperature. All these methods are easy to apply and give immediate confirmation of the patient's clinical and respiratory conditions.

Regarding the monitoring of the thoracopulmonary mechanics, of a noninvasive type, the *"respiratory inductive plethysmography"* (RIP) or with the *"electrical impedance tomography"* (EIT) can be used.

The RIP measures, constantly over time, the Tidal Volume (TV), the inspiratory time (Ti), the expiratory time (Te), the inspiratory time/total time ratio (Ti/Ttot), the tidal volume/inspiratory time ratio (TV/Ti), the respiratory rate (RR), the minute volume (V/m'). But, by simultaneously evaluating the volumetric variations of the thorax and abdomen, it also highlights any thoraco-abdominal asynchronisms that may have an unfavorable effect on the global ventilation of the patient [7, 8] (Fig. 6.5).

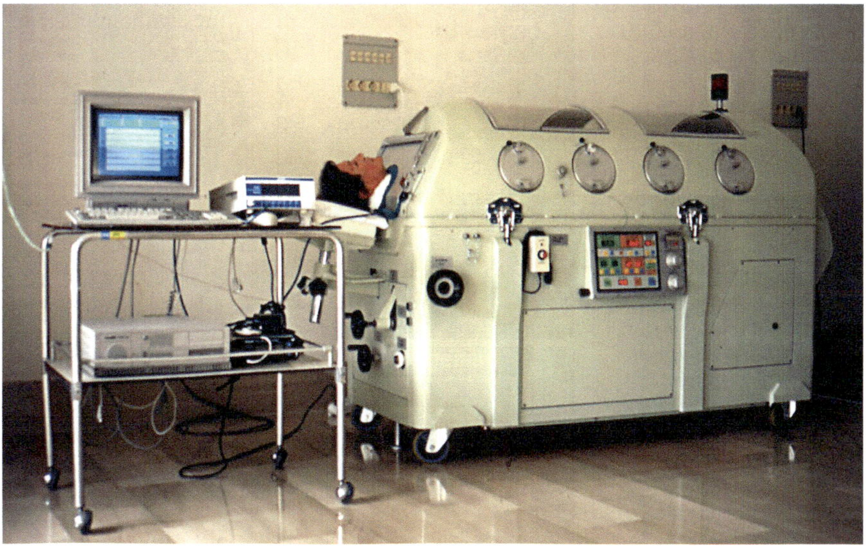

Fig. 6.5 Bloodless monitoring by "respiratory inductive plethysmography" (RIP). In this case the patient, placed inside an iron-lung, is under continuous control of the excursions of the thorax and abdomen, detectable in the form of waves and numerical values which confirm the correctness and effectiveness of the mechanical ventilation

The (EIT) measures, through sensors placed inside a chest strap, the thoracic electrical impedance [9], allowing the observation of the movement of internal sections through dynamic images similar to those of a CT scan. The superiority in definition and image quality of the latter is indisputable, but the portability and practicality of the EIT, as well as the cost, certainly make it interesting for bedside monitoring. The same EIT is of valid help in recognizing poorly ventilated or hyperventilated areas of the chest, in evaluating the district asynchronisms (Fig. 6.6b) and in monitoring possible areas of alveolar recruitment or atelectasis by varying the settings on the ventilator. In extrathoracic mechanical ventilation it is certainly an important monitoring modality because, unlike machine monitoring, it allows to visualize the dynamic ventilatory response of the patient and the reactions of internal sections of the chest during the application of the respirator. Thoracic impedance analysis, after appropriate calibration, also makes it possible to evaluate the percentage of Tidal Volume of each single thoracic quadrant, called ROI, which participates in the overall Tidal Volume (Fig. 6.6a).

The comparison between volume or pressure curves detected by the ventilator, compared with those detected on the patient with RIP or EIT allows a finer adjustment of the settings on the machine to obtain better therapeutic results. If you want even more detailed data on the ventilation trend during NPV or BCV, you need to approach the upper airways with the sensors. If we consider pulse oximetry (O_2 Sat) as a measure of the patient's oxygenation, we must consider "capnography" [10] as a method that allows us to evaluate correct ventilation. This method, initially used

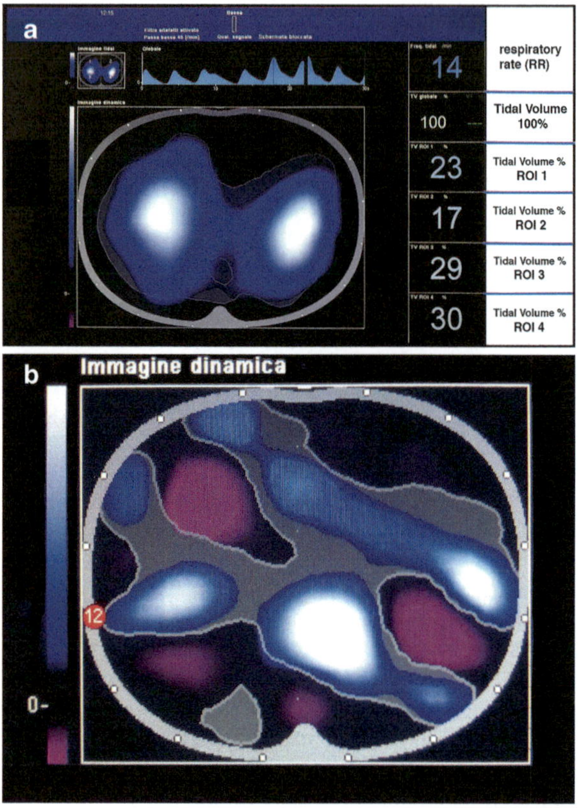

Fig. 6.6 Up high (**a**) the images that can be detected with "electrical impedance tomography" (EIT) highlight the characteristics and participation rates in global ventilation (TV) of lung areas called "ROI" in a subject undergoing NPV. Note how a large part of the global VT, in the extrathoracic negative ventilation mode, unlike, generally, what happens in intrathoracic positive pressure ventilation (PPV), is supported by the posterior lung zones (ROI 3 and 4). Below (**b**) is shown, in particular, the extreme inhomogeneity and complete ventilatory asynchronism in a subject suffering from severe emphysematous COPD, in spontaneous breathing, before being subjected to NPV

in the Intensive Care Unit to evaluate, act by act, the emission of carbon dioxide during invasive mechanical ventilation, was based on data provided by a transducer placed near the tracheal tube (mainstream). In more recent times, the devices, increasingly smaller and even portable, have been also equipped with internal CO_2 detectors which, using appropriate probes, aspirate air samples near the upper airways (sidestream) to reconstruct the end-tidal curves CO_2. There is a delay of a few seconds in the analysis of the carbon dioxide emitted with the ventilatory acts, but, basically, the monitoring is more than valid to understand whether the lung ventilator is doing its job well or if the patient responds properly to the extrathoracic mechanical ventilation.

If, on the other hand, we want to place an oronasal or face mask on the patient's face, almost all the monitoring used in mechanical positive pressure ventilation can be carried out.

The patient's face is surely limited in its complete freedom, however, while respecting the noninvasiveness, additional values can be obtained in the study of ventilatory monitoring. The pressures inside the airways cannot be measured, since a real ventilatory circuit is not being used, instead only a mask, however, both curves of the in-expiratory flows and those of the lung volumes can be measured. This can also be done with portable spirometers.

At this point, the monitoring would be even more complete since, in addition to the variations in volumes and pressures detected in the extrathoracic air of the ventilator, we could compare these with the variations in flows and volumes mobilized by the patient being treated. The further addition of equipment such as RIP or EIT would allow to have full control of almost all the patient's ventilatory mechanics.

6.3.4 Invasive Patient Monitoring (2nd Level)

If a more in-depth evaluation of the patient's ventilatory mechanics is necessary and in particular to obtain the measurement of the *"esophageal pressure"* (P_{es}) and, indirectly, of the *"pleural pressure"* (P_{pl}) and of the *"transpulmonary pressure"* (P_L), it would be necessary to place a balloon-tipped catheter in the esophagus. This measurement would allow the evaluation of the pressor action of the NPV on the patient's chest and, if dynamically combined with the simultaneous variations in volume, would provide a curve of the dynamic lung compliance and would also facilitate studies on the ventilatory work. Furthermore, esophageal pressure has also been suggested as a guide in ventilatory management in subjects with lung damage [11]. The same curve can be obtained by intubating the patient and connecting him to a second ventilator that can show ventilator loops. In fact, when noninvasive extrathoracic mechanical ventilation is combined with synchronized positive pressure ventilation, the measurements and curves detectable by both ventilators are obtained at the same time. But most importantly, based on this data, we can operate on each individual machine to obtain the best ventilation profile for the patient.

An evaluation of the effect of NPV on the abdomen and indirectly on the diaphragm can be obtained with the introduction of a bladder catheter to which a pressure transducer has been applied. The measurement can be obtained after filling the empty bladder with 50 mL of saline using the mid-axillary level as a reference line [12]. In a study carried out by Konstantinos Raymondos et al. [13], a reduction in abdominal pressure with an average of 20.5 mmHg was highlighted in subjects suffering from ARDS and subjected to negative mechanical ventilation.

If, during NPV, rises the need or desire to monitor the cardiac index, the intrathoracic blood volume index, the extravascular pulmonary water index and the variation in stroke volume by means of thermal dilution, the *"PiCCO"* system can be used by inserting a catheter into an artery [14].

More complex investigations such as the study of the pulmonary arterial system by means of the introduction of a Swan-Ganz catheter are not excluded.

Although currently not present on any ventilator, future control of extrathoracic mechanical ventilation (BCV or NPV) as well as optimal man-ventilator synchronization could be achieved with the implementation of *"Neurally Adjusted Ventilatory Assist"* (NAVA). In this case, it would be necessary to insert an esophageal tube, equipped with particular sensors, which would intercept the patient's spontaneous inspiratory drive at the level of the esophageal cardias and, thus, control the ventilator according to the patient's needs.

6.4 Settings

The regulation of the NPV or BCV ventilator is based on the interface of the machine with the patient and on the adjustment operations to be carried out to obtain effective mechanical ventilation.

The use of an iron-lung type ventilator forces the patient to lie down and hermetically close the box at the level of the patient's neck. The same thing happens with the "*Exovent*" ventilator, even if the material used for the closure at neck level is softer and more biocompatible; and furthermore, the patient can also assume a semi-sitting or side-lying position. The neck closure prevents or makes it very difficult to treat tracheostomized patients. Instead, in patients undergoing ventilation with a cuirass, by appropriately shaping its upper part, it is possible to create a space that gives free access to the tracheostomy tube. Also in this case it is possible to carry out mechanical ventilation in a sitting position.

Once the ventilator has been applied to the patient, the first settings to be defined will be the levels of negative pressure to be delivered, the inspiratory and expiratory times, any possible pause at each reversal of the ventilatory cycle and the ventilatory frequency. The initial ventilatory rate settings should be equal to or slightly less than the patient's spontaneous ventilatory rate.

It will be the volumetric increase of the inspiratory act (TV) and, therefore, of the volume/minute (V/m') which will produce a better oxygenation and a progressively lower need, on the part of the patient, to maintain an initial high ventilatory frequency. In this case, consensually, this frequency on the ventilator can be progressively reduced. The latter (this frequency), if the patient is connected to the machine with a sensor that will act as an inspiratory trigger, will be controlled directly by the patient's spontaneous respiratory rate. All of this, of course, in the presence of an awake and cooperative patient, while in the case of a patient with sensory numbness or even in a coma, it will be the doctor who adjusts all the ventilator settings and, in this case, the ventilation will be of the "controlled type."

The adjustments on the inspiratory and expiratory times or on the I/E ratio and the pressure level to be established will be a consequence of the patient's pathophysiological and clinical knowledge, as normally occurs with the use of ventilators which release a positive pressure into the airways.

The initial negative pressures must be low (between 10 and 15 cm/H_2O) in order to make the patient easily adapt to the machine. Subsequently, the negative pressure values can be increased (usually between 20 and 30 cmH_2O) in order to obtain better efficacy from mechanical ventilation. In any case, bear in mind that the patient, having his head free, will be able to speak and report to us, moment by moment, the progress of his ventilatory treatment and any needs he may have.

It must be remembered that preset extrathoracic negative pressure values do not exactly correspond to the positive pressure values of a machine acting directly on the airways. This is explained by the fact that, to obtain the same pressure, flow or volume changes within the chest, negative ventilation must first address the "*Chest Elastance*" (E_{cw}) and, therefore, lose some strength and effectiveness in overcoming it. It will be direct monitoring on the airways or the use of RIP or EIT, as mentioned previously, which will allow, with more precision, to control the entire respiratory cycle, the pressure levels to be delivered and the duration of the treatment.

The machines that deliver a NPV or BCV have pressure transducers, positioned inside the machine or even in the cuirass, which interact with the control system to always have a constant analysis of the entire ventilation cycle and, possibly, act as an alarm in case of malfunction. Additional alarms, which can be activated by the patient in case of need, are positioned in the larger ventilators. More recent machines, as in the case of the "*Exovent,*" have various sensors, positioned in several parts of the appliance, to allow more detailed control of the global operation of the ventilator and support different configurations.

6.5 Conclusion

Over the years, noninvasive extrathoracic mechanical ventilation has undergone various improvements and has been enriched with new ventilation modes, facilitated by the use of electronic engineering. This has led to a shift from the original "controlled" ventilation mode to the "assisted" mode, through the use of sensors placed in the upper airways that facilitated human-machine synchronization. Furthermore, in addition to the common ventilation modes present on almost all negative pressure ventilators (*Intermittent Negative Pressure Ventilation* or NPV, *Biphasic Chest Ventilation* or BCV, *Continuous Negative Pressure Ventilation* or CNPV, *Ventilation with Two Levels of Negative Pressure* or NPV-NEEP), new ventilation modes have recently been added with the latest devices, such as the "*High-Frequency Chest Wall Oscillation*" (HFCWO), the "*Cardiac Synchronized Biphasic Chest Ventilation*" (CS-BCV), and the "*Positive + Negative Synchronized Ventilation*" (PNSV). All this has allowed the ventilator to be increasingly adapted to the patient's respiratory needs, increasing the possibilities for intervention, including in diagnostic and surgical settings.

To obtain physiological and clinical information about the patient during mechanical ventilation, monitoring is used, which has been divided into ventilatory machine monitoring and clinical and functional patient monitoring. The collection of all data, which occurs simultaneously with the ventilator treatment, allows for more precise setting of all the ventilator parameters and monitoring of their performance, ensuring that at every stage of its application, the best benefits can be achieved with the least complications.

Although it is an older ventilation method, the introduction of new materials has led to the creation lighter and more compact devices, making them easier to use. Furthermore, with the advent of new and innovative ventilation methods, mostly electronically controlled, BCV is enjoying a new lease of life and is proving capable of having a positive impact in many healthcare settings: from Pediatrics to Medical

Departments, from Pulmonology to Rehabilitation Centers, from Intensive Care Units to Operating Rooms, up to its use in Endoscopic Diagnostics and Radiology.

References

1. Drinker P, Shaw LA. An apparatus for the prolonged administration of artificial respiration. I. A design for adults and children. J Clin Invest. 1929;7:229–47.
2. Gunella G. Treatment of acute on chronic respiratory failure with iron lung: results in a series of 560 cases. Ann Med Physique. 1980;2:317–27.
3. Raymondos K, Ahrens J, Ulrich Molitoris U. Combined negative- and positive-pressure ventilation for the treatment of ARDS. Case Rep Crit Care. 2015;2015:714902.
4. Vincenzi U. A new mode of mechanical ventilation: positive + negative synchronized ventilation. Multidiscip Respir Med. 2021;16(1):788.
5. Al-Saady NM, Fernando SSD, Singer M, Bennett ED. External high-frequency oscillation can replace intermittent pressure ventilation in patients with acute respiratory failure. Intensive Care Med. 1992;18(Suppl. 2):S54, Abstr. 63.
6. Penny DJ, Hayek Z, Rigby ML, Redington AN. Ventilation with external high frequency oscillation around a negative baseline increases pulmonary blood flow after the Fontan operation. Cardiol Young. 1992;2:277–80.
7. De Groote A, Verbandt Y, Paiva M, et al. Measurement of thoracoabdominal asynchrony: importance of sensor sensitivity to cross section deformations. J Appl Physiol (1985). 2000;88(4):1295–302.
8. Caleffi Pereira M, Porras DC, Lunard AC, et al. Thoracoabdominal asynchrony: two methods in healthy, COPD, and interstitial lung disease patients. PLoS One. 2017;12(8):e0182417.
9. Bachmann MC, Morais C, Bugedo G, et al. Electrical impedance tomography in acute respiratory distress syndrome. Crit Care. 2018;22(1):263.
10. Rackley CR. Monitoring during mechanical ventilation. Respir Care. 2020;65(6):832–46.
11. Talmor D, Sarge T, Malhotra A, et al. Mechanical ventilation guided by esophageal pressure in acute lung injury. N Engl J Med. 2008;359:2095–104.
12. De Keulenaer BL, De Waele JJ, Powell B, et al. What is normal intra-abdominal pressure and how is it affected by positioning, body mass and positive end-expiratory pressure? Intensive Care Med. 2009;35(6):969–76.
13. Raymondos K, Molitoris U, Capewell M, et al. Negative- versus positive-pressure ventilation in intubated patients with acute respiratory distress syndrome. Crit Care. 2012;16(2):R37. https://doi.org/10.1186/cc11216.
14. Hofkens P-J, et al. Common pitfalls and tips and tricks to get the most out of your transpulmonary thermodilution device: results of a survey and state-of-the-art review. Anesthesiol Intensive Ther. 2015;47(2):89–116.

7 BCV Applications: Operational Choices and Ventilator Settings

Maria Papaioannou and Georgia Vasileiadou

7.1 Introduction

Ventilation via cuirass has gained attention nowadays as an alternative to noninvasive ventilation through a mask interface. The device used for this approach resembles a piece of armor that covers the torso used by soldiers in the past [1].

With the use of positive pressure during the expiratory phase to force air out of the lungs and negative pressure during the inspiratory phase to actively move the diaphragm downward, biphasic cuirass ventilatory devices support ventilation and contribute to spontaneous breathing [2]. They can also be used in a secretion clearance spectrum for airway clearance, especially for patients with cystic fibrosis, bronchiectasis, and neuromuscular disease. The biphasic cuirass ventilator, as a secretion management tool, is characterized by comfort, effectiveness, and efficiency. The cuirass applying high-frequency oscillatory waves achieves the thinning and advancing of secretions to the large airways. In this mode, it combines with its assisted cough function so as to facilitate expectoration [3].

7.2 Clinical Benefits of BCV

BCV ventilation offers patients several clinical advantages. By increasing the PaO2/FiO2 ratio, it improves the FRC (oxygenation residual capacity). It can be combined with other ventilation methods, such as positive pressure ventilation (PPV), continuous positive airway pressure (CPAP), bilevel positive airway pressure (BIPAP), and high-flow nasal cannula (HFNC), and it also supports more expeditious weaning from PPV. This ventilatory technique helps reverse atelectasis by regulating the flow of secretions from the lungs. It has been demonstrated to lower the rates of

M. Papaioannou (✉) · G. Vasileiadou
1st ICU, General Hospital of Thessaloniki "G. Papanikolaou", Exohi, Thessaloniki, Greece

O. Alibrahim et al. (eds.), *Biphasic Cuirass Noninvasive Ventilation*, Noninvasive Ventilation. The Essentials, https://doi.org/10.1007/978-3-032-20933-7_7

intubation and reintubation and enhance pulmonary compliance and patient adherence to therapy. Biphasic Cuirass Ventilation is used to cure persistent air leaks. It improves cardiac preload and raises cardiac output in terms of the hemodynamic effects [4].

7.3 Indications of BCV Use

Biphasic cuirass ventilation has been used in several pathological conditions, particularly in patients with neuromuscular diseases such as amyotrophic lateral sclerosis (ALS), spinal muscular atrophy (SMA), muscular dystrophy (MD), and Guillain–Barré syndrome who experience acute or chronic respiratory failure because of thoracic restrictive disorders and may be dependent on continuous ventilatory support. The patients frequently exhibit an unproductive cough, difficulties in clearance, airway obstruction, restrictive lung pathology, swallowing challenges accompanied by dysphagia and aspiration, recurrent respiratory infections, disturbances in sleep-related breathing, alveolar hypoventilation, and respiratory failure. This cohort of patients could derive significant advantages from negative pressure ventilation therapy, which would substantially mitigate their symptoms [5].

Moreover, patients who are diagnosed with cystic fibrosis and those who require HFCWO due to thick and copious secretions who present difficulty in removing them may also be assisted by BCV. The respirator is utilized as chest physical therapy, including volume expansion and pulmonary secretion clearance, to enhance the patient's compromised ability to maintain clear airways [6].

The biphasic cuirass ventilation (BCV) device is an alternative respiratory support device for patients with chronic obstructive pulmonary disease (COPD), especially during exacerbations. It may assist in improving their exertional capacity, managing those who present with hypercapnia to effectively remove CO_2, assisting them with the removal of excessive bronchial secretions resulting in reduced hospitalizations, and reducing mortality rates. Additionally, patients with asthma or bronchiolitis who displayed hypoxemia and respiratory distress after receiving BCV therapy exhibited improvement in their WOB, an increase in oxygen saturation, prevention of intubation, and decreased atelectasis [7].

It has been reported to be beneficial in patients suffering from COVID-19 infection who present with acute respiratory failure or those suffering from long-term COVID respiratory symptoms. BCV supports patients by relieving symptoms, improving oxygenation, preventing atelectasis, and prohibiting intubation [2].

Many head and spinal cord injury patients will need assistance with ventilation that may be impaired postinjury as well as clearance of the airways. Utilizing airway clearance systems that have an active cough assistance mode increases patients' lung recruitability, keeping their airway open, and improves lung compliance [4].

BCV can also be used when patients face difficulty in weaning from positive pressure ventilation. Negative pressure ventilation can be implemented in anesthesia in ear, nose, and throat (ENT) procedures; in postoperative procedures (e.g., postcoronary bypass, Fontan, Fallot, post-pneumonectomy); and even in prelung transplant, improving pulmonary thorax compliance and decreasing atelectasis so as to increase tidal volume and lead to the resolution of respiratory failure [4].

7.4 Modes of Cuirass Ventilation

The Biphasic Cuirass Ventilator is a negative pressure, pressure-targeted, time- or pressure-cycled, noninvasive ventilator that works similarly to natural respiration. The patient's chest and abdomen are encased in an air chamber by means of the cuirass shell, which is linked to the ventilator by wide-bore tubing and regulated by means of a pressure monitoring tube [8].

The Biphasic Cuirass Ventilator is comprised of four main modes: Continuous Negative Mode, Control Mode, Respiratory Synchronized Mode, and Secretion Clearance Mode, delivering high-frequency chest wall oscillation (HFCWO) and cough [6].

7.5 Continuous Negative Mode (CNEP)

To improve hypoxemia, alveoli and small airways can be recruited by facilitating the continuous negative mode. Patients experiencing greater work of breathing (WOB) may benefit immensely from it. Moreover, it is applicable to small airway diseases, such as bronchiolitis. It could be used in weaning patients from invasive positive pressure ventilation (PPV), thus decreasing the complications of prolonged mechanical ventilation, or even in combination with PPV to counter side effects [8].

CNEP is usually chosen as the initial support mode, with a minimum support in adults of negative pressure of (−8) cmH_2O. This is then adjusted in decrements of 2 cmH_2O until work of breathing is noted to improve. In most cases, a negative pressure of (−15) cmH_2O is adequate; however, it may be necessary to increase to more negative pressures (e.g., 20 cmH_2O) in response to increased work of breathing or hypoxemia, particularly when significant alveolar recruitment is required [8].

A patient must have sufficient respiratory drive in order to select CNEP as a BCV mode. Reduced PEEP may be necessary when used in conjunction with PPV to prevent an increase in mean airway pressure. For the best result of the implementation, this mode appears to be effective in treating early hypoxemic and hypercarbic respiratory failure [8].

7.6 Control Mode

Complete control over the patient's breathing is available in this mode. When a patient exhibits a weak or no respiratory drive, it is indicated. Selecting this mode of ventilation will enhance patients' breathing if their ABGs are marked by CO_2 retention and/or if their dyspnea is not responsive to CNEP titration. Additionally, to improve compliance and oxygenation, it can be used in the assisting mode with

PPV and BCV rates. It is necessary to set and deliver the mandatory respiratory rate in the control mode. The patients still breathe using their own respiratory muscles. The I:E ratio controls both the inspiratory and expiratory phases. The rate is commenced at 2 above the patient's own spontaneous rate, yet it can slowly be decreased as the respirator takes control of the patient's breathing and the I:E ratio is 1:1 [8].

Using this breathing method, the mean cuirass pressure should always be kept at or below −4. Additionally, it is imperative that the inspiratory and expiratory pressures are in equilibrium at rates exceeding 60 cpm, with a ratio of −15/+15. Additionally, the Δp should consistently exceed 10 cm. To summarize, the pressure ratio should be maintained at or near 3:1 (i.e., −21/+7 or −15/+5) [8].

With the patient's improvement, both the mean cuirass pressure and the rate can be progressively decreased. A titration to CNEP may also be attempted if there is an adequate respiratory drive. In contrast, if there is no improvement and hypoxemia is apparent, a greater negative mean cuirass pressure should be applied. A higher minute breathing rate should be implemented in cases when hypercarbia is detected [8].

Following are the recommended beginning settings for a healthy lung, as seen in cases of neuromuscular diseases, brain and spinal cord injuries, reduced cardiac output, anesthetic ventilation, and postcardiac surgery ventilation [8]:

Inspiratory pressure: −21 cmH_2O
Expiratory pressure: +7 cmH_2O
I:E Ratio: 1:1
The frequency rate is set at 2–4 breaths above the patient's own spontaneous rate.

Ventilator settings for a lung obstruction should comprise [8]:

Inspiratory pressure: −24 cmH_2O
Expiratory pressure: +8 cmH_2O
I:E ratio: 1:1 or 1:2
The frequency rate is set equal to or slightly above the spontaneous respiratory rate

Adjustments to the pressure setting should be implemented if the lung exhibits restrictive characteristics [8]:

Inspiratory pressure: −21 cmH_2O
Expiratory pressure: +7 cmH_2O
I:E ratio: 1:1
Frequency starts at up to 60 cpm (can be increased up to 120 cpm for decreased chest wall compliance)

In order to address the issues of low compliance and volume in ARDS patients' lungs, the following adjustments to the power mode parameters are recommended [8]:

Inspiratory pressure: −30 cmH_2O
Expiratory pressure: +10 cmH_2O
The I:E ratio increases from 2:1 to 6:1
Frequency starts at 40, 50, or 60 cpm and increases as well up to 120 cpm to ensure adequate minute ventilation

The physician should not neglect to decrease both the rate and the mean cuirass pressure when the patient's status improves and even attempt a titration to CNEP if adequate respiratory drive is present. If the patient does not improve or even worsens, the pressure ratio could gradually be increased at 3:1. (e.g., change −21/+7 or −24/+8), and/or the I:E ratio be altered for greater Ti in order to lower mean chamber pressure [8].

7.7 Respiratory Synchronized Mode

This mode instantly adapts to the natural breathing alterations that the patient generates because it is totally synchronized with their own respiration. An initial trigger is created by the patient's inspiratory effort, and an additional trigger is created by the patient's initial expiratory effort. The airways or the cuirass may be the source of this trigger.

In this mode, the support is timed with the patient's own respiratory pattern, so the I:E ratio is set by the physician. The set minimum back-up breath rate will be delivered if the patient's own breath rate falls below the set minimum back-up rate and will give a set I:E ratio of 1:1 until triggered by the patient (the cycle will restart again) [8].

The ventilator identifies dyssynchrony with control mode when there is insufficient respiratory drive and the patient needs breath-to-breath assistance to maintain tidal volume. The ventilator will switch to a backup rate at predetermined pressures in the event of apnea.

It should be taken into consideration to lessen the trigger sensitivity when the patient experiences extended durations at 100% of the trigger percentage, as this may suggest auto cycling. If the trigger percentage is 85% or less, the sensitivity should be increased. In this case, a lower value is equal to greater sensitivity. The pressure ratio should be maintained at or near 3:1 (i.e., −21 / +7 or −15 / +5), as mentioned above [8].

One method of achieving airway triggering is to insert the nasal cannula containing the airway pressure sensor tube into the patient's mouth or nostril. Another option is to utilize a conventional type T airway adapter with a pressure measuring port directly linked to the tracheostomy or endotracheal tube or to place the sensor tube inside a tracheostomy mask and place it over the tracheostomy. It is necessary to observe pressure waves on the graphic display to ensure accurate and constant triggering [8].

The airway trigger is more sensitive. Starting sensitivity should be set at 5 and adjusted for maximum synchronization. Cuirass triggering, on the other hand, is better for extreme respiratory effort and should be started around the sensitivity of 3. Trigger percentage readings should read between 85% and 99%, and sensitivity should be adjusted to achieve this. If the trigger percentage is less than 85%, the sensitivity may need to be increased from 5 down to 4. In case of prolonged periods of trigger percentages of 100%, this could be an indication of auto-triggering. Under these circumstances the sensitivity may need to be decreased from 5 up to 6.

The minimum backup breath rate is 6 per minute, and the maximum backup breath rate is 60 per minute. The backup rate should be set to half of what the patient is breathing after settling on support, usually as a safety net for apnea or hypoventilation. The shallower the patient's breathing, the more sensitive the trigger should be to capture their respiratory effort [8].

Adjusting the range, or the difference between the expiratory and inspiratory pressures in this mode, has an impact on tidal exchange. The patient determines the rate, and the tidal exchange adjusts in accordance with the patient's effort throughout the respiratory cycle [9].

7.8 Secretion Clearance Mode

This mode is used as a chest physiotherapy tool to enhance the clearance of secretion from the lungs and consists of two cycles.

- Vibration Mode, which enhances the loosening of the secretion and
- Cough Mode, which creates a cough-like effect to assist in eliminating the secretion.

Frequency, inspiratory pressure, and time are set for the vibration mode (expiratory pressure is not set as the vibration has a preset amplitude). Frequency, inspiratory and expiratory pressures, I:E ratio, and time are set for the cough mode. The cuirass will vibrate for the set period of time and will incorporate the required coughs within the time set. This whole vibration/cough cycle can be repeated up to 20 times if required [8].

Whenever the patient demonstrates thick secretions or severe atelectasis, it is better to choose lower vibration CPM. For the patients who are dependent on continuous ventilation, shorter durations of vibration should be considered [8].

7.9 Monitoring of BCV

There are four sections on the monitor display. The readings for the cuirass, airway, and ECG data are shown on the left side of each of the top three graphs, which also monitor and display the data. The machine's current mode and standby status are displayed in the top bar. The alarm settings are shown on the right side of the screen, and the main parameter settings are at the bottom [10].

While the unit is operational, three options are accessible [10]:

- mode selection
- parameter configuration
- alarm settings

The respirator features both visual and auditory alerts. The visual alerts are located on the right side of the screen and feature a flashing red LED light on the front panel of the power unit [10].

Three distinct methods exist for displaying alarms on the screen [10]:

- When alarm thresholds are established, the background will be illuminated in green.
- In the absence of established alert restrictions, the background will be accentuated in blue.
- If alert thresholds are established but fall below the acceptable range, the backdrop will be marked in red.

The alarm settings that are available in the biphasic cuirass ventilator are listed below:

- Inspiratory Pressure—Functions as both a high and low limit for inspiratory pressure. Varies from ±1 to 9 cmH_2O from the specified value.
- Expiratory pressure—Functions as both a high and low limit for expiratory pressure. Varies from ±1 to 9 cmH_2O from the specified value.
- Apnea (Duration)—The acceptable amount of time for apnea before an alarm is triggered. The duration varies from 10 to 30 s; the alarm can be deactivated by setting the time to zero.
- High Respiratory Rate—The threshold for maximum respiratory rate prior to alarm activation. Varies from 10 to 120 bpm; the alarm can be deactivated by adjusting the bpm to zero [10].

7.10 Considerations—Contraindications

A correct cuirass size is determined by the patient's weight and size. To further avoid excessive leakage when the cuirass shell is placed on the patient, the proper-size seal needs to be attached to it. Error 21 will sound an alarm when low pressure or leakage is identified by the ventilator. In this case, the provider must ensure that all tubing is in place and the seal is properly adhered to the shell [8]. It is important that any leads, lines, tubes, or drains be positioned within the cuirass so that the seal could not pass over points of their entry. The provider must ensure that the patient's thorax structure will provide a good seal of the cuirass [8]. The patient should be turned and repositioned frequently. It is necessary to rotate posterior pressure points to avoid skin deterioration. To maintain a good seal between the patient's skin and the cuirass, the turning must be restricted to an angle [8].

Because the cuirass is attached to the thorax and abdomen, BCV should not be used in patients who have burns or wounds that are draining. Additionally, by putting a barrier of fabric or clothing between the foam seal and the skin, the patient's risk of developing skin lesions is reduced. When a person is obese (>180 kg) or pregnant, BCV should not be used. Furthermore, it should not be applied in the event of a cardiopulmonary arrest [8].

Negative pressure may potentially worsen upper airway obstruction in patients with unstable airways, obstructive sleep apnea, or other types of soft tissue obstruction. For patients to benefit from BCV, their airways must remain open. This can be achieved with standard airway adjuncts for airway patency or with sufficient stenting pressure from CPAP [8].

In any mode, BCV has the potential to mobilize significant amounts of pulmonary secretions to the upper airway. If a patient requires assistance with secretion evacuation, oral suction should be taken into consideration. Frequent assessments of in-line suctioning or sterile tracheal suctioning are necessary for individuals who are intubated or have a tracheostomy tube in place. In patients undergoing secretion clearance with an artificial airway, suctioning ought to be carried out in the final 10–20 s of the cough assist cycle, if necessary [8].

Patients can still use BCV if they have a jejunostomy or gastroenteric tube in place as long as it is contained within the cuirass shell. Meals or bolus feeds should be given after the secretion clearance to avoid aspiration. Before or during the therapy, there should be a brief pause in continuous feeding during secretion clearance [8].

7.11 Discussion

With the majority of the negative effects of positive pressure therapies avoided, BCV is a therapeutic ventilation intervention that supports the expiratory and inspiratory needs of breathing in a physiologically normal manner. BCV enables patients to consume food, articulate speech, and hydrate while receiving complete respiratory assistance [4].

In patients with severe COPD exacerbations and exacerbated chronic respiratory failure, Carpagnano et al. [11] combined the use of positive and negative ventilation and observed that this approach was well tolerated and superior to the individual modes in patients with ARF and COPD exacerbations [11].

A 2016 cohort study by Minato and colleagues [12] reported that BCV treatment was beneficial for children's moderate bronchial asthma (BA) episodes. It shortened the duration of hospitalization and oxygen administration, significantly stabilized the patients' condition from the day treatment started, and was thought to be advantageous from a health economics perspective [12].

In comparison to positive ventilation, negative-pressure ventilation produced better oxygenation and less lung damage in rabbits, according to Grasso et al. [13]. Since negative pressure is exerted on the chest and abdomen globally, this observation could be explained by more efficient lung volume inflation during both inspiration and expiration [13].

As shown in a retrospective analysis [14] of 41 cases of patients who were ventilated with BCV for acute respiratory failure of various causes, BCV in an ICU would be an equivalent or supportive strategy for recruiting the lung with secretion clearance mode, reducing WOB and dead-space ventilation, and increasing oxygenation [14].

Noninvasive mechanical ventilation (negative pressure ventilation, NPV, or noninvasive positive pressure ventilation, NPPV) was implemented in 258 consecutive patients with acute respiratory failure due to chronic respiratory disorders in a prospective cohort study published in 2004 by Gorini et al. [7]. The majority of this population was able to avoid intubation with this approach, according to the authors, which resulted in fewer complications and a lower mortality rate [7].

A combination of BCV and high-flow nasal oxygenation (HFNO) has been documented in the literature for the treatment of COVID-19 pneumonia patients. This process is considered to be an effective noninvasive method for de-escalating therapy and weaning patients off prolonged NIV [2].

Raymondos et al. [15] conducted a comparison between 2 h of continuous external negative pressure ventilation (CENPV) in a tank respirator, also known as "iron lung," and 2 h of continuous positive pressure ventilation (CPPV). They found that CENPV in a tank respirator enhanced gas exchange in ARDS patients at lower transpulmonary, airway, and intraabdominal pressures, suggesting that it can contribute to treating ARDS patients [15].

7.12 Conclusion

It has been demonstrated that biphasic cuirass ventilation can reduce mortality rates, improve patient comfort, and generally prevent the deleterious side effects of other contemporary ventilation techniques.

References

1. Tada M, Kadowaki T, Tsubouchi Y, Nishikawa E, Iwamoto S, Kobayashi K, Kimura M, Ikeda T, Yano S. Concurrent use of biphasic cuirass ventilation and low-intensity noninvasive positive pressure ventilation. Clin Pulm Med. 2020;27(1):26–9.
2. Almeida Borges J, Esquinas AM. Biphasic cuirass ventilation in the escalation of non-invasive ventilation in COVID-19: case report and review. Monaldi Arch Chest Dis. 2023;93(4) https://doi.org/10.4081/monaldi.2023.2510.
3. Mefford GW. Biphasic cuirass ventilation for airway secretions. In: Esquinas AM, editor. Humidification in the intensive care unit. Cham: Springer; 2023. https://doi.org/10.1007/978-3-031-23953-3_34.
4. What is Biphasic Cuirass Ventilation? Hayek medical. 2024. Available at: https://hayekmedical.com/. Accessed 1 July 2024.
5. Annunziata A, Calabrese C, Simioli F, Coppola A, Flora M, Marotta A, Di Spirito V, Didonna F, Cicalese M, Fiorentino G. Negative-pressure ventilation in neuromuscular diseases in the acute setting. J Clin Med. 2022;11(9):2589.
6. Onweni C, Rashid S, Goswami R, et al. Cuirass ventilation: an alternative home-based modality for chronic respiratory failure. Home Health Care Manag Pract. 2020;32(1):40–4.
7. Gorini M, Ginanni R, Villella G, Tozzi D, Augustynen A, Corrado A. Non-invasive negative and positive pressure ventilation in the treatment of acute on chronic respiratory failure. Intensive Care Med. 2004;30(5):875–81.
8. Application of the HAYEK BCV. Hayek Medical. 2024. Available at: https://hayekmedical.com/. Accessed 1 July 2024.

9. Leonard R, Mefford GW. Biphasic cuirass respirator: an approach based on normal ventilation. Respir Ther J Respir Tech. 2014;9(5):24–8. Available at: https://www.respiratorytherapy.ca/pdf/RT-9-5-ON14-R5.pdf.
10. Ghani S. RTX Respirator, Ventilator Handouts, Revision 1. 2005. Available at: chrome-extension://efaidnbmnnnibpcajpcglclefindmkaj/, https://media.gosh.nhs.uk/documents/RTX_Respirator.pdf. Accessed 4 July 2024.
11. Carpagnano GE, Sabato R, Lacedonia D, Di Gioia R, Saliani V, Vincenzi U, Foschino-Barbaro MP. New non invasive ventilator strategy applied to COPD patients in acute ventilator failure. Pulm Pharmacol Ther. 2017;46:64–8.
12. Minato TM, Okada KO. Investigation of the efficacy of biphasic cuirass ventilation for children hospitalized with a moderate bronchial asthma attack. Pediatr Pulmonol. 2016;51(S43):Proceedings #K59, p S83.
13. Grasso F, Engelberts D, Helm E, Frndova H, Jarvis S, Talakoub O, McKerlie C, Babyn P, Post M, Kavanagh BP. Negative-pressure ventilation: better oxygenation and less lung injury. Am J Respir Crit Care Med. 2008;177(4):412–8.
14. Kotani T, Sato T, Sato Y, Tanabe H, Ozaki M. The role of biphasic cuirass ventilation in acute respiratory failure. Am J Respir Crit Care Med. 2007:A435.
15. Raymondos K, Molitoris U, Capewell M, Sander B, Dieck T, Ahrens J, Weilbach C, Knitsch W, Corrado A. Negative- versus positive-pressure ventilation in intubated patients with acute respiratory distress syndrome. Crit Care. 2012;16(2):R37.

Biphasic Cuirass Ventilation: Advantages, Contraindications, and Complications

8

Erika Pineda, James Baxter, Vanessa Marthia, and Omar Alibrahim

8.1 Introduction

Negative pressure ventilation (NPV) has evolved from when it was first introduced in 1929 by Drinker and Shaw [1]. Their contributions supported the treatment of acute poliomyelitis. Over the decades, NPV devices have become more readily available and portable, allowing ease for administration of NPV. With improvements in the equipment, its use has continued to play a beneficial role in patients with acute and chronic respiratory disorders, from bronchiolitis in children to chronic obstructive pulmonary disease (COPD) in adults. Recent literature supports the use of Biphasic cuirass ventilation (BCV) in children with Fontan circulation and other cardiac surgeries. It has also been reported useful in palliative medicine, as short-term or long-term home treatments in patients with multiple conditions.

Given the recent interest in BCV as a feasible option to provide NPV not only in the hospital but in the out-of-hospital setting, it is crucial to become familiar with this fairly unexplored modality. This chapter will review the advantages and indications (including in pediatric acute and chronic respiratory failure and cardiac disorders, such as postcardiac surgery). We will also discuss considerations for patient selection, short-term vs long-term use, disadvantages, side effects, monitoring, and contraindications for use.

E. Pineda (✉) · J. Baxter · V. Marthia
University at Buffalo, Buffalo, NY, USA
e-mail: jbaxter@upa.chob.edu; vmarthia@upa.chob.edu

O. Alibrahim
Pediatric Critical Care Medicine, Duke University Hospital, Durham, NC, USA
e-mail: omar.alibrahim@duke.edu

O. Alibrahim et al. (eds.), *Biphasic Cuirass Noninvasive Ventilation*, Noninvasive Ventilation. The Essentials, https://doi.org/10.1007/978-3-032-20933-7_8

8.2 Advantages

NPV is a non-invasive form of respiratory support, and when administered via the biphasic cuirass ventilator, in addition to its overall compact size and ease of use, it provides many benefits to patients. It eliminates complications and decreases the costs associated with intubation and conventional mechanical ventilation while decreasing the length of hospitalizations [2–4]. Management of respiratory failure in infancy and childhood leading to intubation can result in significant complications peri-intubation, such as tube mispositioning, hypoxemia, and adverse hemodynamic effects leading to cardiopulmonary arrest [5]. Furthermore, mechanical ventilation use in the pediatric population has been associated with increased risk of lower respiratory tract infections, mucus plugging, atelectasis, and ICU neuromyopathy [6]. In the pediatric population, some studies suggest that BCV as a noninvasive respiratory support modality decreases the fraction of inspired oxygen (FiO_2) requirements and increases carbon dioxide (CO_2) clearance within hours of its use and is associated with a lower likelihood of intubation [2, 7].

BCV supports ventilation by applying negative pressure onto the chest wall, assisting lung rccoil as well as exhalation. This active form of exhalation is unique to this modality of ventilation. In a prospective multicenter cohort study investigating variables predictive of NPV failure, the response rate to NPV was found to be equivalent to other forms of noninvasive ventilation (NIV) [8]. BCV has also been used successfully in small children with beneficial effects on the cardiopulmonary circulation, deemed hemodynamically safer than previous NPV devices. The application of negative pressure onto the chest wall increases transpulmonary pressure, recruiting areas of atelectasis, leading to dilation of pulmonary capillaries and improving preload to the heart, therefore augmenting cardiac output [9, 10].

NPV offers several other clinical advantages. One of its key benefits is preserving essential physiological functions such as speech, cough, and swallow. This supports natural patient behavior and comfort, provides ease of suctioning, and allows for enteral nutrition [11]. Furthermore, patients are able to participate in their care by coughing, taking deep breaths, and swallowing, all of which assist in lung recruitment [2]. Notably and in alignment with patient-centered care, using BCV allows for intact communication between patients and care providers.

Additionally, the noninvasive nature of BCV provides better comfort and reduces the need for sedatives and analgesics compared to invasive ventilation. A key clinical advantage of NPV over positive pressure ventilation, given its ability to simulate natural lung movements, is the decreased risk of barotrauma or volutrauma.

NPV may be used in those who are unable to tolerate a facial mask due to facial deformity, claustrophobia, or excessive oral secretions [11]. NIV respiratory support modalities such as bilevel or continuous positive airway pressure (i.e., BIPAP or CPAP) require tightly fitting masks that may not accommodate all-sized patients. These interfaces can precipitate anxiety and make secretions and/or emesis problematic. Delivering extrathoracic negative pressure ventilation without engaging the face or airway is an alternative strategy without the risks of invasive ventilation or NIV [12]. This form of ventilation is especially effective in young children and is

Table 8.1 Advantages of negative pressure ventilation use

Advantages
Comfort
Maintains normal swallowing, feeding, and speech
Access to oral and nasal secretions
Reduced risk of aspiration
Ease of use
Suitable for patients who are unable to tolerate facemasks, have claustrophobia, or have facial abnormalities
Decreases risks of positive pressure ventilation (e.g., barotrauma, reduced venous return)
Less need for sedation
Provides chest physiotherapy

safe to use in conjunction with other modalities for noninvasive support, such as high-flow nasal cannula (HFNC) [12]. Lastly, it can provide rapid alternating positive and negative pressures to the chest as physiotherapy to aid in secretion clearance, similar to cough assist devices [12]. The advantages of negative pressure ventilation are listed in Table 8.1.

8.3 Patient Selection

8.3.1 Acute Respiratory Failure

NPV has been shown to be effective at treating multiple disease states that cause acute respiratory failure. The subatmospheric pressure generated by NPV is applied to the anterior chest wall, opening airways and creating negative pressure in the alveoli. The resulting effect is a pressure gradient that drives oxygen to the alveoli for gas exchange. In addition, NPV creates excursion of the diaphragm, which ultimately augments a patient's natural respiration. This form of noninvasive ventilation can be used alone or in conjunction with other noninvasive modalities.

In parenchymal diseases such as bronchiolitis and pneumonia, the pressure gradient created by NPV helps rerecruit collapsed and/or consolidated alveoli. The benefit of NPV in these particular disease processes was described in a retrospective cohort of 118 children with bronchiolitis and pneumonia in a single center. NPV has been shown to successfully lower oxygen requirements within the first hour of initiating the intervention [3]. A single-center retrospective study of 233 critically ill patients with acute respiratory failure found that 70% of the patients did not need escalation to any form of positive pressure ventilation after being supported by NPV/BCV. The use of NPV was also associated with a 28% decline in the annual percentage of PICU admissions requiring intubation, 3 years after introducing the use of NPV in children with acute respiratory failure, and only a 3% rate of complications [12]. Invasive positive pressure ventilation can be associated with adverse complications including increased length of hospital stay, exposure to sedation with potential ICU delirium and withdrawal, risk for barotrauma, ventilator-associated lung infections, and postintubation trauma [6]. Given the risks associated with invasive positive pressure ventilation, it is reasonable to expect that NPV can help prevent these adverse effects. Additionally, in children with asthma, NPV has been shown to improve oxygenation and decrease the work of breathing [13].

In the neonatal population, NPV has been shown to allow for a reduction in oxygen requirement after starting treatment in respiratory distress of the newborn [11]. Furthermore, a few case reports have shown a role in the use of this non-invasive treatment in patients with congenital diaphragmatic hernia [14].

8.3.2 Chronic Respiratory Failure

Many medical conditions resulting in chronic respiratory failure can benefit from the use of NPV. Historically speaking, negative pressure ventilation was used for patients who suffered poliomyelitis. While these patients received NPV via large devices known as "iron lungs", the advent of newer, smaller, and easier-to-use devices has allowed patients with various neuromuscular diseases to benefit. Neuromuscular diseases are characterized by weakness of the respiratory muscles, which ultimately can limit diaphragmatic excursion and thus limit the negative pressure the body can generate for breathing. Although positive pressure ventilation is commonly used for patients with neuromuscular diseases, the use of NPV is beneficial as it assists with augmenting their own natural breathing and eases their ability to inspire using the body's natural muscles. NPV is a feasible treatment option for patients who depend on respiratory support for prolonged periods throughout the day [15].

NPV has been shown to be beneficial in adults with chronic obstructive pulmonary disease (COPD), by increasing ventilation and decreasing hyperinflation and work of breathing in a state characterized by progressively worsening airway obstruction, increasing atelectasis, and alveolar damage. Huang et al., followed 129 patients with COPD in a prospective study over a 5-year period in Taiwan. One group received support of NPV with an unsupervised home exercise program, and the second group only received an unsupervised home exercise program. The investigators found that pulmonary rehabilitation with NPV reduced yearly decline of lung function, exacerbations, hospitalization rates, and improved medical costs [16].

Cystic fibrosis causes thick secretions with subsequent mucus plugging of the airways and alveoli, resulting in impaired ventilation and gas exchange. In this setting, NPV may be beneficial, however, more research is needed to help guide clinicians on how to best deploy its use.

8.3.3 Cardiac Disorders

NPV has shown great benefit for a large number of patients with cardiac conditions. NPV creates negative intrathoracic pressure, which facilitates venous return, increasing RV preload, and facilitates alveolar recruitment, decreasing RV afterload [17]. The physiologic changes that occur with the increase in negative intrathoracic pressure are particularly beneficial in patients with right-sided cardiovascular pathologies.

NPV is frequently used after repair of right-sided heart lesions, as it has been shown to improve cardiac output, increase stroke volume, and improve pulmonary and systemic vascular resistances after repair of such lesions as Tetralogy of Fallot [18]. Post-Fontan patients are subject to decreased cardiac output secondary to decreased venous return. Subsequently, post-Fontan physiology has also been shown to benefit from negative pressure ventilation [19]. The application of NPV in post-Fontan patients increases pulmonary blood flow and improves cardiac output [20, 21]. Ultimately, any condition that can benefit from increased venous return and therefore preload, may benefit from the use of NPV. Shime et al., assessed changes in hemodynamics and gas exchange in 16 infants and children after surgery for congenital heart defects by applying continuous negative external pressure (CNEP) with a cuirass. They concluded that by applying CNEP prophylactically immediately after extubation, there was a decrease in right ventricular load and improved arterial oxygenation [22]. Cardiac output is improved by lowering mean thoracic pressure which maximizes the venous return to the heart [23]. There is no increased intrathoracic pressure as is seen in traditional modes of positive pressure ventilation. In patients with right heart failure, negative pressure ventilation supports functional residual capacity by decreasing the afterload of the right ventricle and increasing the pulmonary blood flow. This optimizes oxygenation and alveolar ventilation [12] (*Please refer to* Chap. 26 *for further details related to the use of NPV in cardiac patients*).

Phrenic nerve palsy is a known complication postcardiac surgery, and one that can often lead to respiratory failure. While many of these patients require positive pressure ventilation, either via noninvasive or invasive ventilation, some ultimately require tracheostomies for chronic ventilation. Although positive pressure ventilation is the primary form of noninvasive treatment used for this condition, NPV has also been shown to be helpful as an alternative to current therapies [7].

8.3.4 Short Term Versus Long Term Use

As discussed, NPV can be utilized for acute or chronic respiratory conditions. Acutely, NPV via BCV or other modalities, can offer a form of respiratory support to patients in acute respiratory failure to overcome numerous respiratory illnesses and potentially avoid intubation. Typically, NPV via BCV can only be applied to the chest wall continuously for a few days before skin irritation and breakdown develops. In those with acute respiratory failure who are ultimately intubated, NPV can be used to wean from positive pressure ventilation. It can be used in conjunction with other respiratory support modalities (i.e., high flow nasal cannula, CPAP, or

BiPAP) to support patients postextubation and help avoid the need for reintubation.

Chronic respiratory conditions such as COPD, central hypoventilation syndromes, and neuromuscular disorders can also benefit from long-term use of NPV, [11] but 24-h use is often impractical from a logistical standpoint. However, it can be used in short durations each day, or overnight while sleeping, to help support those with chronic respiratory conditions.

8.4 Disadvantages

There is little published data on the complication rates of NPV in the general pediatric population, but overall complications seem to be rare. The majority of side effects of NPV come from stable, chronically ventilated patients. The most common side effects are poor compliance, upper airway obstruction, and musculoskeletal pain. Although NPV delivered via BCV is portable, its use restricts motion and may cause back pain. In more severe cases, rib fractures and pneumothorax have been reported [11]. Some of the most common reported pediatric complications include hypothermia, skin irritation at contact points, and upper-airway obstruction [4].

There have been reports of gastroesophageal reflux and aspiration due to the application of negative pressure on the tone of the lower esophageal sphincter. These effects can be minimized via the use of metoclopramide [24]. Other treatments that may help include the routine use of GI prophylaxis and placement of a

Table 8.2 Side effects of negative pressure ventilation use via the biphasic cuirass ventilator

Side effects
Poor compliance
Hypothermia
Musculoskeletal pain
Skin irritation at contact points
Agitation requiring sedation for application and/or continued use
Aspiration
Gastroesophageal reflux
Rib fractures/pneumothorax
Upper airway obstruction

nasogastric or nasoduodenal tube for enteral feedings. A summary of the side effects of negative pressure ventilation is presented in Table 8.2.

8.5 Monitoring Parameters

We recommend frequent assessments, at least every 4–6 h, to evaluate the integrity of the skin for breakdown or signs of pressure injuries. Although, in children there is a lower incidence of interface-related skin ulcers or compromise, likely due to the foam padding on the BCV which allows for less irritation and moisture trapping than the plastic seal on NIV devices [12]. In addition, due to concerns for hypothermia while on BCV we recommend frequent temperature assessments.

Patients should also be assessed for tolerance of BCV. Although the device is not particularly uncomfortable in its use, it does cause significant restrictions in patients which may lead to agitation as they should remain supine while the device is in place. In our clinical practice, in pediatric patients, we resort to the use of intravenous dexmedetomidine for sedation as needed. We recommend frequent assessments for comfort level and synchrony during delivery of NPV. Some patients might only need sedation with induction, as that is when the peak of discomfort tends to occur.

8.6 Contraindications

Any musculoskeletal condition that causes an abnormal shape of the thorax, such as kyphoscoliosis, or severe obesity is a relative contraindication to NPV, as the cuirass requires a tight seal over the chest wall.

Absolute contraindications for the use of NPV include open skin lesions or burns on the chest or abdomen and rib fractures or any other trauma to the thorax, as these can potentially worsen. NPV should not be used in patients with recent surgeries to the chest or abdomen, as it can create undue pressure and irritation on the surgical sites, and potentially harm the area of the body [11]. Any form of upper airway obstruction (i.e., obstructive sleep apnea) is a contraindication to using NPV since negative extra-thoracic pressure can ultimately worsen these obstructions [11]. Lastly, lack of upper airway protection is a strong contraindication for the use of NPV due to the risk of aspiration and new onset or worsening upper airway obstruction in unconscious patients or those with bulbar dysfunction. However, a retrospective study reporting the effects of NPV use in adult patients with acute respiratory failure in the setting of neuromuscular disease utilized nasogastric tubes and/or oropharyngeal airways to minimize the risk of aspiration and upper airway obstruction in the obtunded and comatose patients [11]. Although risk may be mitigated in selected cases and under close monitoring, caution is advised. Risk of aspiration continues to be a concern in unconscious or neurologically impaired patients, and for purposes of this chapter, will be listed as an absolute contraindication, as more

Table 8.3 Contraindications of negative pressure ventilation use

Contraindications	
Absolute	Relative
Open skin lesions	Abnormal chest wall
Rib fractures/thoracic trauma	Severe obesity
Recent chest/abdomen surgery	Uncooperative patients
Lack of upper airway protection	Claustrophobia
Upper airway obstruction	

supportive data in the pediatric population can be presented. The contraindications of negative pressure ventilation are listed in Table 8.3.

8.7 Conclusion

Despite the need for more robust, controlled trials, NPV represents a valuable and underutilized tool in the armamentarium for managing pediatric respiratory failure, particularly offering unique advantages for patients with cardiac pathophysiology. Increased familiarity with its advantages, contraindications, and complications, as outlined in this chapter, may promote its appropriate use and stimulate further research.

References

1. Drinker PSL. An apparatus for the prolonged administration of artificial respiration. I. A design for adults and children. J Clin Invest. 1929;7:229–47.
2. Corrado A, Gorini M, Villella G, De Paola E. Negative pressure ventilation in the treatment of acute respiratory failure: an old noninvasive technique reconsidered. Eur Respir J. 1996;9(7):1531–44.
3. Nunez CA, Hassinger AB. Predictors of negative pressure ventilation response in pediatric acute respiratory failure. Respir Care. 2020;65(1):91–8.
4. Deep A, De Munter C, Desai A. Negative pressure ventilation in pediatric critical care setting. Indian J Pediatr. 2007;74(5):483–8.
5. Kerrey BT, Rinderknecht AS, Geis GL, Nigrovic LE, Mittiga MR. Rapid sequence intubation for pediatric emergency patients: higher frequency of failed attempts and adverse effects found by video review. Ann Emerg Med. 2012;60(3):251–9.
6. Sood S, Ganatra HA, Perez Marques F, Langner TR. Complications during mechanical ventilation-A pediatric intensive care perspective. Front Med. 2023;10:1016316.
7. Raine JSM, Mok Q, Shinebourne EA, Southall DP. Negative extrathoracic pressure ventilation for phrenic nerve palsy after paediatric cardiac surgery. Br Heart J. 1992;67:308–11.
8. Antonelli M, Conti G, Moro ML, Esquinas A, Gonzalez-Diaz G, Confalonieri M, et al. Predictors of failure of noninvasive positive pressure ventilation in patients with acute hypoxemic respiratory failure: a multi-center study. Intensive Care Med. 2001;27(11):1718–28.
9. Gorini M, Ginanni R, Villella G, Tozzi D, Augustynen A, Corrado A. Non-invasive negative and positive pressure ventilation in the treatment of acute on chronic respiratory failure. Intensive Care Med. 2004;30(5):875–81.

10. Sills JHCW, Pietz J. Continuous negative pressure in the treatment of infants with pulmonary hypertension and respiratory failure. J Perinatol. 1989 Mar;9(1):43–8.
11. Corrado A, Gorini M. Negative-pressure ventilation: is there still a role? Eur Respir J. 2002;20(1):187–97.
12. Hassinger AB, Breuer RK, Nutty K, Ma CX, Al Ibrahim OS. Negative-pressure ventilation in pediatric acute respiratory failure. Respir Care. 2017;62(12):1540–9.
13. Stone RCA, Jundos R, Metz R, Whitmore J. Biphasic cuirass ventilation for respiratory distress due to asthma or bronchiolitis. Crit Care Med. 2018;46(1):1160.
14. Davis PJ, Field D. Continuous negative extrathoracic pressure respiratory support for neonates after congenital diaphragmatic hernia repair. Acta Paediatr. 2007;88(10):1156–67.
15. Annunziata A, Calabrese C, Simioli F, Coppola A, Flora M, Marotta A, et al. Negative-pressure ventilation in neuromuscular diseases in the acute setting. J Clin Med. 2022;11(9):2589.
16. Huang HY, Chou PC, Joa WC, Chen LF, Sheng TF, Lin HC, et al. Pulmonary rehabilitation coupled with negative pressure ventilation decreases decline in lung function, hospitalizations, and medical cost in COPD: a 5-year study. Medicine (Baltimore). 2016;95(41):e5119.
17. Alibrahim O, Rehder KJ, Miller AG, Rotta AT. Mechanical ventilation and respiratory support in the pediatric intensive care unit. Pediatr Clin N Am. 2022;69(3):587–605.
18. Shekerdemian LS, Bush A, Shore DF, Lincoln C, Redington AN. Cardiorespiratory responses to negative pressure ventilation after tetralogy of fallot repair: a hemodynamic tool for patients with a low-output state. J Am Coll Cardiol. 1999;33(2):549–55.
19. Shekerdemian LSSD, Lincoln C, Bush A, Redington AN. Negative-pressure ventilation improves cardiac output after right heart surgery. Circulation. 1996;94:49–55.
20. Charla P, Karur GR, Yamamura K, Yoo SJ, Granton JT, Oechslin EN, et al. Augmentation of pulmonary blood flow and cardiac output by non-invasive external ventilation late after Fontan palliation. Heart. 2021;107(2):142–9.
21. Shekerdemian LS, Bush A, Shore DF, Lincoln C, Redington AN. Cardiopulmonary interactions after Fontan operations: augmentation of cardiac output using negative pressure ventilation. Circulation. 1997;96(11):3934–42.
22. Shime NTC, Itoi THS. Continuous negative extrathoracic pressure in children after congenital heart surgery. Crit Care Resusc. 2006;8(4):297–301.
23. Lockhat DLD, Zidulka A. Hemodynamic differences between continuous positive and two types of negative pressure ventilation. Am Rev Respir Dis. 1992;146:677–80.
24. Marino WDPC. Reversal of negative pressure ventilation-induced lower esophageal sphincter dysfunction with metoclopramide. Am J Gastroenterol. 1992;87(2):190–4.

Part III

Clinical Hospital Applications. Pulmonary and Critical Care

Biphasic Cuirass Ventilation Use in Nasal-Face Mask Intolerance

9

Carmine Iermano, Mariangela Calabria, and Arturo Cuomo

9.1 Introduction

In the Bible, God gives life with a breath, sealing in the man's chest that which we call soul.

> … then the Lord God shaped man with dust from the ground and blew into his nostrils a breath of life and man became a living being. [Genesis 2, 7]

The power of life has always been inherent in the breath. It seems obvious that breathing represents an essential activity for living. Therefore, since ancient times, man has attributed unique and even mystical properties to the air and its inhalation. Controlling respiratory exchanges has represented the first and irreplaceable objective in the treatment of respiratory failure.

The incompetence to maintain valid oxygenation and adequate elimination of carbon dioxide (CO_2) represent the cause of organ damage and a limit for the patient's survival. For centuries, man has used practical methods to try saving human lives: such methods are part of history and have been handed down to us from ancient documents. There have been many attempts, since the mid-1800s, to realize mechanical ventilation, but these were not supported by precise scientific elements and/ or adequate physiological knowledge, and therefore symbolized the anecdotal and evolutionary phase of such methods. The lack of adequate and

C. Iermano (✉) · M. Calabria (✉)
Department of Anesthesia, Endoscopy and Cardiology, Istituto Nazionale Tumori "Fondazione G. Pascale" – IRCSS, Naples, Italy
e-mail: c.iermano@istitutotumori.na.it; mariangela.calabria@istitutotumori.na.it

A. Cuomo
Division of Anesthesia, Intensive Care and Pain Therapy, Istituto Nazionale Tumori "Fondazione G. Pascale" – IRCSS, Naples, Italy
e-mail: a.cuomo@istitutotumori.na.it

O. Alibrahim et al. (eds.), *Biphasic Cuirass Noninvasive Ventilation*, Noninvasive Ventilation. The Essentials, https://doi.org/10.1007/978-3-032-20933-7_9

specific instrumentation to adequately assess hypoxemia and hypercapnia, meant that the treatment of respiratory failure was limited to the administration of drugs that modified the threshold and hypercapnic stimulus sensitivity of the respiratory centers.

The advent of *mechanical ventilation* and then of *extracorporeal supports* represented real and undeniable progress in the treatment of respiratory failure regardless of its origin [1].

Until the 1960s, negative pressure ventilation (NPV) was the most widely used mechanical ventilation method. The 1928 saw the first use of the "iron lung", one of the first negative pressure machines used for long-term ventilation [2].

The intrathoracic vacuum, in the original model, caused simultaneous expansion of both the thorax and abdominal cavity, resulting in accumulation of venous blood in the lower abdomen.

It was subsequently improved and then it revolutionized the response to the polio epidemic of the 1940s. Its operation was based on the vacuum pump mechanism, which created a negative pressure causing expansion of the chest wall, a decrease in intrapulmonary pressure, and consequent penetration of ambient air into the lungs.

This process mimics the natural negative pressure in the intrathoracic space [2].

With the development of positive pressure ventilation, the use of NPV in respiratory failure was largely abandoned due to the complexity of device handling and monitoring. However, in recent years, advances in ventilator technology, with improved patient–ventilator interaction and the development of more portable devices with comfortable flexible cuirasses, has once again resulted in the use of cuirass ventilation devices in the intensive care unit (ICU) and in operating rooms, with applications constantly evolving. The latest generation of cuirass ventilators are versatile and can apply many patterns of ventilation achievable with positive pressure devices.

On the other hand, Noninvasive Ventilation (NIV) is still one of the prominent treatments for acute and chronic respiratory failure and an optimal tool to avoid intubation and improve survival in patients with acute or chronic hypoxemic respiratory failure (ARF).

NIV works through various mechanisms. It intermittently blows positive pressure to the airways elevating transpulmonary pressure, increasing tidal volume and decreasing the work on inspiratory muscles and the effort required for breathing in. In this way, NIV increases functional residual capacity, enrolling the greatest number of alveoli also collapsed ones, so decreases atelectasis, shunt, dyspnea, and carbon dioxide retention [3].

NIV has beneficial effects also on the cardiovascular system. In fact, in the condition of euvolemia, it improves left ventricular output by reducing left ventricular afterload and by increasing intrathoracic pressure [3].

NIV can be delivered via various modalities and titrated according to the patient's specific respiratory demand. It is able to decrease healthcare-acquired infections and sepsis: several studies show a considerable reduction in rates of healthcare-acquired pneumonia compared to physiologically similar patients intubated via endotracheal tubes [4].

The main indications for NIV are: acute exacerbation of COPD (Chronic Obstructive Pulmonary Disease) and asthma, acute heart failure, chronic COPD and pulmonary rehabilitation, OSAS (Obstructive Sleep Apnea Syndrome), obesity hypoventilation syndrome, weaning from invasive mechanical ventilation, prevention of postextubation failure in patients previously intubated, chest wall diseases and neuromuscular diseases, palliative care and do-not-intubate patients, miscellaneous (very old patients, community-acquired pneumonia, and bridge to transplantation).

However NIV, including noninvasive variable positive airway pressure ventilation and continuous positive airway pressure (CPAP), is associated with high failure rates due, in most cases, to patient discomfort. In particular, the choice of the interface and the ventilatory setting adopted play a key role in the success of respiratory assistance [4].

Currently, we can count six main classes of interfaces, each one in different sizes: the oronasal mask, the nasal mask, the full-face mask, the nasal prongs, the mouthpieces, and the helmet. The *nasal mask* is experienced as one of the less claustrophobic devices with a low risk of aspiration, it allows to speak, to cough and to expectorate, but it can lead to a high incidence of leaks if it has not a good grip on the patient face with uncomfortable eye or nasal irritation due to air stream. On the other hand, the *full face mask* is a good choice for protuberant facial features, does not cause ulcer pressure on the nasal bridge even if it can cause on the forehead or chin and leads to low air-leaks but is one of the most claustrophobic devices, especially in anxious patients making it difficult to communicate and worsening ventilatory performance [4].

So these devices, although the prevention with antidecubitus products, often cause distressing and painful pressure ulcers that need a long time to heal, when their use is prolonged (Fig. 9.1). In the latter, sedation seems to be the option to allow better tolerability, but it is not always possible because NIV needs collaborative patients to work properly.

Otherwise literature shows that a rotating strategy, whenever possible, can be a good alternative not only to avoid skin lesions but also to increase NIV tolerance [5].

The patient–ventilator interaction is another crucial aspect to achieve improvements in gas exchange. When NIV starts, it is essential to explain to the patients what they are experiencing so they don't offer resistance to air flow. Asynchrony is a condition in which the patient's own breathing drive does not line up with the mechanical support of the ventilator, resulting in a scarce fitting, opposition, and poor NIV tolerance [6]. In the latter, we need constant monitoring because oxygenation may worsen with consequent hypercapnia and acidosis.

Literature shows that ineffective efforts are more frequently observed with the helmet while double triggers are more recurrent with mask [7].

In this context, the ventilation modality plays a crucial role to have better NIV's tolerability: the pressure support ventilation (PSV) is more comfortable than volume controlled ventilation (VCV) [4].

Another significant factor for NIV intolerance is inadequate air humidification causing upper airway mucosa dryness, oral mucosa ulcers, and nasal congestion.

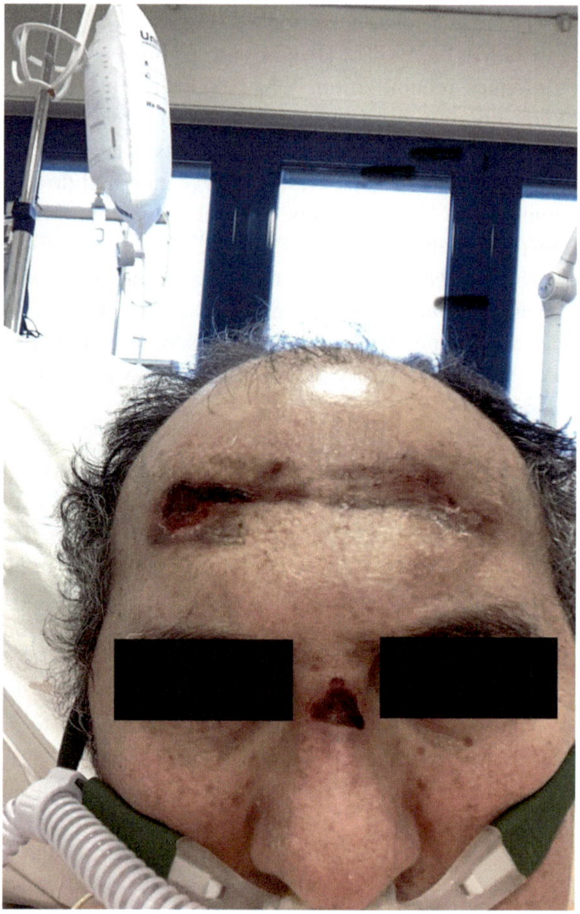

Fig. 9.1 Photo taken from the personal archive of Dr. C. Iermano

Moreover, the surrounding noise, especially when NIV is delivered through a mask or helmet, may be annoying for patients who need to wear earplugs [4].

Anyway intolerance consequent to pain, discomfort, claustrophobia, agitation, or prolonged use could lead to NIV failure [4].

On the other hand, Biphasic Cuirass Ventilation (BCV) is a noninvasive ventilation that uses different interfaces, among them a cuirass is a shell-like unit that creates *negative pressure* on the chest using a combination of a fitted wrap and a soft air chamber. Different sizes and shapes of the shells are available even for babies. Some are customized to fit the patient's body. The negative pressure is produced inside the shell, while the edges have to be adherent to the patient's body to avoid air leaks and generate the pressure variations on the chest. The cuirass is connected to the ventilator and acts through different modality of ventilation [8].

This mode of noninvasive respiratory support, thanks to advances in technology, offers portability and comfort, the patient's face is not covered, so he can converse, eat, and even cough.

The device enables inspiration generating a negative pressure within the chest and provides expiration delivering positive pressure around the chest wall. In this way, the cuirass is able to recruit collapsed airways resulting as a good tool for improving oxygenation, clearing carbon dioxide (CO2), weaning patients from ventilatory support, and in special conditions increasing cardiac output [9].

The candidates to NPV are usually patients with intolerance to NIV via nasofacial mask. NPV is also beneficial in young patients and children who have undergone complex cardiac reconstructive surgery due to the potential effects on cardiopulmonary circulation (Table 9.1).

Particularly, NPV seems to play an important role, when there are contraindications or intolerance to NIV via nasal-face mask ventilation such as:

- Facial trauma, facial deformities, or anatomical abnormalities that prevent proper mask fit
- Recent upper airway or upper gastrointestinal surgery
- Hemodynamic instability, severe hypotension or shock
- Impaired consciousness or inability to protect airway due to the risk of aspiration
- Copious secretions or active vomiting
- NPV allows fibrobronchoscopy to be performed for therapeutic and diagnostic procedures without disconnection from the ventilator
- Palliative cases (in end-of-life or end-of-life cancer patients, for example).

Its application is varied. For example, in patients who are already receiving NIV, BCV reduces the requirements for pressure support and inspired oxygen and increases chest expansion with enhanced CO2 removal. In this context, fits as an

Table 9.1 Description of advantages and disadvantages of NIV vs. BCV

NIV		BCV	
Advantages	Disadvantages	Advantages	Disadvantages
Increase alveolar recruitment Inspiratory muscle unloading Increased FRC and lung compliance Improved gas exchange Decreased LV preload Decreased transmyocardial pressure Decreased LV afterload Improved cardiac output	Discomfort due to: Fixing system Ventilatory setting Humidification Noise Position of the patient Psychological distress Anxiety Fear Pain Facial pressure ulcers	Preservation of physiological functions(conversate, eat, cough etc) Portability and comfort Improvement of quality life in palliative patients Weaning from dependence on external ventilatory support (especially in NMDs) Utilization in case of intolerance to NIV via mask ventilation Use in haemodynamic instability Use in chest physiotherapy and secretion clearance	Not indicated in severe obesity, severe kyphoscoliosis, rib fractures, recent abdominal surgery Lack of protection of the upper airways Upper-airway obstruction due to the downfall of the tongue on the posterior pharyngeal wall Lack of expertise in many centers

alternative tool for de-escalation and weaning from prolonged noninvasive ventilation therapy, with the added benefit of bypassing many side effects [10].

Even SHNEERSON [11] suggested that for neuromuscular disorders the cuirass may be sufficient to overcome ARF for some patients and can also be effective in weaning patients from intermittent positive pressure ventilation (IPPV) via endotracheal tubes.

Nowadays the prevalence of NMDs (Neuromuscular Disorders) is significantly increased and so does the demand for minimally invasive ventilatory support in order to carry on terminal cares at home or in a cozy hospice. In NMDs, the diaphragm and respiratory muscles are affected. The evolution of disease includes difficulty breathing, muscle weakness till patients are bedridden, ineffective coughing, swallowing, and last respiratory distress [9].

Among NMDs, amyotrophic lateral sclerosis (ALS) is a neurodegenerative and incurable disease that affects both the upper and motor neurons, causing progressive muscular weakness with inevitably respiratory insufficiency and consequently death. Palliative therapy is the only possibility of treatment. In this setting, the cuirass system is an easy device, could be the best choice for long term ventilation in medical home care, may be comfortably worn by patients, avoiding harm due to the insufficient compliance of patients to NIPPV's (Noninvasive Positive Pressure Ventilation) devices or to prevent their negative side effects (air leaks, subcutaneous emphysema, pressure ulcers, etc.).

In fact, literature reports a poor tolerance with NIV delivered via the nasal mask due to air loss that often occurs when the device does not properly fit to the patient's face. It results in dry mouth, poor patient–ventilator interaction and ineffective ventilation. Besides, it could be difficult to handle the optimal fixing system that has to maintain the interface in place during NIV and to prevent air leaks [4].

Major air leaks cause patient–ventilator asynchrony. In fact in this scenario, the ventilator delivers an increased inspiratory assistance that could result in a worse patient's workload, increased intrathoracic pressure and sometimes catastrophic complications [4].

Hino et al., described a case of a boy with nemaline myopathy who developed tension pneumothorax while undergoing NIPPV. The patient developed a persistent air leak after pleurodesis, causing a lower NIPPV inspiratory pressure and requiring additional respiratory support without development of high airway pressures that may aggravate pneumothorax. In this interesting case, with the biphasic cuirass ventilation the air leak was resolved [12].

The literature shows that NIPPV can cause in specific types of patients a barotrauma, impairing the treatment.

Furasawa et al., reported a case of subcutaneous and mediastinal emphysema in a 39-year-old woman with late-onset Pompe disease in the course of NIPPV and increased airway pressure. In this case, BCV alone caused dyspnea and hypoxia, instead a synergy of cuirass ventilation (control mode) and NIPPV (assist/control mode),was able to decrease the inspiratory pressure and to resolve the subcutaneous and mediastinal emphysema with increased thoracic compliance. Thus, a combination of cuirass ventilation and NIPPV is a brilliant strategy for managing barotrauma that may occur during NIPPV in a respirator-dependent patient [13].

BCV seems to play an interesting role also in reducing length of stay for NMDs patients. Jackson et al. investigated the long-term efficiency of nocturnal cuirass-assisted ventilation in twenty five patients with scoliosis or kyphosis, after a thoracoplasty and with neuromuscular disease. They showed that nocturnal cuirass-assisted ventilation plays a role in long-term management of patients with neuromuscular and skeletal chest wall disorders. In fact, the median amount of time spent in hospital declined from 15 days per patient in the first year after initial discharge with cuirass-assisted ventilation, to between 3 and 5.5 days per patient in subsequent years [14].

Another relevant role of NPV is due to a HFCWO (High Frequency Chest Wall Oscillation) modality. It can be applied in frequencies up to 1200 oscillations per minute, for improvement of oxygenation, clearing of carbon dioxide or for mobilization of secretions from peripheral airways like occurs with chest physiotherapy. This ventilation modality applying cyclical negative and positive (biphasic) pressure is able to assist in coughing and secretion clearance from the airways [15].

This ventilation modality is extremely effective in disorders like Cystic Fibrosis where serious mucociliary dysfunction, causes copious secretions and prohibits clearing inhaled particles and mucus, and thereby predisposes them to recurrent infections. The cuirass ventilator's "secretion clearance" mode is a successful modality that through vibration consent to mobilize and thin out the mucus from the respiratory system of patients. It then uses its assisted cough function to help expelling fluid secretions, decreasing patient susceptibility to recurrent infections [9].

A proper use of NPV is in the presence of maxillofacial injuries (skeletal components, dentition, or soft tissues of the face) resulting from trauma to the maxillofacial region. Maxillofacial accidents are becoming more frequent and severe. The severity and pattern of the maxillofacial trauma depend on the anatomic site of trauma, the energy, and the direction of the force unleash to the face. Facial trauma can result in superficial wounds, abrasions, facial bone fractures, and may occur in combination with other systemic injuries like head, cervical spine, chest, abdomen, and extremities, prompting a multidisciplinary approach for their handling [16].

In this setting, patients may need a long of stay in ICU undergoing surgeries and then may need equally long periods of weaning from invasive ventilation. So NIPPV with a nasal-face mask is contraindicated, due to the lack of device adherence to the face and due to the damage that positive pressure may cause. Cuirass ventilation by placing a shell (the cuirass) on the anterior chest and upper abdomen bypasses the upper airway and allows unrestricted access for surgery in the larynx and the trachea without risk of hypercapnia associated with apneic techniques, in selected patients for example in patients who previously had complications because of repeated tracheal intubations resulting in postsurgery stenosis [17]. In addition, the long ICU stay may result in major susceptibility to pulmonary infections that need daily fibrobronchoscopy, so BCV allows it to be performed without recurrent logoff from the respiratory support.

Newly, BVC is expected to have an important growth in the perioperative management of complex airway surgeries, opening up new perspectives. During airway surgeries like vocal cord polyp excisions or vocal cord augmentation, BCV as a mode of ventilation, can clear the need for tracheal intubation or other invasive airway maintenance techniques. This is very helpful in various airway surgeries where the surgical team needs to have unhindered access to the airway [18].

Besides, in case of recent upper airway or upper gastrointestinal surgery, where positive pressure may damage surgical anastomosis, NPV represents a valid alternative to ensure adequate ventilation without serious side effects.

Do not underestimate that NPV also has an impact on the cardiovascular system. The effects of positive pressure ventilation on the cardiovascular system are mediated by the increase in transpulmonary pressure, which results in increased pulmonary vascular resistance and in a reduction of venous return in conditions of euvolemia, in a substantial reduction of left ventricular afterload and a potential positive effect on left ventricular stroke volume. However, positive-pressure ventilation (PPV) also results in complex cardiovascular interactions. More often than not, these interactions impede blood flow through ventilated lungs and reduce global cardiac output [19].

Whereas PPV decreases venous return, cuirass ventilation reduces intrathoracic pressure, allowing for increased venous return to the heart and subsequent increase in cardiac output [20].

Specifically, Shekerdemian et al. demonstrated that NPV had hemodynamic advantages over conventional PPV after cardiac surgery in pediatric patients, as demonstrated by a notable improvement in cardiac output [21].

BCV improves the quality of life of palliative patients, like pediatric patients [22], NMDs patients, or oncologic patients by allowing them to continue daily life in their own home, conserving their mobility and communication with family.

Biphasic cuirass ventilation is highly recommended in the long-term respiratory support of patients with respiratory failure from various etiologies. The easy skills required to use this device is a plus that makes it a special tool for hospice or home-based palliative care. Patients can spend in a familiar environment the remaining life. Chronic nocturnal hypoventilation is subsets of ALS (amyotrophic lateral sclerosis) patients with normal or only moderately impaired bulbar function but with considerable symptoms, literature shows that BCV has been shown to prolong survival in addition to improving the quality of life [9].

BCV represents, as we have seen, a more physiological mode of ventilation, very similar to spontaneous respiration, also very useful from the psychological point of view. In fact, it represents a very valuable alternative to NIV in patients who show an intolerance of psychological nature to the adherence to NIV in nasofacial mask.

In fact, among patients suffering from chronic neuromuscular diseases that require NIV, it is possible to highlight psychological damage, which worsen their symptoms with aggravation of the disease itself and reduced adherence to the NIV [23].

In patients with neuromuscular diseases, anxiety and depression lead to increased periods of dyspnea and hospitalization due to worsening of their respiratory performance, as well as a deterioration of quality of life with an increased risk of death [24, 25].

9.2 Conclusions

In conclusion, we can surely assert that in the presence of "intolerance" to the nasal-face mask, BCV represents an excellent alternative to a noninvasive positive pressure ventilation (NIPPV) by avoiding the various side effects like literature shows. In patients with acute and chronic respiratory failure, the use of BCV improves lung function and offers many advantages over NIPPV due to its portability and easy management, also improving quality of life especially in end of life patients. So, with advances in ventilator technology and the development of comfortable flexible cuirasses, the role of negative pressure ventilation must be reconsidered whenever there are conditions. It is advisable to spread of this technique for using both in ICU and operating rooms.

Competing Interests The authors have no conflicts of interest to declare that are relevant to the content of this chapter.

References

1. Tobin MJ. Principles and practice of mechanical ventilation. 1st ed. New York: McGraw Hill; 1994.
2. Gorham J. A medical triumph: the iron lung. Respir Ther. 1979;9(1):71–3.
3. Criner GJ, Gayen S, Zantah M, Dominguez Castillo E, Naranjo M, Lashari B, Pourshahid S, Gangemi A. Clinical review of non-invasive ventilation. Eur Respir J. 2024;64(5):2400396.
4. Cammarota G, Simonte R, De Robertis E. Comfort during non-invasive ventilation. Front Med. 2022;9:874250.
5. Antonaglia V, Ferluga M, Molino R, Lucangelo U, Peratoner A, Roman-Pognuz E, et al. Comparison of noninvasive ventilation by sequential use of mask and helmet versus mask in acute exacerbation of chronic obstructive pulmonary disease: a preliminary study. Respiration. 2011;82:148–54.
6. Carlucci A, Pisani L, Ceriana P, Malovini A, Nava S. Patient-ventilator asynchronies: may the respiratory mechanics play a role? Crit Care. 2013;17:R54.
7. Longhini F, Colombo D, Pisani L, Idone F, Chun P, Doorduin J, et al. Efficacy of ventilator waveform observation for detection of patient-ventilator asynchrony during NIV: a multicentre study. 2017;3:00075.
8. Thomson A. The role of negative pressure ventilation. Arch Dis Childh. 1997;77:454–8.
9. Onweni C, Rashid S, Goswami R, et al. Cuirass ventilation: an alternative home-based modality for chronic respiratory failure. Home Health Care Manag Pract. 2019;32(1):40–4.
10. Almeida Borges J, Esquinas AM. Biphasic cuirass ventilation in the escalation of non-invasive ventilation in COVID-19: case report and review. 2023;93(4).
11. Shneerson JM. Assisted ventilation. 5. Non-invasive and domiciliary ventilation: negative pressure techniques. Thorax. 1991;46(2):131–5.
12. Hino H, Suzuki Y, Ishii E, Fukuda M. Biphasic cuirass ventilation for treatment of an air leak after pneumothorax in a patient with nemaline myopathy: a case report. J Anesth. 2016;30:1087–90.
13. Furusawa Y, Yamamoto T, Oya Y, Miyama K, Suzuki J, Murata M. (2010) Treatment of subcutaneous and mediastinal emphysema with cuirass ventilation in a patient with Pompe disease undergoing non-invasive positive pressure ventilation. Clin Neurol 50:306-310.
14. Jackson M, Kinnear W, King M, Hockley S, Shneerson J. The effects of five years of nocturnal cuirass-assisted ventilation in chest wall disease. Eur Respir J. 1993;6(5):630–5.

15. Linton DM. Cuirass ventilation: a review and update. Crit Care Resusc. 2005;7(1):22–8.
16. Khan TU, Rahat S, Khan ZA, Shahid L, Banouri SS, Muhammad N. Etiology and pattern of maxillofacial trauma. Plos One. 2022;17(9):e0275515.
17. Kristensen MS, Hesselfeldt R, Schmidt JF. Modern cuirass ventilation for airway surgery: unlimited access to the larynx and trachea in anaesthetised patients. Br J Anaesth. 2023;131(4):e106–9.
18. Bodhey A, Bodhey M, Shallik NA, Al Nadhari M, Griess HF, Al Ani O, Sainuddin S, Thomas KP, ElHanfi O, Jose S, Nair A. Biphasic cuirass ventilation for airway surgeries: a comprehensive review. Cureus. 2024;16(12):e75477.
19. Corp A, Thomas C, Adlam M. The cardiovascular effects of positive pressure ventilation. BJA Educ. 2021;21(6):202–9.
20. McBride WT, Ranaldi G, Dougherty MJ, Siciliano T, Trethowan B, Elliott P, Rice C, Scolletta S, Giomarelli P, Romano SM, Linton DM. The hemodynamic and respiratory effects of continuous negative and control-mode cuirass ventilation in recently extubated cardiac surgery patients. J Cardiothorac Vasc Anesth. 2012;26(5):873–7.
21. Shekerdemian LS, Bush A, Lincoln C, Shore DF, Petros AJ, Redington AN. Cardiopulmonary interactions in healthy children and children after simple cardiac surgery: the effects of positive and negative pressure ventilation. Heart. 1997;78(6):587–93.
22. Bosch-Alcaraz A. Non-invasive ventilation improves comfort in pediatric palliative care patients. Enfermeria Intensiva. 2014;25(3):91–9.
23. Pungchompoo W, Suwan P, Kunapun S, Pungchompo S, Tungpunkom P. Experiences of symptoms and health service preferences among older people living with chronic diseases during the last year of life. Int J Palliat Nurs. 2019;25:129–41.
24. Pooler A, Beech R. Examining the relationship between anxiety and depression and exacerbations of COPD which result in hospital admission: A systematic review. Int J Chron Obstruct Pulmon Dis. 2014;9:315–30.
25. Leander M, Lampa E, Rask-Andersen A, Franklin K, Gislason T, Oudin A, Svanes C, Torén K, Janson C. Impact of anxiety and depression on respiratory symptoms. Radiother Oncol. 2014;108:1594–600.

Biphasic Cuirass Ventilation: Long-Term Effects in Pulmonary Hypertension and Cardiac Function

10

Elisa Salsano, Oriana Rossi, and Martina Spavone

10.1 Introduction

Pulmonary hypertension (PH) is a pathophysiological disorder that can involve multiple clinical conditions and is associated with a variety of cardiovascular and respiratory diseases. The definitions for PH are based on hemodynamic assessment by right heart catheterization (RHC). Pulmonary hypertension is defined by a mean pulmonary arterial pressure (mPAP) greater than 20 mmHg.

All age groups are affected. Present estimates suggest a PH prevalence of ~1% of the global population. Due to the presence of cardiac and pulmonary causes of PH, prevalence is higher in individuals over 65 years of age. Globally, left heart disease (LHD) is the leading cause of PH. Lung disease, especially chronic obstructive pulmonary disease (COPD), is the second most common cause. Regardless of the underlying condition, developing PH is associated with worsening symptoms and increased mortality [1].

Biphasic cuirass ventilation (BCV) is a form of noninvasive extrathoracic mechanical ventilation system that supports spontaneous breathing by utilizing a pressure source capable of providing both positive and negative pressure. Use of BCV improves dramatically gas exchange and cardiac function in patients with pulmonary hypertension (PH).

E. Salsano (✉)
Geriatric and Intensive Geriatric Care Unit, San Giuseppe Moscati Hospital, Avellino, Italy
e-mail: elisa.salsano@aornmoscati.it

O. Rossi
Medical Department, University Aldo Moro, Bari, Italy

M. Spavone
Geriatric Department, University of Naples Federico II, Naples, Italy

O. Alibrahim et al. (eds.), *Biphasic Cuirass Noninvasive Ventilation*, Noninvasive Ventilation. The Essentials, https://doi.org/10.1007/978-3-032-20933-7_10

10.2 Oxygenation and Lung Perfusion in BCV

Lung inflation occurs when the difference between pressure inside versus outside the lung overcomes tissue and airway factors that impede distension. The transpulmonary pressure represents the difference between the pressure in the alveolus (i.e., inside the lung) versus that in the pleural cavity (i.e., outside the lung). With positive-pressure ventilation (PPV), the transpulmonary pressure is increased by making the alveolar pressure more positive; conversely, with negative-pressure ventilation (NPV), the transpulmonary pressure is increased by making the pleural pressure more negative.

Biphasic cuirass ventilation (BCV), is a form of noninvasive extrathoracic mechanical ventilation. It consists of a cuirass and a pressure source capable of providing both positive and negative pressure, which supports spontaneous breathing in a more physiological manner compared with positive pressure ventilation.

Grasso et al. demonstrated that, compared to PPV, negative pressure ventilation resulted in greater functional residual capacity (FRC) and in a better oxygenation. NPV may distend lungs in a different manner compared with positive pressure, resulting in more homogeneous ventilation, less injury, and superior oxygenation. Furthermore, they demonstrated that when negative pressure was applied using a device applied only to the chest (Curiass; Breasy Medical Equipment, Ltd., London, U.K.) and positive pressure was applied in the usual way, global lung perfusion was significantly greater with the negative-pressure chest device than with PPV [2].

The NPV can have very different hemodynamic effects compared with positive pressure ventilation. In general, positive pressure decreases ventricular afterload and preload. Negative pressure applied only to the chest [3], in contrast to that applied to the whole body, could conceivably augment right ventricular preload and thereby increase lung perfusion and improve oxygenation. This could be particularly important where the circulation is critically dependent on right ventricular filling (e.g., hypovolemia or restrictive diseases). This phenomenon was confirmed in the study of Grasso et al. demonstrating no change in cardiac output when negative pressure was applied using the whole-body device, but a significant increase when negative pressure was applied with curiass [2].

10.3 Clinical Use in Pulmonary Hypertension of BCV

The first studies of Negative pressure ventilation (NPV) and pulmonary Hypertension (PH) were conducted in newborn after the Fontan operation [4]. NPV has been shown to improve oxygenation and increases pulmonary blood flow in infants with persistent PH [5].

Yoko sato et al., reported in their study that BCV decreased pulmonary artery pressure (PAP) in patients with secondary pulmonary hypertension (PH) due to chronic respiratory failure. In this study, they investigated the effect of BCV on pulmonary circulation to determine the mechanism of PAP's decreasing. Fifteen patients with PH caused by chronic respiratory failure were included, none had dehydration and none had received vasodilator therapy. PH was defined as mean PAP (mPAP) >20 mmHg determined by right heart catheterization (RHC). Serum levels of N-terminal proB-type natriuretic peptide (NT-proBNP) were obtained before and after the BCV trial. The decrease of NT-pro BNP and of mPAP were statistically significant [6].

BCV may exert its beneficial effects by improving circulatory function particularly in patients with end-stage chronic lung disease in which structural and functional alterations of pulmonary vessels can lead to secondary pulmonary hypertension (PH) or cor pulmonale.

This may be explained by the fact that BCV may improve oxygenation and reduce pulmonary vascular resistance (PVR). There are two possible mechanisms through which it improves pulmonary hypertension (PH):

First, BCV may directly improve thoracic mobility, increasing ventilation volumes and allowing for comfortable respiration in patients with restrictive lung disease. With BCV, the pressure support provided during both inspiration and expiration correlates with decreased work of breathing and more comfortable respiration.

Secondly, BCV may decrease the work of breathing by modulating the interaction between respiration and circulation. In this way, BCV may reduce cardiac load, thereby decreasing the excess work of breathing associated with chronic lung disease and lowering N-terminal probrain natriuretic peptide (NT-proBNP) levels that indicates reduced afterload in the right ventricle and/or ventricular adaptation to stress.

Furthermore, the use of BCV at home, after appropriate training with a 1-day session, could potentially increase physical exercise capacity and cardiac compensation in this patient, leading to an improvement in quality of life, increased resistance to physical effort, and reduced rehospitalizations.

BCV may directly improve thoracic mobility. However, many studies have shown tidal volume and minute volume increase with the use of NPV or BCV in healthy volunteers [7, 8], as well as in patients with chest wall diseases [9] and COPD [10]. Previous studies have demonstrated that negative pressure ventilation relieves the diaphragm and other respiratory muscles in COPD patients [10, 11]. Extrathoracic negative pressure directly affects expansion of the thoracic cage by stretching the diaphragm and intercostal muscles for inspiration. Improvement of thoracic mobility increases ventilation volumes and allows for comfortable respiration in restrictive lung disease patients. Extrathoracic positive pressure during expiration assisted may increase elastic recoil of the chest wall.

10.4 Conclusion

Actually, the mainstay of treatment for pulmonary hypertension are supplemental oxygen, diuretics, digitalis, and anticoagulants. More recent therapeutic options including proteinoids, endothelin receptor antagonists, and phosphodiesterase-5 inhibitors, but the efficacy of these newer agents remains controversial.

The literature provides evidence that applying Biphasic cuirass ventilation (BCV) can improve gas exchange and cardiac function, not only in adult patients with acute exacerbations of chronic respiratory failure and secondary PH, but also in restrictive lung disease patients.

Therefore, BCV could represent a promising approach for treating PH caused by chronic lung diseases, although further studies are needed to define the duration, frequency, and long-term effects of its use in a larger sample size.

References

1. Humbert M, et al. Guidelines for the diagnosis and treatment of pulmonary hypertension: Developed by the task force for the diagnosis and treatment of pulmonary hypertension of the European Society of Cardiology (ESC) and the European Respiratory Society (ERS). Endorsed by the International Society for Heart and Lung Transplantation (ISHLT) and the European Reference Network on rare respiratory diseases (ERN-LUNG). Eur Heart J. 2022;43(38):3618–731. https://doi.org/10.1093/eurheartj/ehac237.
2. Grasso F, Engelberts D, Helm E, Frndova H, Jarvis S, Talakoub O, McKerlie C, Babyn P, Post M, Kavanagh BP. Negative-pressure ventilation: better oxygenation and less lung injury. Am J Respir Crit Care Med. 2008;177:412–8. https://doi.org/10.1164/rccm.200707-1004OC.
3. Borelli M, Benini A, Denkewitz T, Acciaro C, Foti G, Pesenti A. Effects of continuous negative extrathoracic pressure versus positive endexpiratory pressure in acute lung injury patients. Crit Care Med. 1998;26:1025–31. https://doi.org/10.1002/ppul.1950170305.
4. Shekerdemian LS, Bush A, Shore DF, Lincoln C, Redington AN. Cardiopulmonary interactions after Fontan operations: augmentation of cardiac output using negative pressure ventilation. Circulation. 1997;96:3934–42. https://doi.org/10.1161/01.CIR.96.11.3934.
5. Sills JH, Cvetnic WG, Pietz J. Continuous negative pressure in the treatment of infants with pulmonary hypertension and respiratory failure. J Perinatol. 1989;9:43–8.
6. Yoko Sato, Takuma Asakura, Noriyuki Saeki, Kazutetsu Aoshiba, Toru Kotani. Biphasic cuirass ventilation decreased the indices of pulmonary circulation in patients with secondary pulmonary hypertension. Eur Respir J. 2011;38(Suppl 55):2288. https://doi.org/10.1007/s00540-016-2172-7.
7. Glerant JC, Jounieaux V, Parreira VF, Dury M, Aubert G, Rodenstein DO. Effects of intermittent negative pressure ventilation on effective ventilation in normal awake subjects. Chest. 2002;122:99–107. https://doi.org/10.1378/chest.122.1.99.
8. Hirasawa J, Arizono S, Taniguchi H, Ogawa T, Watanabe F, Hasegaw R. Relationship between intermittent negative pressure level and tidal volume during biphasic cuirass ventilation in normal subjects [in Japanese]. Nihon Kokyuki Gakkai Zasshi. 2011;49:990–2.
9. Kinnear W, Petch M, Taylor G, Shneerson J. Assisted ventilation using cuirass respirators. Eur Respir J. 1988;1:198–203. PMID: 3164275
10. Gigliotti F, Spinelli A, Duranti R, Gorini M, Goti P, Scano G. Four-week negative pressure ventilation improves respiratory function in severe hypercapnic COPD patients. Chest. 1994;105:87–94. https://doi.org/10.1378/chest.105.1.87.
11. Corrado A, Gorini M, Villella G, De Paola E. Negative pressure ventilation in the treatment of acute respiratory failure: an old noninvasive technique reconsidered. Eur Respir J. 1996;9:1531–44. https://doi.org/10.1183/09031936.96.09071531.

11 Biphasic Cuirass Non-invasive Ventilation. Neuromuscular Disorders

Giuseppe Fiorentino and Anna Annunziata

Abbreviation

ALS	Amyotrophic lateral sclerosis
BCV	Biphasic cuirass ventilation
HFO	High-frequency oscillation
IMV	Intermittent mandatory ventilation
mPPV	Mask-positive-pressure ventilation
NMDs	Neuromuscular diseases
NPV	Negative pressure ventilation
PPV	Positive-pressure ventilation
SIMV	Synchronized IMV
VC	Vital capacity

11.1 Introduction

Negative pressure ventilation (NPV) is a helpful intervention for patients with neuromuscular diseases (NMDs) experiencing chronic or acute respiratory failure (ARF). This technique saw common practice in the 1950s, principally to care patients with respiratory compromise resulting from a neuromuscular disease, poliomyelitis. Advances in technology have led to the design and creation of more user-friendly NPV devices, sparking renewed interest in its application. A thorough understanding of available respiratory support methods, including their indications, contraindications, and potential adverse effects, is crucial for tailoring treatment plans to the complexities of each patient's condition.

G. Fiorentino (✉) · A. Annunziata
Respiratory Unit- Monaldi AO Dei Colli, Naples, Italy

O. Alibrahim et al. (eds.), *Biphasic Cuirass Noninvasive Ventilation*, Noninvasive Ventilation. The Essentials, https://doi.org/10.1007/978-3-032-20933-7_11

Biphasic cuirass ventilation (BCV) refers to the use of a portable external thoracic shell that creates a cover around the anterior chest and generates negative pressure which can assist with breathing. Various modes exist, including controlled biphasic ventilation, continuous negative pressure, and high-frequency oscillation, all of which can be applied when traditional invasive methods of positive pressure ventilation are not possible. Previously described applications include heart failure or lung disease requiring chest physiotherapy, acute respiratory failure to assist intubated patients in weaning from respiratory support, and respiratory compromise from neuromuscular defects.

11.2 Respiratory Pathophysiology of Neuromuscular Disease

NMDs certainly progress and impact the respiratory system. Respiratory muscle weakness, frequently combined with variations in the chest wall and lung mechanics, reduces vital capacity (VC) and cough effectiveness. The degree of VC reduction varies extensively from mild, such as in hemidiaphragm paralysis, to severe, as seen in advanced amyotrophic lateral sclerosis (ALS). NMDs can also affect bulbar muscles, swallowing, sleep quality that result in acute or chronic ventilatory failure, together with recurrent aspiration and pneumonia. Hypoventilation is a frequent observation, and while upper airway obstruction can occur, it is often not due to central respiratory drive issues. The presence of obstructive sleep apnea or severe obesity may contraindicate NPV, because of the risk of upper airway collapse, and device size limitations. When respiratory support is deemed necessary, offering a variety of interface options and pulmonary ventilation techniques is important [1]. In patients with NMD experiencing respiratory failure often require continuous (24-hour) respiratory support, and NPV can be a useful component of a comprehensive strategy, also alternating with other ventilation modalities as needed. NPV is often contemplated for patients who are unable to tolerate pressure positive NIV due to different motivations such as facial abnormalities, claustrophobia, or difficulties managing airway secretions [2]. Given its potential impact on cardiopulmonary circulation, NPV may be beneficial in patients, especially children, with complex cardiac conditions. However, in certain conditions, such as Duchenne muscular dystrophy where significant cardiac alterations are common, positive pressure treatment during non-invasive ventilation could pose a risk to hemodynamic alteration, NPV is more secure in the management [3]. Due to its appliance, the thoracic traction produced by negative pressure is unsuitable for patients with thoracic fractures. Severe kyphoscoliosis or recent abdominal surgery can also make the interfaces unusable. Though technological advancements have enhanced NPV, specific guidelines for its use persist indefinite.

11.3 Biphasic Cuirass Ventilation (BCV) in Patients with Neuromuscular Disorders

BCV assists ventilation by producing negative pressure to the thorax intermittently or continuously. This technique trusts on generating negative pressure externally to the chest, which expands the lungs and facilitates airflow movement. This cuirass is supporting by a piston pump which can provide ventilation up to high frequencies and baseline negative pressure is produced from a vacuum pump. This machine can behave as a conventional negative pressure ventilator at frequencies of 2 Hz. Tidal volume increases in proportion to the negative pressure span generated within the cuirass and minute ventilation is related to the tidal volume and respiratory frequency. At above a frequency of 2 Hz, however, the BCV oscillator performs more as a high-frequency oscillator and oxygenation is realized essentially by diffusion. The inspiratory and expiratory phases can be accurately managed by regulating the negative air pressure, allowing for complete or partial control over the patient's breathing patterns. Frequencies of up to 15 Hz can be obtained with this machine and frequency, inspiratory and expiratory pressures, and I:E ratio are performed for individual patients. The capacity of the machines to oscillate in high frequency (up to 1200 cycles per minute) followed by deep breaths and positive expiratory pressure (artificial cough) facilitates the clearance of secretions. Lung compliance, lung volumes and gas exchange are well maintained, and patients are comfortable using the flexible cuirass [4–6]. Older NPV methods depend on the thorax's natural recoil during expiration, which limits ventilation frequency to about 30 breaths per minute. The tidal volume achieved is generally proportional to the difference between peak and trough pressures during inspiration. More recent NPV systems generate fluctuating pressure against a consistent negative expiratory pressure. Patients with respiratory failure due to muscle weakness may use BCV to delay the requirement for invasive procedures such as intubation or tracheostomy [5].

11.4 NPV Interfaces in NMD

The interfaces for NPV are as follows: Iron Lung, Poncho, and Cuirass [4–6].

- *Iron Lungs*: Iron lungs encase the body up to the neck. Early models created an intrathoracic vacuum that expanded both the chest and abdominal cavities, resulting in venous blood pooling in the lower abdomen. Using a vacuum pump, they produce negative pressure to enlarge the chest wall, reducing intrapulmonary pressure and consenting ambient air to flow into the lungs.
- *Cuirass*: A shell-shaped device that fits around the chest with fabric straps. Many sizes and shapes of shells are available that allow to accommodate even patients. Some are customized to perfectly fit the patient's body. The cuirass applies negative pressure on a lower surface, but compared to the poncho, it can assist the patient during the exhalation phase patient's body. Cuirass ventilation maximizes the gradient of venous return to the heart by depressing mean intrathoracic pres-

sure, developing a better cardiac output compared with positive pressure ventilation at matched FRC and tidal volumes. In contrast, when the whole body up to the neck is enclosed in a negative pressure chamber, the ambient pressure around the body is subatmospheric, the airway opening is atmospheric, and this is hemodynamically correspondent to the ambient pressure being atmospheric and the airway opening pressure above atmospheric.

- *Poncho*: A jacket-like device that creates negative pressure. The pressure is delivered inside a poncho-shaped suit, which the patient must wear, closed at the neck, wrists, and ankles with straps that ensure airtightness. The empty space between the suit and the patient's body is guaranteed by a metal/plastic net connected to a supporting plane placed at the back. The poncho is often made with GORE-TEX and is available in different sizes.

11.5 NPV Modes

Ventilator can work in many different patterns [4–6]:

- Controlled biphasic ventilation is analogous to intermittent mandatory ventilation (IMV), with the patient able to take breaths easily when wanted between the mandatory breaths.
- Continuous negative pressure is like to CPAP and can be set at any pressure around the baseline to increase the FRC as necessary.
- Synchronized Biphasic Cuirass Ventilation (BCV). Cuirass-triggered breaths are similar to the spontaneous breaths in the synchronized IMV (SIMV).
- High-frequency oscillation (HFO) can be applied in frequencies up to 1200 oscillations per minute, for the realization of oxygenation, reduction of carbon dioxide, or secretion mobilization from the lung periphery as it occurs with chest physiotherapy. A major benefit of externally applied cyclical negative and positive (biphasic) pressure is the ability to assist in coughing and secretion clearance from the airways.
- Cardiac synchronized. A new addition to the various modes of cuirass ventilation is the capacity to time the ventilatory cycle to accord with the cardiac cycle. This is done by sensing the electrocardiograph signals to drive the negative pressure ventilator rate and timing. This mode of ventilation has reported benefits in specific cardiac diseases, enhancing cardiac output and during MRI scanning. In fact, in highly sensitive magnetic resonance scanning of the heart and thorax, cardiac and ventilatory interaction often interferes with clear imaging.

11.6 Clinical Application

The application of BCV in the treatment of NMDs has been shown to prolong survival in addition to improving the quality of life for subsets of ALS patients with normal or only moderately impaired bulbar function. This mode of respiratory support offers portability and comfort and, since the patient's face is not covered, conversation, eating, and even coughing can proceed unhindered.

Clinical applications real world is:

- Acute Respiratory Failure: NPV can be used in acute settings to support patients with sudden respiratory problems due to neuromuscular weakness.
- Chronic Respiratory Failure: It can also be used long-term to manage chronic respiratory insufficiency in patients with neuromuscular disorders.
- Home Ventilation: NPV can be an option for home ventilation, especially for patients who cannot tolerate other forms of noninvasive ventilation. Biphasic cuirass ventilation has demonstrated favorable outcomes in the long-term respiratory support of patients with NMDs. Noninvasive ventilation techniques like cuirass ventilation improve the quality of life of palliative patients by allowing for continued mobility and communication while affording them the option of managing their condition in the home.

Alexander et al. reported 10 patients with DMD, in which the symptoms were totally relieved and $PaCO_2$ was lowered below 50 mmHg by mechanical ventilation treatment in the hospital. Subsequently, on an outpatient basis, these patients utilized a combination of different ventilatory devices (both NPV and PPV). On these customized therapeutic regimens, the patients were able to carry out their activities of daily living in an independent fashion [7].

In 1981, Garay described the long-term effect of the application of NPV at home in a pivotal study carried out on eight patients with alveolar hypoventilation syndromes due to poliomyelitis and scoliosis. After the reversal of severe hypercapnia, all patients were discharged and maintained at home for an average period of 10 years, utilizing NPV provided by a tank ventilator or pneumowrap. The 5-year survival was 100% [8]. Splaingard in 1985 reported 20 years of experience using NPV at home to ventilate 40 patients with neuromuscular disease. The purpose of the study was to determine the costs, complications, and clinical outcomes of this form of respiratory support. Emerson tank respirators were used mainly during sleep, and intermittent positive pressure breathing machines were used by 98% of patients, with an average equipment cost of $2700 annually. Patients in whom NPV was initiated on an elective rather than emergency basis saved an average of $12,000 during their initial hospitalization. Life-table analysis showed a 5-year survival of 76% and a 10-year survival of 61%. Complications were minor and occurred at an average rate of less than one per year per patient at home on NPV. Failure to achieve satisfactory NPV in nine patients was associated with age or severe thoracocervical scoliosis, which prevented proper fitting of the NPV [9]. The ventilator-management protocol followed over 12 yrs. in 23 patients with Duchenne muscular dystrophy (DMD) and six polio survivors with chronic respiratory failure (CRF) secondary to the late effects of poliomyelitis or postpolio syndrome has been reported by Curran [10]. After the onset of respiratory failure, patients with DMD continued to show a classic course of progressive, generalized muscle weakness and a steadily declining vital capacity from an average of 0.48–0.34 L. The DMD group required an average increase of 0.95 h in their daily use of assisted ventilation, provided by a tank ventilator, per year. Their overall average length of survival was increased from 19 years 9 months to 25 years 9 months. The 5-year survival was 76%. Schiavina reported the clinical course in 31 patients with chronic respiratory failure due to neuromuscular or chest-wall disorders treated at home for 6 months with NPV. Ventilatory assistance during the night was provided by poncho wrap or pneumowrap. The average duration of mechanical ventilation was 8 hours per day at the beginning of the follow-up period. Some patients needed to increase the number of hours of ventilation because of a significant decrease in vital capacity and an increase in the level of dyspnea. Five patients underwent polysomnographic studies before and during NPV. The recording during NPV showed a general improvement in all but one patient in the quality and the structure of sleep with an increase in sleep efficiency and in the percentage of the rapid eye movement phase. This happened despite an increase in the number of arousals associated with the appearance of obstructive apneas. However, the level of desaturation caused by obstructive events was lower than that caused by central events in the baseline recording. At the end of the 6-month follow-up period, the survival was 87% [11].

Jackson determined that long-term nocturnal cuirass ventilation benefited those with neuromuscular and skeletal chest wall disorders. They investigated the 5 yrs. effectiveness of cuirass-assisted ventilation and examined whether mortality and morbidity could have been predicted at the time of admittance. Twenty-five patients were commenced on nocturnal cuirass-assisted ventilation between 1983 and 1985, 10 with scoliosis or kyphosis, 8 with a thoracoplasty, and 7 with neuromuscular disease. Mean pretreatment vital capacity was 30% of predicted, and $Paco_2$ was 62 mmHg. Nocturnal cuirass-assisted ventilation has a role in the long-term management of patients with neuromuscular and skeletal chest wall disorders. Fifteen patients were alive 5 years later. Two had discontinued assisted ventilation, both dying soon afterwards, and three had been changed to intermittent positive pressure ventilation. $Paco_2$ in the survivors had risen from a mean of 46 mmHg after one year to 52 mmHg after 5 years but remained significantly less than at presentation [12].

A study by Baydur on the long-term effects of NIV in patients with musculoskeletal disorders has described 46 yrs. of experience in 79 patients submitted to home ventilatory assistance with NPV (tank respirator or cuirass in 31 cases) or mask-positive-pressure ventilation (mPPV) (in 48 patients). The proportion of patients that reported a positive outcome, in terms of improved sense of well-being and independence, was greater with mPPV than NPV (67 versus 29%), and in the subgroup of patients with poliomyelitis, the number of tracheostomies was greater with NPV than mPPV. It is important to stress, however, that the population treated with NPV and mPPV was not homogeneous in terms of age, diagnosis, and pulmonary function. Furthermore, the duration of home mechanical ventilation in patients treated with NPV was much greater than in those with mPPV (24 versus 3.2 yrs).

From these studies, although uncontrolled, it appears that NPV has been used successfully for long-term home mechanical ventilation in patients with neuromuscular and chest wall disorders. NPV devices, however, are more cumbersome and difficult to use than recent home PPV devices. Although direct comparisons between the efficiency of NPV and mPPV are rare, in patients with muscular dystrophy and bulbar weakness NPV tends to predispose patients to obstructive apneas during sleep. This is probably due to the absence of coordination between upper airway muscle activity and the ventilator cycle. For these reasons, NPV has been largely supplanted by mPPV in the last decade. In experienced hands, NPV remains a second choice to be used in patients who, for technical or other reasons, cannot be offered mPPV. It has been reported that brief discontinuation of mPPV in some patients who were affected by chronic hypercapnic respiratory failure, due to intolerable nasal irritation or upper airway congestion, is associated with significant worsening of the arterial blood gas tensions. In these cases, and other clinical conditions, such as facial deformity or lack of teeth, NPV should be used as an alternative to mPPV.

Annunziata investigates the use of negative-pressure ventilation (NPV) for managing ARF in NMD. It details the history, interfaces (iron lung, poncho, cuirass), and modes of NPV, and identifies suitable candidates as those intolerants to noninvasive positive pressure ventilation. The article highlights NPV's potential benefits in preserving physiological functions and aiding weaning while acknowledging limitations like the lack of upper airway protection.

In the literature, there is a report of a patient with nemaline myopathy who had been on respiratory support by PPV since the age of 6 years. At the age of 11 years, he developed a persistent air leak after tension pneumothorax. The use of PPV improves patients' respiratory symptoms and quality of life, and pneumothorax is a relatively rare complication of mPPV. The patient was successfully treated with BCV. This method has some advantages: compared with PPV, there is no direct pressure on the lung, there is less barotrauma, and there is equal or greater ventilation with less dead space and more pulmonary perfusion. First, the negative pressure generated within the cuirass supports continuous inspiration, and the positive pressure within the cuirass assists expiration. BCV applies pressure over the thorax; the lung expansion is also done without direct positive pressure in the airways. In a rabbit model, the transpulmonary pressure generated by BCV was consistently lower than that generated for a comparable level of NIPPV. In that same model, samples of inflated lungs were fixed after a 2.5-h period of ventilation for histologic scoring and showed a lower lung injury score for BCV than for PPV. There may be less barotrauma with BCV than with PPV. Second, the patient maintained adequate respiration, although the respiratory function examination could not be performed because of his condition in this case. In the same animal model described above, the lung volume and dead space were improved, as shown by computed tomography. In addition, the tidal volume of the patient may be supported by BCV, as in a previous case. Finally, the application of BCV may benefit the hemodynamic condition of the patient with pneumothorax under restrictive physiology due to neuromuscular disease. There are also effects on ventricular preload and afterload. BCV applied only to the chest can augment the preload; in contrast, NIPPV decreases it. Pneumothorax increases the afterload. NIPPV could decrease it if NIPPV applies sufficient positive pressure and increases lung volume during inspiration, as well as increasing the capacity of pulmonary vessels due to inflation.

Notably, Hino suggested BCV as a useful alternative to PPV delivered through a nasal mask, face mask, or nasal plugs. Noninvasive positive pressure ventilation is still comparatively intrusive and, in this case, BCV proved advantageous in resolving a persistent air leak in a patient who was a high-risk surgical candidate and had developed tension pneumothorax while on NIPPV.

11.7 Advantages and Limitations of NPV

Limits of NPV have to be considered: firstly, the lack of protection of the upper airways, and secondly, upper-airway obstruction due to both the downfall of the tongue on the posterior pharyngeal wall and the lack of inspiratory upper-airway muscle activation. These problems are particularly relevant in comatose patients, in those with neurological disorders associated with bulbar dysfunction (e.g., bulbar amyotrophic lateral sclerosis), and in patients affected by apnea during sleep. In unconscious patients with normal bulbar function, the placement of a nasogastric tube and the positioning of an oropharyngeal airway can reduce the problem of aspiration pneumonia and upper-airway closure due to the collapse of the tongue.

The intermittent upper-airway collapse leading to obstructive apnea is a potential risk associated with NPV in patients affected by neuromuscular diseases. This complication was first recognized several decades ago: the glottic closure was observed in normal subjects hyperventilated in iron lungs and was thought to represent a protective reflex against hyperventilation. The lack of preinspiratory activation of upper-airway muscles predisposes these structures to collapse when exposed to negative pressure. Hill et al. observed some clustering of disordered breathing events during REM sleep in Duchenne muscular dystrophy patients during NPV when the breathing pattern was irregular and the upper-airway tone was reduced.

The major advantage of NPV is the preservation of physiological functions, such as speech, cough, swallowing, and feeding. These aspects are very relevant for patients who are continuously ventilated, and who may be dependent on respiratory support before or after the acute event. Moreover, NPV, unlike positive-pressure ventilation (facial or total-face interfaces are generally used in acute settings), allows fibro bronchoscopy to be performed for various procedures without interruption from the respiratory support.

11.8 Use in Palliative Medicine

Somewhat surprisingly, cuirass ventilation applications in palliative care are relatively new. However, the minimal technical skill required to operate these devices makes it an ideal addition to home hospice or home-based palliative care for properly selected patients. Its noninvasive nature allows patients to continue to talk, eat, and interact with family members without the interference of face masks or tubes. Equally important is that one can quickly choose to discontinue therapy if it proves ineffective or is no longer desired, unlike chronic PPV via tracheostomy (Fig. 11.1).

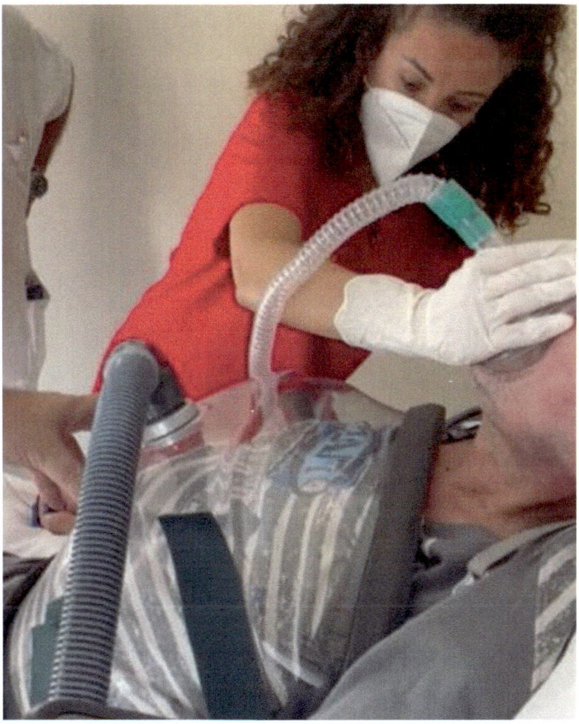

Fig. 11.1 Palliative use con HF combinated

11.9 Weaning from Invasive Ventilation

Advantages have been displayed from the use of cuirass ventilation in patients who are already intubated and receiving positive pressure ventilation. When the biphasic extrathoracic pressures are applied, the necessities for pressure support are undoubtedly reduced and physiological increases in oxygenation and cardiac output are realized. Especially where adaptive positive pressure ventilatory modes are used, the requirements for inspired pressure support can be seen to drop progressively and quickly. It is easy to demonstrate that biphasic cuirass ventilation allows rapid weaning from invasive positive pressure support. Spontaneously generated tidal volumes increase with enhanced CO_2 removal and reduced inspired oxygen requirements. In problematic ventilatory weaning, where the limiting aspect for weaning is inspiratory muscle weakness in a system with pulmonary compliance and airway resistance relatively normal, it makes good sense in any awake, cooperative patient to try cuirass ventilation to achieve earlier weaning from positive pressure ventilation and extubation. This will make the patient's life immediately more pleasant with the ability to talk, eat, and breathe freely around the mandatory negative pressure breaths. It should also decrease the occurrence of ventilator-associated pneumonia and laryngeal damage. Patients can then be moved to a step-down or intermediate care facility, or even home until muscle strength recovers (Fig. 11.2).

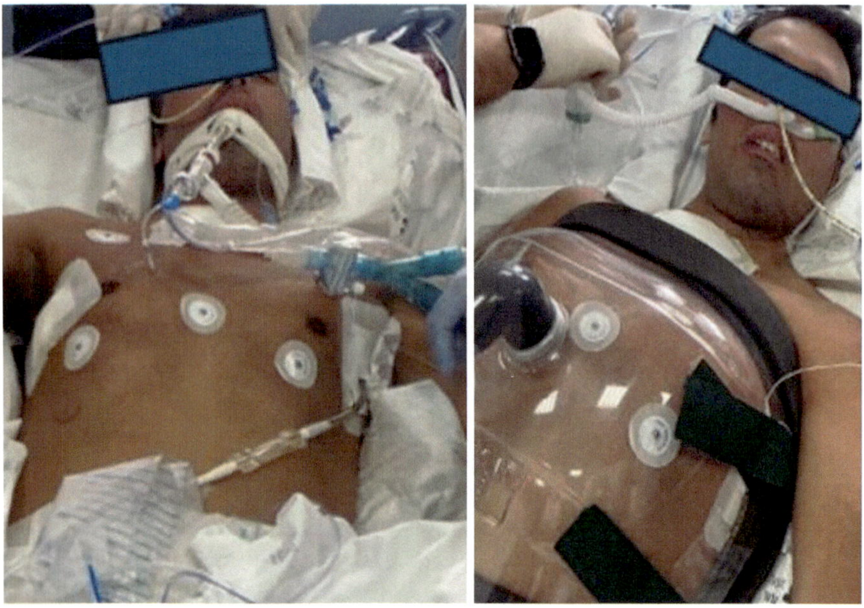

Fig. 11.2 Weaning with the negative pressure use

11.10 NPV in Chest Physiotherapy and Secretion Clearance

This is a physiotherapy tool used to enhance the clearance of secretions from the lungs using two alternating modes. This is realized by high-frequency oscillations (up to 1200 oscillations per minute) around a negative baseline followed by an artificial cough that has a prolonged inspiratory phase trailed by a forced short expiratory phase. Clearing of airway secretions can be improved by cuirass ventilation when used in high-frequency oscillations followed by supra-normal inspiratory to expiratory excursions. NPV-cuirass ventilation, when used in high-frequency oscillations followed by larger-than-normal inspiratory to expiratory excursions is used to improve the clearing of airway secretions. This sequential procedure can be programmed into the modern-day cuirass ventilator and applied at regular intervals to the patient either with or without continuous biphasic ventilation as required [16]. Normally, in our experience, there is the use of NPV and cough assistance together in a manual activity (Fig. 11.3).

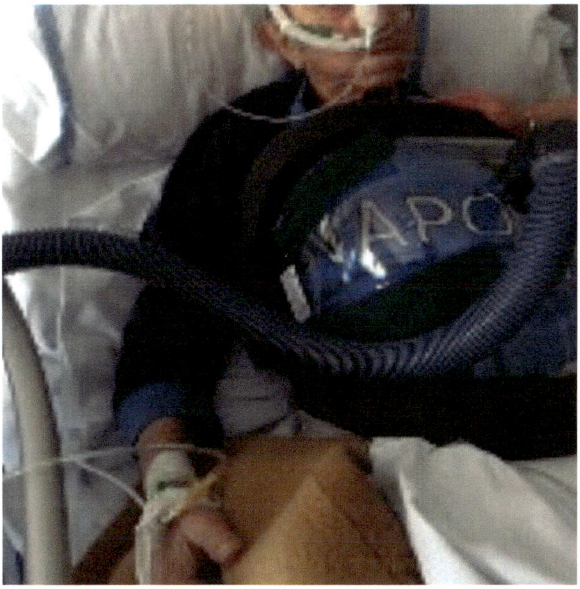

Fig. 11.3 Combinate use of cough assist and negative ventilation

11.11 Monitoring the use of NPV

During the establishment of negative pressure ventilation, it is important to ensure that there is adequate gas exchange; when there is no arterial line this is best achieved by using oxygen saturation and end-tidal carbon dioxide monitoring. For chronic use oxygen saturation monitoring alone is most used.

11.12 Problems, Potential Complications, and Limitations of NPV

A common complication of cuirass ventilation, regardless of whether or not the device has biphasic capabilities, is skin irritation and abrasions that can become niduses for infection. The cuirass ventilator wraps tightly around the chest, in close proximity to the skin. Older cuirass devices were especially prone to falling off patients and damaging skin, making them less than ideal for long-term use. The main disadvantages of NPV relate to the use of cuirass: physical access to the patient for nursing care may be restricted and, despite being transparent, accurate assessment of chest wall movement and signs of respiratory distress may be difficult. Though it is desirable to obtain a good seal around the patient, one has to be careful to protect the skin at contact points minimize skin injury and avoid venous obstruction (Fig. 11.4). There needs to be a means of access to the child or infant for monitoring purposes while maintaining ventilation, and a mechanism permitting rapid release of the patient from the ventilator if necessary. The biggest problem in the use

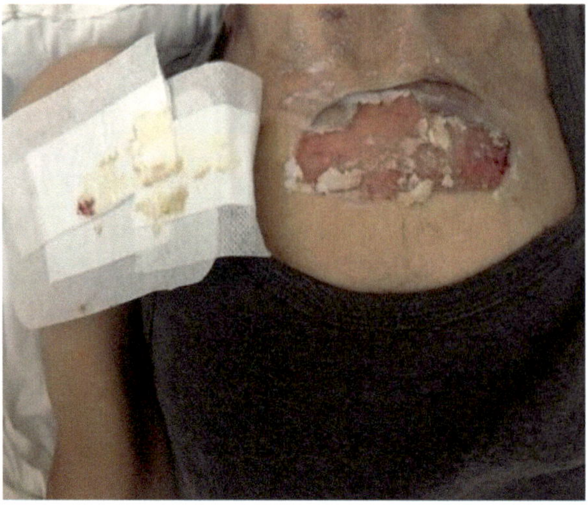

Fig. 11.4 Pressure skin lesion from continuous use of the corais

NPV, however, is that of extrathoracic upper airway obstruction. Ventilation is thought to be related to suppression of the normal preinspiratory activation of upper airway muscles, rendering upper airway structures floppier and more susceptible to passive closure. There is a possibility of reflux and aspiration correlated with dynamic effects on the lower esophageal sphincter. Obstruction is more likely during REM sleep when the breathing pattern is irregular and upper airway tone is reduced. When the difficulty with upper airway obstruction is recognized, it is manageable either by the addition of nasal continuous positive airway pressure or by the application of an alternative method of mechanical ventilation, for example, positive pressure ventilation with a nasal mask.

11.13 Conclusion

NPV appears to be a promising modality to deliver NIV for a selected group of patients. The potential benefits of NPV include reduced airway complications, improved pulmonary parenchymal inflation at reduced airway pressures, improved hemodynamic thereby reduced cardiovascular compromise, decreased sedation requirements, and improved enteral nutrition. NPV can be utilized by patients with chronic respiratory failure, who, for a variety of reasons, are unable to tolerate noninvasive positive-pressure ventilation or are dependent on mechanical ventilation 24 hours a day.

Bibliography

1. Benditt JO. Respiratory care of patients with neuromuscular disease. Respir Care. 2019;64(6):679–88. https://doi.org/10.4187/respcare.06827. PMID: 31110036.
2. Boentert M, Wenninger S, Sansone VA. Respiratory involvement in neuromuscular disorders. Curr Opin Neurol. 2017;30(5):529–37. https://doi.org/10.1097/WCO.0000000000000470. PMID: 28562381.

3. McBride WT, Ranaldi G, Dougherty MJ, Siciliano T, Trethowan B, Elliott P, Scolletta S, Giomarelli P, Romano SM, Linton DM. Haemodynamic effects of negative pressure ventilation. Br J Anaesth. 2011;106(3):420. https://doi.org/10.1093/bja/aer018. PMID: 21317236.
4. Brochard LJ. Mechanical ventilation: negative to positive and back again. Crit Care Clin. 2023;39(3):437–49. https://doi.org/10.1016/j.ccc.2022.12.002. PMID: 37230549.
5. Shneerson JM. Assisted ventilation. 5. Non-invasive and domiciliary ventilation: negative pressure techniques. Thorax. 1991;46(2):131–5. https://doi.org/10.1136/thx.46.2.131. PMID: 2014494; PMCID: PMC462978.
6. Linton DM. Cuirass ventilation: a review and update. Crit Care Resusc. 2005;7(1):22–8. PMID: 16548815.
7. Alexander G, Gerhardt T, Brancalari E. Hyaline membrane disease. Comparison of continuous negative pressure and nasal positive airway pressure in its treatment. Am J Dis Chest. 1979;133:1156–9.
8. Garay SM, Turino GM, Goldring RM. Sustained reversal of chronic hypercapnia in patients with alveolar hypoventilation syndromes. Long-term maintenance with non-invasive nocturnal mechanical ventilation. Am J Med. 1981;70(2):269–74. https://doi.org/10.1016/0002-9343(81)90761-0. PMID: 6781339.
9. Splaingard ML, Frates RC Jr, Jefferson LS, Rosen CL, Harrison GM. Home negative pressure ventilation: report of 20 years of experience in patients with neuromuscular disease. Arch Phys Med Rehabil. 1985;66(4):239–42. https://doi.org/10.1016/0003-9993(85)90157-1. PMID: 3885906.
10. Curran FJ, Colbert AP. Ventilator management in Duchenne muscular dystrophy and postpoliomyelitis syndrome: twelve years' experience. Arch Phys Med Rehabil. 1989;70(3):180–5. PMID: 2647055.
11. Schiavina M, Fabiani A, Gunella G. External negative pressure ventilation techniques. Monaldi Arch Chest Dis. 1994;49(6):516–21. PMID: 7711706.
12. Jackson M, Smith I, King M, Shneerson J. Long term non-invasive domiciliary assisted ventilation for respiratory failure following thoracoplasty. Thorax. 1994;49(9):915–9. https://doi.org/10.1136/thx.49.9.915. PMID: 7940434; PMCID: PMC475193.
13. Baydur A, Gilgoff I, Prentice W, Carlson M, Fischer DA. Decline in respiratory function and experience with long-term assisted ventilation in advanced Duchenne's muscular dystrophy. Chest. 1990;97(4):884–9. https://doi.org/10.1378/chest.97.4.884. PMID: 2182299.
14. Annunziata A, Calabrese C, Simioli F, Coppola A, Flora M, Marotta A, Di Spirito V, Didonna F, Cicalese M, Fiorentino G. Negative-pressure ventilation in neuromuscular diseases in the acute setting. J Clin Med. 2022;11(9):2589. https://doi.org/10.3390/jcm11092589. PMID: 35566729; PMCID: PMC9101364.
15. Hino H, Suzuki Y, Ishii E, Fukuda M. Biphasic cuirass ventilation for treatment of an air leak after pneumothorax in a patient with nemaline myopathy: a case report. J Anesth. 2016;30(6):1087–90. https://doi.org/10.1007/s00540-016-2250-x. Epub 2016 Sep 19. PMID: 27644222.
16. Ikeda M, et al. Respiratory physiotherapy with assistance of biphasic cuirass ventilation for patients with neurological disease on tracheostomy positive pressure ventilation. J Neurol Sci. 381:599.
17. Shah PS, Ohlsson A, Shah JP. Continuous negative extrathoracic pressure or continuous positive airway pressure compared to conventional ventilation for acute hypoxaemic respiratory failure in children. Cochrane Database Syst Rev. 2013;2013(11):CD003699. https://doi.org/10.1002/14651858.CD003699.pub4. PMID: 24186774; PMCID: PMC6464907.

Biphasic Cuirass Ventilation Stable COPD Patients

12

María José Antona Rodríguez

12.1 Introduction

12.1.1 Context of Stable COPD

Chronic obstructive pulmonary disease (COPD) represents a major global health burden, associated with substantial morbidity and mortality [1]. It is characterized by persistent and largely irreversible airflow limitation, encompassing two key pathological components: chronic obstructive bronchiolitis (small airway disease) and emphysema [1]. Although cigarette smoking remains the principal risk factor, only 20–30% of smokers develop clinically significant COPD, suggesting critical roles for genetic predisposition and environmental exposures [2].

Clinically, COPD presents with characteristic symptoms such as dyspnea, chronic cough, and sputum production. Many patients also experience acute worsening of symptoms (exacerbations), often triggered by respiratory infections or environmental pollutants [3]. These pathophysiological alterations lead to air trapping, dynamic hyperinflation, and exertional dyspnea, significantly impairing functional capacity [1].

Current therapeutic strategies primarily rely on bronchodilators, with inhaled corticosteroids reserved for patients with eosinophilic inflammation. However, no pharmacological interventions, aside from smoking cessation, have been shown to modify the disease's natural progression [4]. The underlying mechanisms include chronic corticosteroid-resistant inflammation, accelerated pulmonary aging, and defective repair mechanisms—largely driven by oxidative stress [1]. Collectively, these features profoundly impair daily activities, social participation, and emotional well-being, contributing to a marked decline in health-related quality of life.

M. J. A. Rodríguez (✉)
Servicio de Neumología, Hospital de Zafra, Zafra, Badajoz, Spain

O. Alibrahim et al. (eds.), *Biphasic Cuirass Noninvasive Ventilation*, Noninvasive Ventilation. The Essentials, https://doi.org/10.1007/978-3-032-20933-7_12

12.1.2 Limitations of Current Treatments

Despite therapeutic advances—particularly with long-acting bronchodilators (LAMAs and LABAs)—significant unmet needs persist in the management of stable COPD. Two of the most critical limitations include the inability to reverse respiratory muscle dysfunction and the limited efficacy of current therapies in preventing exacerbations [5].

Exacerbations, even when infrequent, have major clinical implications. They accelerate lung function decline, reduce physical activity, and negatively impact mental health. In a landmark natural history study by Suissa et al. (n = 73,106), mortality following the first COPD-related hospitalization reached 50% at 3.6 years and 75% at 7.7 years [6]. More concerning, the risk of subsequent exacerbations rises exponentially: it triples after the second event and increases 24-fold by the tenth, with inter-exacerbation intervals shrinking from 5 years (between the first and second) to under 4 months (between the ninth and tenth) [6].

Current maintenance therapies present three major limitations:

- *Limited impact on exacerbation progression*: While symptoms may improve, current regimens do little to prevent the acceleration of disease that typically follows the second exacerbation [6].
- *High postexacerbation mortality*: Mortality rates peak at 40 deaths per 10,000 patient-days during the first week after hospitalization, largely unaffected by conventional bronchodilator therapy [6].
- *No modification of disease trajectory*: To date, no pharmacotherapy has been shown to alter the natural history of COPD; smoking cessation remains the only intervention with proven disease-modifying effects [6].

Noninvasive positive pressure ventilation (NIPPV) remains the standard of care for acute hypercapnic respiratory failure but shows limited efficacy in stable COPD. Patient adherence is often poor due to discomfort from the facial mask, aerophagia, and poor synchrony with spontaneous breathing efforts. Moreover, NIPPV does not directly address respiratory muscle dysfunction or the inherent limitations of positive pressure physiology.

These shortcomings underscore the urgent need for alternative modalities that target exacerbation prevention, respiratory muscle support, and posthospital care—beyond symptomatic relief alone.

12.1.3 Introduction to Biphasic Cuirass Ventilation

Biphasic Cuirass Ventilation (BCV) is a novel noninvasive negative-pressure ventilation modality designed to more closely mimic physiological respiration by cyclically applying external thoracic pressure [7]. Initially developed for patients with neuromuscular disorders (e.g., Duchenne muscular dystrophy and spinal cord injury), BCV has shown promise in enhancing alveolar ventilation while circumventing complications associated with positive pressure devices [8].

The system utilizes a hermetically sealed thoracic cuirass that alternates between negative inspiratory pressure (−15 to −30 cmH_2O) and positive expiratory pressure (+5 to +10 cmH_2O). This biphasic mechanism supports diaphragmatic function and reduces the work of breathing by an estimated 35–40% compared to conventional positive-pressure ventilation [9].

Preliminary data suggest that BCV may benefit patients with stable COPD—particularly those with chronic hypercapnia ($PaCO_2$ >50 mmHg) who are unable to tolerate NIPPV [10]. Observational studies report improvements in gas exchange (reductions in $PaCO_2$ by 6–12 mmHg) and functional exercise capacity (increases in 6-minute walk distance) [11]. In a 2022 multicenter cohort ($n = 87$), adherence to BCV reached 78%, compared to 52% for BiPAP, largely due to greater patient comfort and avoidance of mask-related side effects [12]. However, the Global Initiative for Chronic Obstructive Lung Disease (GOLD) guidelines highlight that BCV's role in stable COPD remains investigational and requires validation through randomized controlled trials [13].

12.2 Objective of This Chapter

This chapter aims to critically examine the physiological rationale and emerging clinical evidence supporting the use of Biphasic Cuirass Ventilation (BCV) in stable COPD, with particular emphasis on:

- *Physiological mechanisms*: How BCV improves gas exchange and reduces respiratory muscle load in comparison with traditional invasive and noninvasive ventilation strategies [10, 12].
- *Clinical evidence*: A review of current studies demonstrating BCV's impact on hypercapnia, exercise tolerance, and quality of life—highlighting key outcomes such as mean reductions in $PaCO_2$ (6–12 mmHg) and gains in 6-minute walk distance (20–40 meters).
- *Practical applicability*: An analysis of BCV's potential integration into current COPD management algorithms, considering its strengths (adherence, safety profile) and limitations (equipment availability and technical training requirements).

In addition, we will identify current knowledge gaps—particularly the lack of long-term randomized data—and propose future research directions for BCV in stable COPD.

12.3 Justification for Focusing on Stable COPD

Exploring the role of mechanical ventilation with Biphasic Cuirass Ventilation (BCV) in stable COPD is timely and clinically relevant for several reasons:

- *Unmet clinical needs*: Patients with stable COPD, particularly those with chronic hypercapnia and frequent exacerbations, represent a subgroup with limited effective options. Conventional therapies often fail to address respiratory muscle fatigue or impaired ventilatory mechanics, key factors in disease burden and progression.
- *Intolerance to existing ventilatory support*: Many patients cannot tolerate positive pressure ventilation due to interface discomfort, poor synchrony, and gastrointestinal side effects. BCV offers a mask-free alternative that may improve adherence and comfort.
- *Potential to reduce exacerbations and hospital readmissions*: By improving alveolar ventilation and reducing carbon dioxide retention, BCV may help break the cycle of frequent exacerbations and prevent posthospitalization deterioration, key objectives in stable COPD management.
- *Alignment with current research priorities*: There is growing interest in nonpharmacological interventions that address the systemic consequences of COPD and improve patient-centered outcomes This approach offers a physiologically rational and patient-centered strategy for optimizing care in individuals with advanced COPD, particularly in those for whom conventional pharmacological or ventilatory interventions have proven inadequate.

12.4 Clinical Benefits for COPD Patients

BCV offers several advantages specifically valuable for COPD management:

1. Improved Gas Exchange
   - Effectively reduces CO_2 retention, a major challenge in COPD
   - Transient improvements in SpO_2 observed after each BCV session
   - More efficient CO_2 clearance than conventional methods due to active exhalation phase
2. Physiological Advantages
   - Maintains and redevelops respiratory muscles that often atrophy with respiratory failure and mechanical ventilation
   - Avoids impairment of cardiac function commonly seen with positive pressure ventilation
   - Provides more homogenous lung inflation with less hysteresis compared to positive pressure ventilation
3. Secretion Management
   - Incorporates High Frequency Chest Wall Oscil
   - lation (HFCWO) to mobilize secretions.
   - Includes cough assist mechanism to enhance expectoration
   - More effective than vest therapies which may induce atelectasis

4. Patient Comfort and Quality of Life
   - Noninvasive and mask-free, avoiding facial skin breakdown
   - Allows patients to eat, speak, and drink during ventilation
   - Can be used at home, enabling continuity of care

12.4.1 Practical Considerations for COPD Treatment

Clinical domain	Implementation guidelines	Technical notes
Treatment session	Start with 30 min per day and progress to 60 min sessions as tolerated.	Initial settings often use negative pressure of −15 to −25 cmH_2O and positive pressure of 3–10 cmH_2O.
Device selection	Available in both adult and pediatric sizes: 4 adult sizes 7 pediatric sizes.	Weight: 6.2 kg. Battery life: 4 h of continuous use approx. Modern units are fully computerized and portable.
Pressure settings	Acute exacerbations: Insp: −20 to −25 cmH_2O Exp: +8 to +10 cmH_2O Stable COPD: Insp: −15 to −20 cmH_2O Exp: +3 to +5 cmH_2O	I:E ratio 1:2 to 1:3 (normally) Backup rate: 12–16 bpm
Safety monitoring	Continuous waveforms display Automatic pressure release if leak >15% Mandatory pre/post ABG for first 3 sessions (especially critical for patients with baseline $PaCO_2$ >55 mmHg)	Avoids barotrauma risk associated with positive pressure ventilation Does not require sedation unlike many positive pressure approaches Reduce infection risk compared to invasive methods

12.4.2 Evidence in COPD Management

Clinical studies have demonstrated the therapeutic potential of Biphasic Cuirass Ventilation (BCV) across various COPD presentations:

- Acute Respiratory Failure:
  - BCV shows comparable efficacy to noninvasive positive pressure ventilation (NIPPV) in preventing intubation, with superior patient tolerance [14]
  - Observational data reveal significant improvements in gas exchange (PaO_2/FiO_2 ratio increase of 32%) within 2 hours of initiation [15]
- Chronic Respiratory Failure:
  - A multicenter study (n = 43) demonstrated sustained reductions in $PaCO_2$ (mean −7.2 mmHg, $p < 0.01$) after 3 months of nightly BCV therapy [16]
  - Associated with 42% reduction in hospitalization days compared to standard care [16]

- Weaning Difficulties:
  - Case series show 78% success rate in transitioning COPD patients from invasive ventilation when BCV was used as bridge therapy [17]
  - Maintains equivalent gas exchange with 30% lower work of breathing versus pressure support ventilation [18]
- Pulmonary Hypertension: In patients with COPD-associated PH (mPAP >25 mmHg), BCV sessions produced:
  - 17.6% reduction in mean pulmonary artery pressure (27.2 → 22.4 mmHg) [19]
  - 14.3% improvement in cardiac index (2.8 → 3.2 L/min/m^2) [19]
  - 38% decrease in NT-proBNP levels ($p = 0.003$) [19]

12.4.3 How BCV Works in COPD

Component	Technical specifications	Physiological effect in COPD
Device Setup	Hermetically sealed cuirass shell covering chest/upper abdomen. Connected to a programmable ventilator.	Noninvasive interface avoids facial mask discomfort. Allows normal speech and eating during therapy.
Inspiration Phase	Negative pressure generation: −15 to −25 cmH_2O Chest wall expansion	Mimics natural diaphragmatic breathing Reduces inspiratory muscle work by 35–40% Improves ventilation-perfusion matching
Expiration Phase	Positive pressure application: 3–10 cmH_2O Active exhalation assistance	Counters auto-PEEP and air trapping Reduces dynamic hyperinflation Decreases expiratory muscle effort
Control Parameters	Respiratory rate: 6–1200 cycles/min Adjustable I: E ratio (1:1 to 1:4) Tidal volume titration	Customizable ventilation matching disease severity Optimizes CO_2 removal while preventing volutrauma Maintains synchrony with patient's breathing pattern
Unique Advantages	Negative pressure physiology Mask-free interface Biphasic pressure control	Better tolerated than NIV (78% vs 52% adherence) Reduces $PaCO_2$ by 6–12 mmHg Improves 6MWD by 20–40 meters

***

12.5 Conclusion and Future Perspectives

Biphasic Cuirass Ventilation (BCV) represents a valuable therapeutic option for COPD patients across the disease spectrum, from acute exacerbations to chronic management. Its physiological approach to ventilation addresses key limitations of conventional methods by offering unique advantages:

- Mimics natural breathing through negative pressure.
- Eliminates adherence barriers associated with facial interfaces.
- Reduces both inspiratory muscle load (35–40%) and dynamic hyperinflation.

Moreover, the growing interest in nonpharmacological interventions for COPD (targeting systemic consequences and improving patient-centered outcomes) positions BCV as an innovative paradigm. Its physiological basis warrants systematic investigation in:

1. Mechanisms of action:
   (a) Effects on alveolar recruitment in emphysema.
   (b) Modulation of pulmonary oxidative stress.
2. Clinical outcomes:
   (a) Impact on long-term exacerbation frequency.
   (b) Preservation of diaphragmatic function.
3. Implementation:
   (a) Safe home protocols.
   (b) Patient selection criteria.

BCV emerges as a physiologically rational alternative in advanced COPD, combining technical innovation with patient-centered outcomes. While robust evidence is still needed for full integration into therapeutic algorithms, its potential to transform chronic respiratory failure management is promising.

References

1. Hurst JR, Skolnik N, Hansen GJ, Anzueto A, Donaldson GC, Dransfield MT, et al. Understanding the impact of chronic obstructive pulmonary disease exacerbations on patient health and quality of life. Eur J Intern Med. 2020;73:7–11.
2. Silverman EK, Sandhaus RA. Clinical practice. Alpha1-antitrypsin deficiency. N Engl J Med. 2009;360(26):2749–57.
3. Vogelmeier CF, Román-Rodríguez M, Singh D, Han MK, Rodríguez-Roisin R, Ferguson GT. Goals of COPD treatment: focus on symptoms and exacerbations. Respir Med. 2020;166:105938. https://doi.org/10.1016/j.rmed.2020.105938. Epub 2020 Mar 21.
4. Vestbo J, et al. Global strategy for the diagnosis, management, and prevention of chronic obstructive pulmonary disease. Am J Respir Crit Care Med. 2013;187(4):347–65.

5. McCarthy B, Casey D, Devane D, Murphy K, Murphy E, Lacasse Y. Pulmonary rehabilitation for chronic obstructive pulmonary disease. Cochrane Database Syst Rev. 2015;2015(2):CD003793. https://doi.org/10.1002/14651858.CD003793.pub3. PMID: 25705944; PMCID: PMC10008021.
6. Suissa S, Dell'Aniello S, Ernst P. Long-term natural history of chronic obstructive pulmonary disease: severe exacerbations and mortality. Thorax. 2012;67(11):957–63. https://doi.org/10.1136/thoraxjnl-2011-201518. Epub 2012 Jun 8. PMID: 22684094; PMCID: PMC3505864.
7. Corrado A, Gorini M. Negative-pressure ventilation: is there still a role? Eur Respir J. 2002;20(1):187–97.
8. Chatwin M, Toussaint M, Gonçalves MR, et al. Airway clearance techniques in neuromuscular disorders. Respir Med. 2018;136:98–110.
9. Hill NS, Carlisle C, Kramer NR. Effect of a noninvasive ventilation trial in COPD. Respir Care. 2012;57(12):2045–52.
10. Ambrosino N, Vagheggini G. Noninvasive ventilation in exacerbated COPD. Eur Respir Rev. 2020;29(157):200001.
11. Garuti G, Bagatti S, Verucchi E, et al. Physiological effects of BCV in hypercapnic COPD. Pulmonology. 2022;28(3):198–206.
12. Réminiac F, Vecellio L, Heuzé-Vourc'h N, et al. Adherence comparisons between BCV and NIV in COPD. Respir Med Res. 2022;81:100899.
13. Global initiative for chronic obstructive lung disease (GOLD). Global strategy for prevention, diagnosis and management of COPD: 2023 Report.
14. Corrado A, Gorini M, Ginanni R, et al. Negative pressure ventilation versus conventional mechanical ventilation in the treatment of acute respiratory failure in COPD patients. Eur Respir J. 1998;12(3):519–25. PMID: 9762779.
15. Gupta D, Nath A, Agarwal R, Behera D. A prospective randomized controlled trial on the efficacy of noninvasive ventilation in severe acute asthma. Respir Care. 2010;55(5):536–43. PMID: 20420727.
16. Toussaint M, Chatwin M, Soudon P. Mechanical ventilation in Duchenne patients with chronic respiratory insufficiency: clinical implications of 20 years published experience. Chron Respir Dis. 2007;4(3):167–77. PMID: 17711917.
17. Younes M, Kun J, Webster K, Roberts D. Response of ventilator-dependent patients to different levels of pressure support and proportional assist. Am J Respir Crit Care Med. 2002;165(6):819–24. PMID: 11897650.
18. Gorini M, Corrado A, Villella G, et al. Physiologic effects of negative pressure ventilation in acute exacerbation of chronic obstructive pulmonary disease. Am J Respir Crit Care Med. 2001;163(7):1614–8. PMID: 11401882.
19. Ambrosino N, Vagheggini G. Noninvasive positive pressure ventilation in the acute care setting: where are we? Eur Respir J. 2008;31(4):874–86. PMID: 18378782.

Biphasic Cuirass Ventilation- Chest Wall Disorders+

13

Mostafa Elshazly, Marwa Sayed Daif,
and Samar Hamed Farrag

13.1 Introduction

The respiratory pump's main component is the chest wall, which is made up of the rib cage, belly, spine, and respiratory muscles. At all lung volumes, the elastic forces of the lung encourage passive inward recoil, whereas the elastic forces of the chest wall encourage passive outward recoil. Normally, the chest wall has a high compliance, which opposes that of the lung. As a result, the labor of breathing is minor when the respiratory muscles expand a healthy chest wall (in the same direction as the chest wall resting posture). However, when problems tighten and reduce the compliance of the chest wall, the work of breathing might increase dramatically [1].

While diseases of the neuromuscular and chest wall systems are rare in isolation, they together make up a significant category of illnesses that can result in chronic ventilatory failure. This is most noticeable in scoliosis, kyphosis, following a thoracoplasty, muscular dystrophies such as Duchenne muscular dystrophy (DMD), myotonic dystrophy, postpoliomyelitis, and motor neurone disease. If bulbar function is reduced, tracheostomy ventilation may be required; nevertheless, noninvasive ventilation is recommended in other conditions. Positive pressure procedures utilizing nose and face masks are typically the initial choice, however negative pressure ventilation is an option.

M. Elshazly (✉)
Faculty of Medicine, Cairo University, Cairo, Egypt

M. S. Daif
Faculty of Medicine, Ain Shams University, Cairo, Egypt

S. H. Farrag
Faculty of Medicine, Cairo University, Cairo, Egypt

O. Alibrahim et al. (eds.), *Biphasic Cuirass Noninvasive Ventilation*, Noninvasive Ventilation. The Essentials, https://doi.org/10.1007/978-3-032-20933-7_13

There are no randomized controlled trials on the indications for initiating noninvasive ventilation, but it is usually provided if there are symptoms of nocturnal hypoventilation or right heart failure in the presence of elevated carbon dioxide tension in arterial blood ($PaCO_2$) at night or, more commonly, during the day.

There is no evidence to show that providing "prophylactic" ventilatory support before the onset of ventilatory failure is beneficial. Careful patient selection is crucial, especially when dealing with progressive neuromuscular disorders like motor neurone disease.

While there are no randomized controlled trials on the effectiveness of noninvasive ventilation in these conditions, studies have indicated improved quality of life, physical activity, hemodynamic normalization of blood gases, and slight improvements in physiological measures such as vital capacity and maximal mouth pressures.

Survival in chest wall disorders is 90% at 1 year and 80% at 5 years, and similar figures have been obtained in nonprogressive neuromuscular conditions. However, even with sufficient noninvasive ventilatory support, survival may be limited if the underlying illness is worsening, especially if it affects the bulbar muscles [2].

Acute respiratory failure can exacerbate chronic hypoventilation and pose a life-threatening consequence for patients suffering from neuromuscular disease or diseases of the chest wall. Standard management includes oxygen supplementation, physiotherapy, cough assistance, and, whenever needed, antibiotics, and intermittent positive pressure ventilation. In many centers, non-invasive mechanical ventilation (NIV) using full-face, buccal, or nasal devices has become standard procedure.

Hypercapnic ventilatory failure can occur in most thoracic skeletal illnesses. These share similar physiological characteristics, most notably a restrictive ventilatory dysfunction and poor chest wall compliance. Hypercapnia develops first during sleep and then during physical activity. In general, sternal illnesses rarely cause respiratory failure, unless there is a severe fracture combined with multiple rib fractures resulting in a flail section.

A thoracoplasty is the most frequent rib defect that causes respiratory failure. Severe ventilatory failure can be caused by scoliosis and, less frequently, a kyphosis with severe deformity; however, other spinal illnesses, like ankylosing spondylitis, never result in this consequence [3].

The respiratory drive is intrinsically normal in these conditions, but the mechanical abnormalities prevent it from being translated into a normal degree of lung inflation and deflation. Ventilation/perfusion matching is normally intact, but hypercapnia occurs when the force that the respiratory muscles can generate is overwhelmed by the additional burden placed on them by the respiratory system's lower compliance. During rapid eye movement (REM) sleep, the increased exertion of breathing and decreased respiratory muscle activity cause hypercapnia to appear before it develops during the deeper stages of nonrapid eye movement (NREM) sleep and subsequent waking.

Some respiratory muscle activity persists even during REM and stages 3 and 4 NREM sleep, so that partial rather total respiratory support is usually required.

Considerable experience has been gained over the last 15–20 years in noninvasive ventilation for chest wall disorders, but despite this there are no randomized controlled studies on its effectiveness or indications. However, the existing research implies that the ventilatory requirements fluctuate slightly between the circumstances.

13.2 Kyphoscoliosis

Kyphoscoliosis is a spinal condition defined by rotation of the spinal axis, sagittal plane curvature (kyphosis), and lateral curvature of the spine (scoliosis). It is a common spinal deformity, its prevalence in the United States ranging from 1 in 10,000 people for severe deformities to 1 in 1000 people for mild deformities [1]. The etiology of kyphoscoliosis is unknown for the majority of cases (85% classified as idiopathic), with the rest of cases due to either neuromuscular disease (paralytic or secondary) or is congenital.

The severity of the spinal deformity is assessed by measuring the "Cobb's angle" on a radiograph of the spine. Two imaginary lines that are parallel to the top and bottom vertebrae of the kyphotic or scoliotic curve intersect to generate this angle. The more severe the malformation, the larger the Cobb's angle. Respiratory symptoms are linked to angles more than 100°, while respiratory failure is linked to angles greater than 120°.

13.3 Pectus Excavatum

Pectus excavatum is a congenital chest wall deformity in which the sternum and the adjacent costal cartilages are excessively depressed. The degree of depression is assessed with chest computed tomography scan by measuring the ratio of the transverse to anteroposterior diameter of the rib cage at the level of the deepest sternal depression (Haller index). A ratio > 3.25 indicates significant deformity [4].

13.4 Thoracoplasty

Thoracoplasty was primarily performed in the 1940s and 1950s in the preantituberculous chemotherapy era; this surgical procedure represented the standard approach to control pulmonary tuberculosis. The surgery composed of different combinations of rib removal, rib fracture, phrenic nerve resection, or lung compression by filling the pleural space with foreign material (i.e., ping pong balls) [4].

Very few people who had undergone the procedure are still alive. The severity of the restrictive defect as a result of thoracoplasty was often comparable to that seen in kyphoscoliosis and was related to the number of ribs removed, prior lung resection, presence of fibrothorax, pulmonary fibrosis secondary to underlying granulomatous disease, or the intentional phrenic nerve damage [1].

13.5 Ankylosing Spondylitis

Ankylosing spondylitis affects approximately 0.1% of the general population and is more common in males than in females, with a ratio 16:1. The disease etiology is unclear. There is a genetic predisposition for Ankylosing spondylitis, as 95% of white population with ankylosing spondylitis have the HLA-B27 antigen [5].

It is a chronic multisystemic illness that affects extra-articular organs like the heart and lungs in addition to inflaming the spinal, sacroiliac, and peripheral joints. Clinically, patients present in late adolescence or early adulthood, with back pain and/or morning stiffness due to involvement of sacroiliac joints, which is worse in the morning or after prolonged rest. Onset of symptoms above the age of 45 is rare. About 30% of individuals with AS have involvement of a peripheral joint or non-granulomatous anterior uveitis, 25% of patients suffer from Aortitis and dilatation of the aortic root [6].

13.6 Flail Chest

Flail chest is defined as a double fracture of three or more adjacent ribs, or a combination of sternal and rib fractures resulting in a flail segment of the rib cage and respiratory failure. Flail chest can occur in up to 15% of adults with chest wall trauma. The diagnosis of flail chest can readily be made in spontaneously breathing individuals by observing the paradoxical inward motion of the flail segment of the rib cage during inspiration [1].

13.7 Obesity

Obesity is defined by body mass index (BMI) > 30 Kg/m^2 that is associated derangements in chest wall mechanics and the control of breathing with consequent respiratory morbidity. Obesity causes a decrease in lung volumes, respiratory drive, and respiratory muscle strength, and increase in the work of breathing. Despite these limitations, most morbidly obese patients remain eucapnic; this is known as "simple obesity". However, a subgroup of morbidly obese individuals may develop hypercapnia which is referred to as obesity hypoventilation syndrome [7].

13.8 Pathophysiology

Under normal circumstances the end-expiratory lung volume which is referred to as "functional residual capacity" represents balance point between the elastic recoil pressures of the chest wall and the lung wall. The work of breathing during inspiration is generated to overcome elastic forces, which are related to volume change; resistive forces, which are related to airflow; and inertia, which is related to the initial force required to move tissues and air (not considered significant under normal conditions) [8].

In chest wall disorders, there is great reduction of chest wall compliance, and the lung functions at a lower FRC, thus greater inspiratory force is required to overcome the chest wall stiffness (due to the increased elastic load placed on the respiratory muscles) without producing very great changes in the trans-pulmonary pressure (lung distending pressure) resulting in increased work of breathing, the oxygen cost of breathing that may be three to five times of that seen in healthy individuals, as well as alveolar hypoventilation. The resulting inspiratory muscle compromise (due to the increased workload) decreases ventilatory reserve and predisposes the respiratory muscles to fatigue and contributes to respiratory failure in these patients [9].

One of the adaptive mechanisms to overcome the chest wall stiffness, and the increased elastic load posed on inspiratory muscles is the increased respiratory drive that is usually elevated in these individuals and correlates with the disease severity. However, the increase in neural drive does not necessarily result in increased alveolar ventilation as the stiff chest wall and the exhausted respiratory muscles will limit any augmentation in alveolar ventilation. Another mechanism is a rapid shallow breathing pattern with low tidal volumes, shortened inspiratory time, and an increased respiratory rate [9].

These changes in breathing pattern can cause the work per breath to be decreased. Second, the ratio of the pressure needed to inhale to maximum static inspiratory pressure (a measurement of inspiratory muscle strength) is reduced, that theoretically lessens the incidence of inspiratory muscle fatigue and respiratory failure. However, this adaptive breathing pattern may promote atelectasis, causing hypoxemia, and may lead to a further reduction of lung compliance [10].

In flail chest, the mechanism of respiratory compromise is different from other chest wall disorders. Under normal conditions, during inspiration, pleural pressure becomes sub-atmospheric, that causes lung inflation and—theoretically—a rib cage deflation. The uncoupled flail segment from the remainder of the chest wall, becomes subjected to the deflationary effect of subatmospheric pleural pressure, that is unopposed by the factors that promote rib cage expansion (contraction of intercostal muscles and diaphragm) [1].

Consequently, the flail segment moves paradoxically (inwards) during inspiration. During expiration, with the relaxation of inspiratory muscles, the pleural pressure becomes more positive, and the flail segment moves outwards.

The pathogenesis of respiratory failure in flail chest is complex than being caused by paradoxical movement of flail segments during breathing cycle. One contributing factor is pain that can significantly impair cough effectiveness, cause regional atelectasis, intercostal muscle spasm. Another factor is that flail chest may increase the elastic load imposed on the intercostal muscles through development of regional or generalized atelectasis (due to splinting and pain). Associated conditions related to chest wall trauma such as pulmonary contusion would increase the elastic load, work of breathing, and the oxygen cause of breathing as well. All these combined factors causing increased work of breathing, respiratory muscle exhaustion, hypoxemia (due to atelectasis), and pulmonary contusion, all predispose these patients to respiratory muscle fatigue and respiratory failure [10].

13.9 Noninvasive mechanical ventilation (NIV)

Noninvasive Ventilation had two basic modes of providing mechanical ventilation.

1. Volume-targeted ventilation
2. Pressure-targeted ventilation

In volume-targeted ventilation, the operator sets the tidal volume to be delivered and the duration of inspiration (Ti). The ventilator generates whatever pressure is necessary to deliver the set volume within this time.

The inspiratory and expiratory pressures are adjusted by the operator in pressure-targeted ventilation. In this mode, the volume of air the patient receives is a function of the impedance to inflation of the lungs and chest wall and the inspiratory time. The Ti should be long enough to attain the desired volume and inserted at a frequency that gives the patient enough time to exhale completely.

Patient who had any Chest wall diseases may have two problems as mentioned before in inspiration and also expiration mechanics, so they need both volume and pressure targeted ventilation as type of Biphasic Noninvasive mechanical ventilation is best type for this group of patients in most time if have no contraindication for NIV as whole.

The biphasic cuirass ventilation (BCV) device is an alternative respiratory support device for patients with chronic respiratory failure. Some consider the device a "forgotten" technique of supporting ventilation, although it is portable, lightweight, and simple to use. Biphasic cuirass ventilation can also be utilized to quickly revive patients in severe respiratory distress, and it requires little technical expertise to operate. Biphasic cuirass ventilation can be used by the patient's caregiver in the house, making it a feasible option to other types of mechanical ventilation (e.g., BiPAP) for patients receiving home hospice or palliative care [11].

Indications of NIV in Chest wall diseases as when mechanics of respiratory muscles affected as discussed before lead to:

Acute hypercapnic respiratory failure
Obstructive sleep apnoea
Neuromuscular diseases
Central sleep apnoea
Obesity hypoventilation syndrome
Refractory cardiogenic pulmonary edema

Contraindications for NIV in Chest wall diseases as patient may also have:

The contraindications to treatment with noninvasive ventilation in chest wall disorders are like those with other conditions. They encompass a lack of motivation and an incapacity to apply headgear, cuirass, or jacket. Psychological factors, such as claustrophobia, may be important. Extensive or severe no respiratory disease, such as disseminated cancer, may limit the value of non-invasive support:

Severe facial deformity
Facial burns
Fixed upper airway obstruction
Facial trauma
Copious secretions

13.10 Types of Ventilatory Support Needed in Chest Wall Diseases

13.10.1 Noninvasive Positive Pressure Ventilation

A nasal mask is usually preferable to a full-face mask or a mouthpiece. Patients with chest wall disorders are no more prone to complications, e.g., nasal ulcers, mask displacement, air leaks, or upper airway obstruction, from this type of treatment than those with other disorders. Either pressure- or volume-preset ventilation is likely to be effective. A peak inspiratory pressure of 20–25 cmH2O is often required with pressure-preset ventilation and an inspiratory time of 0.8–1 s with an expiratory time of 2 s.

Considering the rapid respiratory frequency that these subjects adopt, a sensitive triggering system with a short response time is necessary. Positive end expiratory pressure is not essential, apart from in some bilevel pressure-support systems in which it is mandatory to flush the dead space but may be useful at a level of 2–4 cmH2O. Supplemental oxygen is seldom necessary unless the oxygen tension in arterial blood (PaO2) cannot be restored.

13.10.2 Negative Pressure Ventilation

A cuirass or jacket (poncho) form of negative pressure ventilator is always preferred over a tank ventilator. However, these ventilators have the drawback of requiring the subjects to remain sedentary and have a limited range of motion throughout the night.

This is particularly problematic with a kyphosis, where the sharp angulation of the spine can become uncomfortable. Molding a cuirass may also prove challenging for individuals with severe thoracic scoliosis. Negative pressure ventilation is a form of pressure-preset ventilation but is only widely available in the controlled mode because triggering is only present with a limited range of modern tank ventilators.

This can cause incoordination between the ventilator and the patient and upper airway obstruction may develop due to the negative pressure applied to the airway. The inspiratory and expiratory times are like those required for positive pressure ventilation [3].

13.10.3 Patient Selection

Noninvasive ventilation has been proposed in the following situations. Asymptomatic high-risk patients. Patients with a vital capacity of 1–1.5 L, scoliosis developing before the age of 8 years and a high thoracic curve are at risk of developing respiratory failure, usually in the fourth or fifth decade. These patients should be promptly identified and advised of the symptoms that indicate nocturnal hypoventilation. Due to the often-subtle nature of ventilatory failure, they should be monitored over an extended period.

Ventilatory failure may present as an emergency either during an acute illness, such as a chest infection, or following symptoms suggestive of nocturnal hypoventilation over the preceding weeks. Bifrontal headaches in the morning, abrupt awakenings from sleep, uneven breathing patterns when asleep, and excessive daytime sleepiness are symptoms of nocturnal hypoventilation.

Theoretically, treating those who are susceptible to hypercapnic respiratory failure could postpone the development of respiratory failure and avoid the associated consequences. The only evidence about this comes from those with Duchenne muscular dystrophy (DMD) in whom it was found that "prophylactic" ventilatory support was associated with a worse rather than improved survival. The cause of this is unclear but it may have been due to over confidence during respiratory infections in the ventilator subjects, which led them and their carers to seek help too late.

There is no evidence of any benefit of noninvasive ventilatory support if the carbon dioxide tension in arterial blood (PaCO2) while breathing air remains normal. A normal PaCO2 while awake, associated with a high PaCO2 during sleep, could be an indication for nocturnal ventilatory support, but again there is no evidence of this.

In practice, the decision whether to start noninvasive support in these situations usually depends on the severity of the physiological abnormalities that are detected during sleep, in particular, the degree of hypoxia and hypercapnia, and the presence or absence of complications such as polycythemia or a high pulmonary artery pressure. Early ventilation may be helpful for people with scoliosis and poliomyelitis if there is evidence of nocturnal hypoventilation without aberrant arterial blood gas tensions while they are awake. This is because timely relief of excessive muscle activity may stop, slow down, or even reverse the progression of the postpoliomyelitis syndrome. Abnormal blood gas tensions during the day. If hypercapnia is present during the day as well as at night, but without symptoms or any complications such as polycythemia or pulmonary hypertension, the indication for treatment is stronger than with nocturnal hypercapnia alone, but there is little evidence from large or controlled studies to support noninvasive positive-pressure ventilation (NPPV) in this situation.

Abnormal diurnal blood gas tensions and symptoms. Hypercapnic respiratory failure and right heart failure can be indicated by symptoms such as growing shortness of breath on exercise, physical exhaustion, sleepiness, and ankle edema, all of which can be addressed with ventilatory assistance. When there is no hypercapnia throughout the day, the symptoms are uncommon, and a combination of symptoms is the main reason to begin NPPV. It has been recommended—though not based on any published data—that ventilatory support be started when there are symptoms with either PaCO2 ≥ 45 mmHg or more than 5 min spent asleep with arterial oxygen saturation (SaO_2) ≤ 88%.

13.10.4 Tracheostomy Ventilation

Tracheostomy-intermittent positive-pressure ventilation (T-IPPV) is more frequently used in countries (e.g. France) than others (e.g. Italy and the UK). It should be considered in patients with a high level of ventilatory dependency (near 24 h) but is most relevant in individuals with severe swallowing problems, resulting in aspiration. Discharge of T-IPPV patients from hospital is more complex than NPPV recipients but can be achieved efficiently in well-experienced units.

13.10.5 Biphasic Cuirass Ventilation (BCV)

A cuirass is a shell-like unit that creates negative pressure on the chest using a combination of a fitted casing and a soft bladder. It is an adaptation of the sensationalized "iron lung" albeit compacted into a much smaller device. The iron lung was first used in 1928 and was one of the first negative pressure machines used for long-term ventilation.1 In the original model, the intrathoracic vacuum caused simultaneous expansion of both the chest and abdominal cavities, resulting in pooling of venous blood in the lower abdomen.

However, it was refined and revolutionized the response to the 1940s polio epidemic. It works by producing negative pressure through a vacuum pump mechanism, which stretches the chest wall. This results in a decrease in both the intrapulmonary pressure and the amount of ambient air that enters the lungs.

This process mimics the natural negative pressure in the intrathoracic space.

Similarly, biphasic cuirass ventilation (BCV) offers mechanical support for patients suffering from respiratory failure. Although BCV is not a novel ventilatory device, its applications in current palliative care may expand caregivers' capability to provide airway management—particularly in patients with neuromuscular disorders (NMDs; for example, amyotrophic lateral sclerosis [ALS]) or other conditions where chronic respiratory insufficiency exists.

This respiratory support method is comfortable and portable, allowing the patient to speak, eat, and even cough without obstruction because their face is not covered. [3]

13.10.6 Physiology and Design of BCV

Previous applications of the cuirass device include external high-frequency oscillation (EHFO), external chest wall compression (ECWC), external chest wall oscillation (ECWO), and negative pressure ventilation (NPV). Multiple seals and a high-pressure oscillation pump enable respiration in Hayek's redesigned or modified cuirass negative pressure ventilator. The biphasic function of the cuirass device affords users control over the inspiration: expiration ratio (I:E ratio). The patient's chest and upper abdomen are enclosed in a domed plastic shell called a cuirass, which is attached to an external pump.

Because Cuirass ventilators are made to exert equal pressure across the thorax, the lungs can expand evenly and there will be consistent ventilation. The device generates a negative pressure within the chest during inspiration and can be programmed to perform continuous inspiratory assistance. To cause expiration, it then applies positive pressure around the thorax. Its ability to remove carbon dioxide (CO_2), wean patients from external ventilation support, raise cardiac output, and expand collapsed lung regions again is what makes it so effective.

13.11 Modes of Cuirass Ventilation

Depending on the mode being used, Cuirass ventilatory devices have varied degrees of control over both inspiration and expiration. There are five types of cuirass modes: continuous negative pressure, controlled biphasic (also known as intermittent mandatory ventilation, IMV), noninvasive synchronized BCV, high-frequency oscillation, and cardiac synchronization. Like IMV, noninvasive synchronized BCV allows patients to take spontaneous breaths at their own pace and with their own inspiratory and expiratory efforts. The device is then triggered to offer assistance in a manner that is timed to match the patient's respiratory rhythm.

Additionally, the device has a high-frequency oscillation mode (up to 1200 oscillations per minute) that can help with secretion clearance, oxygenation enhancement, and carbon dioxide reduction. These functions can take the place of traditional chest physical therapy. Finally, cardiac synchronized mode uses electrocardiography (ECG) to coordinate the cardiac cycle with the ventilatory cycle, **also known as external ventilatory support**, increasing cardiac output, and re expanding areas of collapsed lung [3].

13.12 Uses of Cuirass Ventilation in Chest Wall Diseases

This easy-to-operate ventilation device can be used for rapid resuscitation of patients in acute respiratory distress, making it a useful tool in emergencies or combat situations. The device's application and restoration of adequate ventilation to the recipient is comparable to traditional intubation and positive pressure ventilation (PPV).

The use of BCV outside of a hospital is possible for first responders and bystanders without medical training with a little technical knowledge or expertise. Moreover, its portable, lightweight construction can be run on rechargeable batteries, allowing for quick, easy transport into challenging situations. It is possible that cuirass ventilation could be utilized to reduce the complications of invasive PPV.

Weaning patients from invasive PPV not only improves their quality of life but also reduces the risk of ventilator-associated pneumonia, laryngeal injury, and respiratory muscle atrophy all of which are associated with prolonged mechanical ventilation.

As medical advances extend the survival of people with terminal diseases, the patient population requiring chronic ventilation will grow; having choices other than tracheostomy and BiPAP would be advantageous.

13.13 Cuirass Ventilation Use in Palliative Medicine

Patients in respiratory failure due to muscle weakness may use BCV to postpone the need for invasive procedures such as intubation or tracheostomy. Such an intervention may enable them to communicate and assist with informed, autonomous decisions regarding their own health care trajectory. Surprisingly, cuirass ventilation uses in palliative care are novel. However, the low level of technical competence necessary to operate these devices makes them a suitable supplement to home care or home-based palliative care for appropriately selected patients. Its noninvasive nature enables patients to continue talking, eating, and interacting with family members without the use of face masks or tubes. Equally important is that one can quickly choose to discontinue therapy if it proves ineffective or is no longer desired, unlike chronic PPV via tracheostomy

Neuromuscular diseases (NMDs) vary in terms of pathogenicity, clinical manifestation, and time course. Most NMDs are genetic and therefore more prevalent in the descendants of specific geographic regions. However, an epidemiological review study published in 2015 showed that, in comparison to 1991, the prevalence of NMDs such as Becker muscular dystrophy, facioscapulohumeral humeral dystrophy, myotonic dystrophy, and Charcot-Marie Tooth disease has increased. The increased prevalence of these illnesses, combined with improved survival rates due to advances in medical care, will drive up demand for minimally invasive ventilatory support. Common symptoms in NMD include muscle weakness, movement limitations, difficulty swallowing, and respiratory distress. As NMDs progress, the diaphragm is frequently impaired, impairing patients' ability to breathe properly. Jackson et al. discovered that long-term nocturnal cuirass ventilation benefitted those with neuromuscular and skeletal chest wall problems. Notably, Hino et al. proposed BCV as a viable alternative to non-invasive positive pressure ventilation (NIPPV)—PPV given using a nasal mask, face mask, or nasal plugs. The use of BCV assisted a high-risk surgical candidate who had acquired tension pneumothorax while on noninvasive positive pressure ventilation (NIPPV) to resolve a persistent air leak. NIPPV is still an intrusive procedure. [12, 13]

13.14 Amyotrophic Lateral Sclerosis

Amyotrophic lateral sclerosis (ALS) is an incurable NMD affecting both the upper and motor neurons, causing progressive muscular weakness and contracture. Patients with ALS exhibit symptoms indicating respiratory insufficiency, which is the most prevalent cause of mortality in this condition. Nevertheless, research has shown that as many as 53% of patients with ALS make no decisions regarding ventilation prior to the onset of respiratory failure.

Mechanical ventilation is known to be an effective means of relieving symptoms of chronic hypoventilation and prolonging life in patients with ALS who have developed respiratory depression. Patients with ALS can use a variety of ways based on where they are during an acute respiratory distress episode, their personal preferences, and if they have upper airway obstruction or thick bronchial secretions. Because ALS is progressive and incurable, palliative therapy is typically the focus of treatment. Chronic nocturnal hypoventilation, for example, is a significant source of symptom burden in this population and can occur long before full-scale respiratory failure develops. [14]

13.15 Other Uses

Cuirass ventilation has been used as an alternative way of ventilation in at least two cases of central alveolar hypoventilation (CAH), a rare condition characterized by respiratory and autonomic system dysfunction.

Patients with CAH are ventilated at night by invasive PPV via tracheostomy. However, tracheostomies can cause recurrent aspiration which fosters pulmonary infections. In these two cases, bronchoscopy was first used to rule out upper airway obstruction prior to BCV conversion as tracheomalacia may develop following prolonged periods of intubation. After a period of overnight SaO2 and end-tidal CO2 monitoring, both patients successfully transitioned to BCV and were able to close their tracheostomies.

Another case report described the successful use of cuirass ventilation in the treatment of a Pompe disease patient who had developed mediastinal and subcutaneous emphysema because of NIPPV.

Further reports still have shown BCV to be especially useful in managing patients with exacerbation of their chronic obstructive pulmonary disease (COPD) complicated by hypercarbic respiratory failure.

Finally, cuirass ventilation may also function as a stand-in for endotracheal intubation in patients with decompensated heart failure. Whereas PPV decreases venous return, cuirass ventilation reduces intrathoracic pressure, allowing for increased venous return to the heart and subsequent increase in cardiac output. Specifically, Shekerdemian et al. demonstrated that cuirass NPV had hemodynamic advantages over conventional PPV following cardiac surgery in pediatric patients, as demonstrated by a notable improvement in cardiac output.

13.16 Complications and Risk of BCV

As outlined above, PPV is an invasive approach that incurs many risks of infection and injury. Cuirass ventilation is a safer solution, though not without risks.

A common complication of cuirass ventilation, regardless of whether the device has biphasic capabilities, is skin irritation and abrasions that can become niduses for infection. The cuirass ventilator wraps tightly around the chest, near the skin. Older cuirass devices were especially prone to falling off patients and damaging skin, making them less than ideal for long-term use. However, contemporary BCV models come in 12 sizes from neonate to adult, allowing for a better fit and for easy adjustment when one treats growing children [3].

13.17 Implications for Home Care

Since the first negative pressure device was introduced in the 1920s, various improvements and advancements have provided patients with a ventilator that is more pleasant, convenient, and simple to use than traditional invasive respirators. Furthermore, these devices may reduce total costs by reducing the cost and problems associated with PPV.

Biphasic cuirass ventilation has demonstrated favorable outcomes in the long-term respiratory support of patients with ALS, cystic fibrosis, NMDs, and chronic respiratory failure from other etiologists.

Noninvasive ventilation techniques like cuirass ventilation improve the quality of life of palliative patients by allowing for continued mobility and communication, while affording them the option of managing their condition in the home [3].

13.18 Outcome and Quality of Life

There are few detailed studies of the impact of NPPV on the quality of life in ALS, and PINTO et al. showed that NPPV did not produce a significant improvement. However, more recent research suggests that considerable gains in quality of life can be obtained despite a persistent deterioration in physical function. It is important that any future work examining this area reviews quality of life over the course of the illness not just at the time ventilatory support is initiated [15].

13.19 Advance Directives

Most patients with ALS and DMD wish to be actively involved with decision-making about their care. Sensitive discussion about the escalation of ventilation support, limits to therapy, and resuscitation status with the patient and family is to be encouraged.

13.20 Conclusions

We should raise awareness regarding cuirass ventilation and its applications in modern health care. Currently, these devices are infrequently used, and there are patients who may benefit BCV being incorporated into their established treatment strategies.

Notably, current research regarding BCV is limited to review articles and case reports, thus making it difficult to standardize BCV use.

Randomized controlled trials are necessary to evaluate fully the efficacy and risks of cuirass ventilators on chest wall diseases, as well as to broaden the scope of their application in palliative medicine in the home.

References

1. Grippi MA, Antin-Ozerkis DE, Dela CS, Kotloff R, Kotton CN, Pack AI. Fishman's pulmonary diseases and disorders, 2-volume set. 6th ed. McGraw Hill Professional; 2022.
2. Shneerson JM, Simonds AK. Noninvasive ventilation for chest wall and neuromuscular disorders. Eur Respir J. 2002;20:480–7.
3. Respiratory Support and Sleep Centre, Papworth Hospital, Cambridge, and Sleep and Ventilation Unit, Royal Brompton and Harefield NHS Trust, London. Correspondence: J.M. Shneerson Respiratory Support and Sleep Centre Papworth Hospital Cambridge CB3 8RE UK Fax: 44 1480830620 E-mail: john.shneerson@papworth-tr. anglox.nhs.uk.
4. Bredin CP. Pulmonary function in long-term survivors of thoracoplasty. Chest. 1989;95(1):18–20.
5. Dougados M, Baeten D. Spondyloarthritis. Lancet. 2011;377(9783):2127–37.
6. Weber U, Lambert RG, Rufibach K, Maksymowych WP, Hodler J, Zejden A, et al. Anterior chest wall inflammation by whole-body magnetic resonance imaging in patients with spondyloarthritis: lack of association between clinical and imaging findings in a cross-sectional study. Arthritis Res Ther. 2012;14(1):R3.
7. Piper AJ, Grunstein RR. Big breathing: the complex interaction of obesity, hypoventilation, weight loss, and respiratory function. J Appl Physiol. 2010;108(1):199–205.
8. Casas A, Pavía J, Maldonado D. Respiratory muscle disorders in chest wall diseases. Archivos de Bronconeumología (English Edition) [Internet]. 2003;39(8):361–6. Available from: https://www.archbronconeumol.org/en-respiratory-muscle-disorders-in-chest-articulo-13050406.
9. Ramonatxo M, Milic-Emili J, Prefaut C. Breathing pattern and load compensatory responses in young scoliotic patients. Eur Respir J. 1988;1(5):421–7.
10. Tzelepis GE, McCool FD, Hoppin FG. Chest wall distortion in patients with flail chest. Am Rev Respir Dis. 1989;140(1):31–7.
11. Home Health Care Manage Pract. 2020;32(1) 40–4 © The Author(s) 2019 Article reuse guidelines: sagepub.com/journals-permissions. https://doi.org/10.1177/1084822319875111 journals.sagepub.com/home/hhc.
12. Jackson M, Kinnear W, King M, Hockley S, Shneerson J. The effects of five years of nocturnal cuirass-assisted ventilation in chest wall disease. Eur Respir J. 1993;6(5):630–5.
13. Hino H, Suzuki Y, Ishii E, Fukuda M. Biphasic cuirass ven tilation for treatment of an air leak after pneumothorax in a patient with nemaline myopathy: a case report. J Anesth. 2016;30(6):1087–90. https://doi.org/10.1007/s00540-016-2250-x.
14. Caroscio JT, Mulvihill MN, Sterling R, Abrams B. Amyotrophic lateral sclerosis. Its natural history. Neurol Clin. 1987;5(1):1–8.
15. Pinto AC, Evangelista T, Carvalho M, Alves MA, Sales Luis ML. Respiratory assistance with a non-invasive ventilator (BiPAP) in MND/ALS patients: survival rates in a controlled trial. J Neurol Sci. 1995;129(Suppl):19–26.

Atelectasis During Biphasic Cuirass Ventilation (BCV): Causes, Diagnosis, Management, and Drawbacks

14

Aneesha Thankamony, Athika M. Sajeer, Marzooq Aslam, Lara A. Ismail, Antonio M. Esquinas, and Nabil A. Shallik

Background and Significance

Biphasic Cuirass Ventilation (BCV) is a form of noninvasive ventilation support that physiologically more accurately mimics breathing than does traditional positive pressure ventilation. The cuirass, which is a shell-shaped garment which goes around the chest wall, is fastened onto a proprietary ventilator, which alternates between periods of negative and positive pressure so that inspiration and expiration are generated.

BCV provides considerable clinical benefit, especially for critically ill or perioperatively managed patients, due to its maintenance of upper airway patency, encouragement of secretion drainage, and minimization of complications of intubation. Atelectasis, or alveolar collapsing, continues, nonetheless, to remain an issue for

A. Thankamony · A. M. Sajeer · M. Aslam
Department of Anaesthesia and Perioperative Medicine, Hamad Medical Corporation, Doha, Qatar
e-mail: AThankamony@hamad.qa; AMohammed51@hamad.qa; MAslam1@hamad.qa

L. A. Ismail
New Giza University, Cairo, Egypt
e-mail: AIBRAHIM3@hamad.qa

A. M. Esquinas
Intensive Care Unit, Hospital Meseguer, NIV in ICU Group, Biomedical Research Institute of Murcia, Pascual Parrilla–IMIB, Murcia, Spain

N. A. Shallik (✉)
Department of Anaesthesia and Perioperative Medicine, Hamad Medical Corporation, Doha, Qatar

Clinical Anaesthesiology Department, Weill Cornell Medical College in Qatar, Doha, Qatar

Clinical Anaesthesiology Department, College of Medicine, Qatar University, Doha, Qatar
e-mail: nshallik@hamad.qa

O. Alibrahim et al. (eds.), *Biphasic Cuirass Noninvasive Ventilation*, Noninvasive Ventilation. The Essentials, https://doi.org/10.1007/978-3-032-20933-7_14

patients managed with BCV. This is especially true for patients with diminished lung compliance, secretion retention, or suboptimal ventilation parameters.

Recognition of atelectasis evolution for BCV helps optimize ultimate outcomes, prevent hypoxemia, and reduce risk for infection. Understanding atelectasis mechanisms, as well as management, permits improved individualization of ventilatory support, such that the benefits of BCV outweigh its liabilities.

Chapter's Objectives

(a) Explore the pathophysiological mechanisms leading to atelectasis during BCV.
(b) Discuss the risk factors contributing to alveolar collapse, including patient positioning, duration of ventilation, and underlying lung pathology.
(c) Review the diagnostic approaches, including imaging and bedside assessment tools such as lung ultrasound.
(d) Evaluate management strategies, including ventilatory adjustments, physiotherapy, and adjunctive measures.
(e) Highlight the limitations of BCV in preventing atelectasis and discuss future research directions for improving patient outcomes.

14.1 Introduction

Biphasic Cuirass Ventilation (BCV) is a form of noninvasive respiratory support modality which breathes the patient physiologically using alternating negative and positive pressure delivered across the thorax. By comparison, when air is delivered into lungs using positive pressure ventilation, respectively, BCV generates a condition of negative extra-thoracic pressure for inhalation and utilizes a positive pressure for support of exhalation. This approach does not entail intubation, preserves upper airway patency, and potentially enhances secretion clearance, and is thus useful in critical care, peri-operative medicine, and pediatrics. [1–3].

Yet, atelectasis, or alveolar collapse, continues to be a concern when using BCV. While BCV is commonly used for alveolar prevention, it might unexpectedly cause alveolar collapse given a set of circumstances. Atelectasis damages oxygen exchange, causes a higher risk for pneumonia, and results in long recoveries [4]. Awareness of how BCV might lead to such a complication helps support the effective and sensible application.

14.2 Mechanisms of Atelectasis During BCV

The pathophysiologic mechanisms for atelectasis with BCV are a combination of ventilatory mechanics and patient physiology.

The second important factor is the reduction of the transpulmonary pressure gradients. The ventilation of the BCV relies on the pressure difference across alveoli and chest wall for ventilation generation. On a very low inspiratory pressure setting, or on a noncompliant cuirass fit, alveoli may not open at all. Partial lung collapse occurs, particularly on the dependent regions of lungs [5].

Inefficient recruitment of alveoli also plays a role, particularly for poorly compliant subjects, i.e., for subjects with acute respiratory distress syndrome (ARDS), pulmonary edema, or obese subjects. Research has shown that, even despite reversal of deteriorating trend of the oxygenation, alveoli remain closed if the resulting negative pressure is not enough [6].

Retention of secretion and airway obstruction are also contributing factors. While mucociliary clearance is enhanced with the help of adjuncts such as cough-assist or percussion modes while using BCV, such a practice is not necessarily routine or regular. This then facilitates the formation of mucus plugging leading to segmental or lobar atelectasis [7].

Lastly, patient position and diaphragmatic mechanics determine the likelihood of collapse. Basal atelectasis is predisposed towards due to supine posture, abdominal distension, or neuromuscular weakness which might limit diaphragmatic excursion, leading to a decrease in ventilation of posterior lung segments [8].

14.3 Risk Factors and Patient Populations

The risk of atelectasis with BCV is multifactorial both on a patient basis and on a technical basis.

It includes obesity, whose chest wall loading results in less efficient negative pressure, and neuromuscular weakness, whose patients do not synchronize adequately with the cuirass cycle. Sedation, prolonged immobilization, and absent cough reflex are also notable contributors [9].

Device- and technique-related risks are ill-fitting cuirasses, less-than-ideal pressure setting, and prolonged shallow tidal volumes that promote microatelectasis with time [10].

Special groups warrant special mention. In children, although BCV permits a noninvasive modality which spares airway trauma, they are at a high risk for secretion retention and rapid desaturation [11]. In critically ill adult patients, particularly those with poor compliance or high secretion load, atelectasis is yet more likely [12].

14.4 Diagnosis of Atelectasis in Patients Receiving BCV

The early diagnosis of atelectasis prevents progressive worsening of hypoxemia and subsequent infection.

Clinically, atelectasis can have oxygen desaturation, tachypnoea, and elevated work of breathing. On examination, some findings are diminished breath sounds or dullness on percussion over affected regions.

Imaging continues at the core of diagnosis. Chest X-ray is frequently the first-choice modality, despite its lack of sensitivity for subtle cases. CT is more specific but seldom a possibility for unstable patients. Lung ultrasonography is progressively being proposed at the bedside. Lung ultrasonography has the capability for recognizing specific patterns like tissue-like echogenicity, immobile air bronchograms, and diminished pleural sliding. Some studies have attested its credibility over chest X-ray, especially for ICU settings and postoperative care [13–15].

14.5 Management Strategies

(a) Optimizing BCV Settings

The first approach to management is through changes in the ventilator setting. An increase in inspiratory negative pressure, sufficient time for expiration, and attainment of a good cuirass seal can decrease the incidence of pulmonary collapse [16].

(b) Adjunctive Measures

Airway clearance is paramount. Bronchoscopy should be used for bulky mucus plugs, but devices for assisting coughing and oscillation modes should aid secretion mobilization. Chest physiotherapy, incentive spirometry, and repetitive turning are cheap but effective measures [17]. Oxygen therapy through high-flow nasal cannula might also enhance oxygenation during optimization of BCV parameters [18].

(c) Patient Positioning

Positioning strategies are very effective at times. Prone or semi-prone positioning can redistribute ventilation for collapsed segments, and prone positioning might have a role for patients with severe posterior atelectasis or accompanying ARDS [19].

(d) Escalation

In worsening atelectasis or respiratory compromise, conversion to conventional positive pressure ventilation may be necessary.

This is particularly true for the severe form of ARDS or hypercapnic/hypoxic unresponsiveness despite alterations in BCV [20].

(e) Pharmacologic Adjunct

The above management gives a mechanical and physical approach, which should be complemented with the addition of pharmacology.

- Mucolytics: The beneficial role of nebulized acetylcysteine or dornase alfa in those with thick, stubborn secretions prone to mucus obstruction.
- Bronchodilators: The patients with concomitant bronchospasm (e.g., COPD, asthma), beta-2 agonists can reduce airway obstruction and indirectly help prevent atelectasis.
- Surfactant Treatment: As a reminder, while more a neonatal/research entity, exogenous surfactant for adult severe ARDS with collapse is a subject of investigation, which could yet have a role for the toughest cases.

14.6 Monitoring and Prevention Protocols

This would provide a practical, actionable framework for clinicians.

- *Proactive Monitoring*: we can follow a protocol for patients on BCV, including:
  - *Regular Auscultation*: To detect new or worsening areas of reduced air entry.
  - *Lung Ultrasound (LUS) Screening*: Propose scheduled LUS exams (e.g., every 12–24 h in high-risk patients) to detect subclinical atelectasis before it causes significant desaturation.
  - *Tidal Volume and Minute Ventilation Checks*: Ensuring that the BCV is generating adequate volumes, not just providing pressure support.
- *Prevention Bundle*: this bundle of care can prevent atelectasis, integrating points from the above points including:

  1. *Cuirass Fit-Check*: Before each shift and after patient repositioning.
  2. *Mandatory Repositioning Schedule*: e.g., turn every 2 h.
  3. *Scheduled "Sigh" or Recruitment Maneuvers*: Using the BCV device itself to periodically deliver a higher negative pressure breath to recruit alveoli (if the device capability exists).
  4. *Routine Adjunct Therapy*: Integration of scheduled chest physiotherapy or cough-assist in high-risk patients.

14.7 Drawbacks and Complications of BCV

Even when BCV provides the benefit of a noninvasive assist, complications become regular.

Technically, limitations comprise air leaks, poor fit, and skin ulcers resulting from prolonged use of the cuirass. Patient–ventilator asynchrony might also occur, particularly for agitated or uncooperative patients [21].

Physiologically, the BCV may not sufficiently recruit in extremely hypoxemic patients, and you might, on some occasions, observe hemodynamic effects, i.e., diminished venous return, because of the negative intrathoracic pressures [22]. These considerations emphasize the necessity for judicious patient choice and close attention.

14.8 Future Directions

More recent work describes enhancements to cuirass design, such as improved seals and light-weighting with ergonomically shaped materials, which could enhance comfort and performance [23]. Further work is examining the integration of BCV with formal physiotherapy and secretion clearance maneuvers for reducing atelectasis [24].

Nonetheless, several questions remain without clear-cut answers. Long-term results for ICU patients, the perioperative role of lung protection for BCV, and the pediatric effectiveness of BCV need answerability based on properly designed clinical trials [25, 26].

A recent comprehensive review by Bodhey et al. highlights the growing evidence for BCV's utility in airway surgeries, underscoring its role in maintaining oxygenation and avoiding intubation, though it also notes the persistent challenge of atelectasis management in this context [27].

The future directions section might be more specific by application of the following suggestions and might be an area of research:

- *Closed-Loop Systems*: We can suggest research into smart BCV systems that could automatically adjust negative/positive pressure levels based on real-time respiratory impedance or EIT (Electrical Impedance Tomography) data to prevent collapse.
- *Standardized Setting Guidelines*: We need evidence-based guidelines on initial pressure settings and titration protocols based on patient phenotypes (obese, neuromuscular, and pediatric).
- *Hybrid Modes*: We need studies investigating hybrid ventilation—for example, combining BCV with High-Flow Nasal Oxygen (HFNO) or with noninvasive positive pressure—to synergistically prevent atelectasis while maximizing comfort and oxygenation.

Key Points for Discussion

- BCV, while protective in many contexts, can predispose to atelectasis if not applied optimally.
- Risk factors are both patient-related and device-related.
- Diagnosis requires vigilance, with lung ultrasound offering a sensitive bedside option.
- Management focuses on optimizing ventilator settings, secretion clearance, and patient positioning.
- In severe cases, transition to positive pressure ventilation remains necessary.

Summary and Conclusion

Biphasic Cuirass Ventilation provides a physiologically favorable, noninvasive approach to ventilatory support. Nevertheless, atelectasis remains a significant potential complication. Understanding the mechanisms, recognizing high-risk populations, and applying timely diagnostic and management strategies are key to preventing adverse outcomes. With continued technological improvements and clinical research, the role of BCV in preventing and managing atelectasis will become clearer and potentially more impactful in critical care and perioperative medicine.

References

1. Egawa T, Ikeda N, Yamamoto T. Effects of extra thoracic mechanical ventilation on pulmonary hypertension secondary to lung disease. J Anesth. 2016;30(4):663–70.
2. Nagase N, et al. Efficacy of biphasic cuirass ventilation in the critical care department. Crit Care. 2010;14(4):R151.
3. Heulitt MJ, et al. Negative pressure ventilation via chest cuirass to decrease ventilator-associated complications in infants with acute respiratory failure: a case series. Respir Care. 2000;45(5):479–84.
4. Hedenstierna G, Edmark L. Mechanisms of atelectasis in the perioperative period. Best Pract Res Clin Anaesthesiol. 2010;24(2):157–69.
5. Ferrer R, et al. Comparative effects of negative- vs. positive-pressure ventilation in surfactant-depleted rabbit lungs. Am J Respir Crit Care Med. 2008;177(12):1374–81.
6. Pelosi P, Croci M, Ravagnan I, et al. The effects of body mass on lung volumes, respiratory mechanics, and gas exchange during anesthesia. Anesth Analg. 1998;87(3):654–60.
7. Hess DR. Secretion clearance techniques: absence of evidence or evidence of absence? Respir Care. 2001;46(11):1296–312.
8. Tusman G, Böhm SH, Warner DO, Sprung J. Atelectasis and perioperative pulmonary complications in high-risk patients. Curr Opin Anaesthesiol. 2012;25(1):1–10.
9. Amato MBP, et al. Driving pressure and survival in the acute respiratory distress syndrome. N Engl J Med. 2015;372:747–55.
10. Yoshida T, et al. Physiologic effects of spontaneous breathing during mechanical ventilation: implications for lung protection. Anesthesiology. 2017;126(6):1037–46.
11. Heulitt MJ, et al. Pediatric negative pressure ventilation experience. Respir Care. 2002;47(6):669–75.
12. Slutsky AS, Ranieri VM. Ventilator-induced lung injury. N Engl J Med. 2013;369:2126–36.
13. Cursino de Moura JF, Oliveira CB, Freire APCF, et al. Lung ultrasound as a diagnostic tool for pulmonary consolidation and atelectasis after cardiac surgery. J Thorac Dis. 2025;17(3):510–20.
14. Mayo PH, Copetti R, Feller-Kopman D. Thoracic ultrasonography: a narrative review. Intensive Care Med. 2019;45:1200–11.
15. Lichtenstein DA. Lung ultrasound in the critically ill. Ann Intensive Care. 2014;4:1.
16. Egawa T, et al. Hemodynamic and respiratory effects of cuirass ventilation in post-cardiac surgery patients. J Card Surg. 2012;27(6):668–74.
17. Stiller K. Physiotherapy in intensive care: towards an evidence-based practice. Chest. 2000;118(6):1801–13.
18. Nishimura M. High-flow nasal cannula oxygen therapy in adults. J Intensive Care. 2015;3:15.
19. Gattinoni L, et al. Prone positioning in acute respiratory distress syndrome. N Engl J Med. 2013;368:2159–68.
20. Brochard L, Slutsky A, Pesenti A. Mechanical ventilation to minimize progression of lung injury in acute respiratory failure. Am J Respir Crit Care Med. 2017;195(4):438–42.
21. Sinderby C, Beck J. Neurally adjusted ventilatory assist in adults. Curr Opin Crit Care. 2013;19(1):56–64.
22. Takata M, et al. Cardiovascular effects of cuirass ventilation: experimental studies. J Appl Physiol. 1991;71(6):2228–35.
23. Nakamura T, et al. Development of next-generation cuirass ventilators. Med Eng Phys. 2019;63:44–51.
24. Hess DR. Respiratory physiotherapy in critical care. Clin Chest Med. 1999;20(2):421–34.
25. Mehta S, Hill NS. Noninvasive ventilation. Am J Respir Crit Care Med. 2001;163(2):540–77.
26. Fauroux B, et al. Non-invasive ventilation in children. Lancet Respir Med. 2016;4(12):998–1010.
27. Bodhey A, Bodhey M, Shallik NA, Al Nadhari M, Griess HF, Al Ani O, Sainuddin S, Thomas KP, ElHanfi O, Jose S, Nair A. Biphasic cuirass ventilation for airway surgeries: a comprehensive review. Cureus. 2024;16(12):e75477. https://doi.org/10.7759/cureus.75477. PMID: 39791051; PMCID: PMC11717378.

15 Biphasic Cuirass Ventilation during Bronchoscopy

Umberto Vincenzi, Leonardo Ciuffreda,
and Massimo Selmi

15.1 Introduction

The history of bronchoscopy begins in 1897 when Gustav Killian, a German otologist, after some experiments made on cadavers and tracheostomized patients, through the use of an esophagoscope, managed to remove a pig bone from the right main bronchus of a patient whom he had accidentally inhaled. The same author, after having removed other foreign bodies, presented the method, called "direkte bronchoskopie", at the 6th Congress of the Society of South German Laryngologists in Heidelberg in 1898 [1].

The method spread to other European countries, but it took about 10 years to make it known overseas. In 1907, Killian went to Pittsburg, invited by the American Society of Otolaryngology, where he met Chevalier Jackson who soon became the father of American broncho-esophagoscopy and who, in the following years, devised variants of the original endoscopic instrument up to proposing a luminous tube to be inserted in the bronchoscope which drastically improved depth vision [2].

In 1929, Philip Drinker and Louis Agassiz Shaw, based on studies of human physiology, presented the first pulmonary ventilator controlled by an electric motor, called "iron-lung" (IL), with the aim of addressing respiratory insufficiency [3]. Since then there has been an increasingly growing development of lung ventilators with evident improvements both in the mechanical field and, in recent decades, also in the electronic field.

It so happened that the first instruments, designed to deal with major problems that could afflict patients with pulmonary diseases, found their first use about a

U. Vincenzi (✉) · L. Ciuffreda · M. Selmi
Operative Unit of Pneumology and Intensive Respiratory Care Unit, "Ospedali Riuniti" University Hospital, Foggia, Italy

O. Alibrahim et al. (eds.), *Biphasic Cuirass Noninvasive Ventilation*, Noninvasive Ventilation. The Essentials, https://doi.org/10.1007/978-3-032-20933-7_15

century ago, although it can also be said that their basic operating principle has always remained the same.

Extrathoracic mechanical ventilation, called "extrathoracic negative pressure ventilation" (ENPV) or "intermittent negative pressure ventilation" (INPV) or more simply "negative pressure ventilation" (NPV), over the years, especially due to the large size of the original IL, lost intervention priorities in favor of ventilation by insufflation of air into the airways, both of the invasive type with the "invasive mechanical pulmonary ventilation" (IMPV) and of the noninvasive type with the "noninvasive ventilation" (NIV).

This happened even if further evolutions of the IL, such as the "portalung" (more transportable and built in light materials), the "poncho" or the "cuirass", decidedly smaller and easier to use, favored their use. With these latest devices, the definition of "biphasic cuirass noninvasive ventilation" (BCV) was also coined.

On the other hand, bronchoscopy also underwent improvements, technological evolutions, and investigations of its equipment.

We can therefore mention: the "transbronchial lung biopsy" with Andersen HA [4], the "transbronchial biopsy of peripheral nodules" with Tsuboi E [5], the conception of the "flexible bronchoscope" with Ikeda S [6], the "bronchoalveolar lavage" with Reynolds HJ [7], the "Transbronchial needle aspiration" (TBNA) with Wang KP [8], the "laser therapy" with Dumon JF [9], the "videobronchoscopy" with Ryosuke O [10], the positioning of the "tracheobronchial stent" with Dumon JF [11], the conception of the "endobronchial ultrasound" with Becker H [12], the "endobronchial valves" in the treatment of emphysema with Toma T [13], the "Real-time electromagnetic navigation bronchoscopy" with Schwarz Y [14], the "Bronchial thermoplasty" for the treatment of severe asthma with Cox G [15], and the "cryobiopsy" with Hetzel J [16].

Now, it is normal to think that, in about a century of life, there has been the opportunity to perform bronchoscopies in subjects who, at the same time, also needed ventilatory assistance and that, over time, there have been methods that reconciled both the needs.

We can broadly divide rigid bronchoscopy from flexible bronchoscopy during extrathoracic noninvasive mechanical ventilation.

15.2 The Rigid Bronchoscope in NPV

Rigid bronchoscopy, despite the advent of flexible bronchoscopy, is still an essential method in particular fields of intervention. This happens more when it is necessary to operate, in an invasive way, mainly on the trachea and on the large airways.

Only in rare cases has it been possible to intervene with a rigid bronchoscope on patients undergoing negative extrathoracic mechanical ventilation using IL and this for two main reasons: (1) it is very difficult to forcefully extend the patient's head, such as to be able to introduce the bronchoscope stiff; (2) the presence, around the neck, of the collar and the rigid closure of the ventilator prevent the free movements of the patient's head and cervico-dorsal rachis and limit the possible need to move the larynx forward when introducing the instrument, with the risk of possible trauma both in the upper airways and in the trachea and main bronchi.

Perhaps these movements will be easier with the marketing of the new "EXOVENT" ventilator, designed in England, equipped with softer and lighter gaskets and with the possibility offered to the patient to be more free, so much so that he can even position himself on his side.

The use of the rigid bronchoscope is decidedly easier in the event of external negative mechanical ventilation with "poncho" or with "cuirass" as the patient has no impediments at the level of the neck and head, has the possibility of moving the trunk and has the free arms. With this type of ventilation, rigid bronchoscopy has been widely used in interventional treatments for tracheobronchial lesions.

Petrella F et al. [17] confirmed that rigid instrument bronchoscopy, in combination with INPV, has proven to be an excellent tool in providing access and control of the airway in patients who require clearing or recalibration of the tracheobronchial axis, resulting from neoplastic or non-neoplastic disease, in the placement of stents, in the treatment of tracheoesophageal fistulas, in the use of laser therapy. They argue that rigid bronchoscopy can still play a role in the diagnosis of endobronchial lesions, when the specimens obtained from flexible bronchoscopy are not sufficient, since the forceps size of the rigid instrument is much larger (Fig. 15.1). Regarding the ventilatory modality these authors state that positive ventilation and jet ventilation do not ensure effective ventilation and safety and both may limit surgical options. They also carry the risk of intraoperative pneumothorax or pneumomediastinum [18].

Natalini G et al. [19] compared INPV, by "poncho", with external high-frequency oscillation (EHFO) on seventy patients undergoing "interventional rigid bronchoscopy" (IRB) for tracheobronchial lesions and found greater hypercapnia, greater acidemia, and greater arterial hypoxemia in subjects undergoing EHFO compared to those treated with INPV. They also found that some patients ventilated with EHFO received inadequate ventilation with the need for increased FiO_2 and manual assisted ventilation [20].

The same author, in collaboration with Cavaliere S, Vitacca M, Ambrosino N and others, confirmed the validity of external negative ventilation by comparing it with "spontaneous assisted ventilation" (SAV) during IRB on patients receiving total intravenous anesthesia. On this occasion, INPV required a smaller amount of opioid

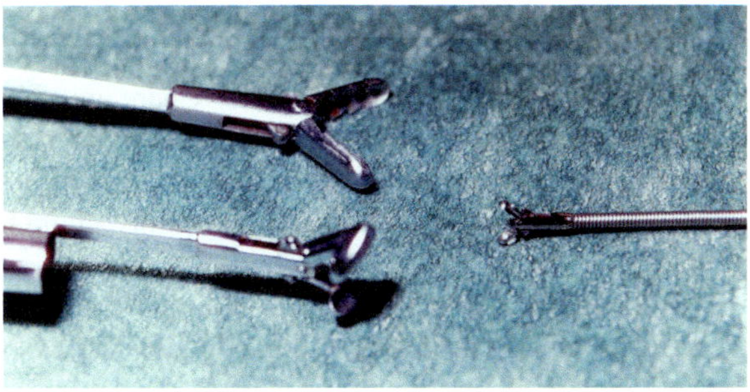

Fig. 15.1 On the left: operating forceps of rigid bronchoscopes. Right: fiberoptic bronchoscope forceps. Note the size difference

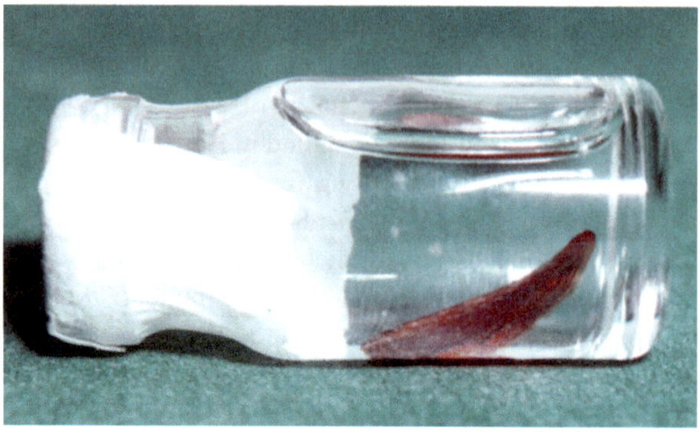

Fig. 15.2 Foreign body removed from the trachea: part of a ladybug

drugs, reduced recovery times, and O_2 requirements, did not lead to respiratory acidosis and excluded the need for manually assisted ventilation. The author concluded by stating that INPV appears a safe, noninvasive and effective ventilatory management during IRB.

Vitacca M. et al. [21] studied, with the "respiratory inductive plethysmography" the possibility of avoiding or reducing apneas and hypoxemia, correlated with respiratory acidosis, in anesthetized and ventilated patients with "poncho" compared to those undergoing ventilation spontaneous assisted. All patients, randomly selected, were treated with endobronchial laser therapy. The results obtained showed, for patients receiving NPV, a reduction in apneas, a reduction in hypercapnia and acidosis, better oxygenation, and a lower need for O_2 therapy.

Hideaki Mori H et al. [22] confirm the choice of BCV over positive pressure ventilation in tracheobronchial stent insertion or removal performed by rigid bronchoscopy.

Surely, in addition to the removal of foreign bodies in the airways (Fig. 15.2), with rigid bronchoscopy the aspiration of the more or less dense endobronchial material is more effective and the possibility of plugging endobronchial hemorrhages with drugs, electrocoagulation, argon plasma coagulation, or cryotherapy.

15.3 The Fibrobronchoscope in NPV

If the use of the rigid bronchoscope requires good dexterity and operating experience, flexible bronchoscopy is less difficult and more practical.

"Flexible bronchoscopy" or "fibrobronchoscopy" (FBO), from its inception, was immediately used in respiratory intensive care units (RICU) and in ICUs, generally to free the airways from bronchial secretions or mucus plugs during ventilation mechanics. When used with the IL there were no problems in its use as the bronchoscope, due to its small caliber and its flexibility, could be introduced both orally and nasally (Fig. 15.3).

It was the preferred tool for doing bronchial toilets, for evaluating the correct ventilation in the ventilator box, for observing the correct positioning of

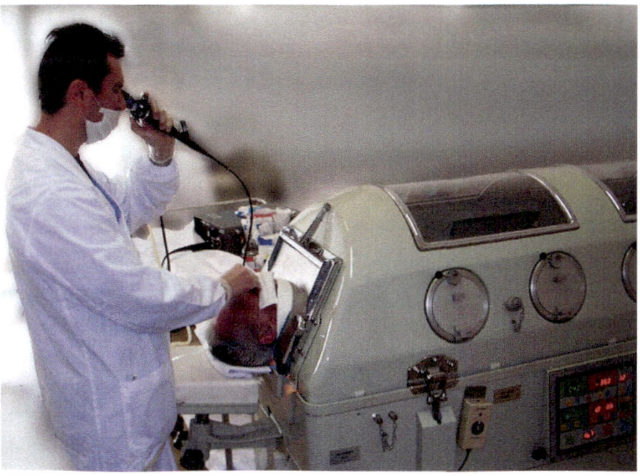

Fig. 15.3 A physician performs bronchoscopy on a patient inside an iron lung in a respiratory ICU setting

esophagogastric tubes in enteral feeding, for checking the correct positioning of previously inserted bronchial stents, for identifying any tracheoesophageal fistulas, to evaluate the possible collapse of the upper airways if, in the expiratory phase, a positive pressure was used (Fig. 15.4)

Todisco T et al. [23], used FBO to remove secretions from the airways, with improvement of oxygenation in 80% of cases, but also to: evaluate situations of bronchomalacia during ventilation with IL, obtain brush-protected samples for bacterial and fungal cultures (with 50% positivity), evaluate the possible compression of the upper airways.

However, these were not the only uses of fiberoptic bronchoscopy during extrathoracic mechanical ventilation.

Various scientific works concerning the study of pulmonary collateral ventilation and in particular the measurement of collateral resistance (Rcoll) have been carried out on animals and humans.

In some of these, fibrobronchoscopy was used, performed in association with contemporary extrathoracic pulmonary ventilation, both positive and negative. The latter was preferred to ventilation by introducing air into the airways as there was the possibility of negatively influencing the pressures, flows, and resistances within the lung tissue to be studied.

In a work done by Cormier Y and Sériès F [24] on dogs anesthetized and ventilated in an IL, it was shown that the resistance to collateral flow (Rcoll) strongly depends on the lung volume. Negative pressure (NEP) increased Functional Residual Capacity (FRC) and reduced Rcoll, while positive pressure (PEP) resulted in a decrease in FRC and an increase in Rcoll.

In another work, done by Cormier Y [25] on mechanically ventilated humans in IL, by wedging a fiberoptic bronchoscope into a right lower lobe subsegmental bronchus and inserting a truncated Swan-Ganz 5f catheter, the author demonstrated a linear relationship, with a 9.8% slope between log Rcoll and $\triangle$ end-expiratory lung volume ($\triangle$EELV). The progressive reduction of Rcoll was closely related to the increase of EELV.

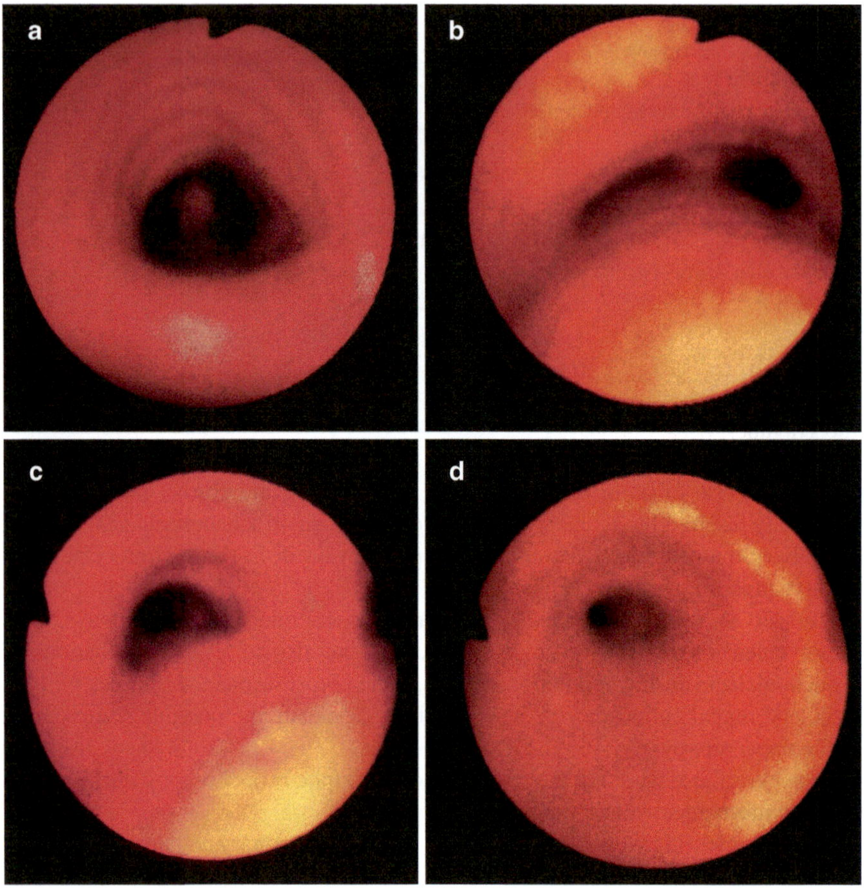

Fig. 15.4 Images of the airways of patients with exacerbated COPD receiving ventilatory treatment with IL. In some patients subjected to extrathoracic mechanical ventilation with positive pressure in the expiratory phase, chronic inflammation and laxity of the bronchial walls can cause real collapse of the bronchial walls and significantly reduce airflow. (**a**) trachea in spontaneous expiration phase; (**b**) anterior collapse of the pars membranacea in expiratory phase with positive pressure of 30 cm. H_2O; (**c**) left main bronchus during spontaneous expiration; (**d**) left main bronchus with concentric collapse in expiratory phase with positive pressure of 35 cm. H_2O

When discussing FBO, it must be remembered that it can have significant negative cardiopulmonary effects (hypoxemia, increased cardiac workload, increased heart rate, blood pressure, and cardiac index), especially in spontaneously breathing and lightly sedated patients. Therefore, the addition of noninvasive mechanical ventilation is often recommended. However, if more demanding procedures need to be performed that require the need to free the upper airways from an oronasal or face mask, the best alternative is precisely NPV or BCV.

It is equally important to consider the caliber of the bronchoscope relative to the lumen of the trachea and the inner lumen of the tracheal tube or laryngeal mask during invasive mechanical ventilation. In the case of a nonintubated patient, the flexible bronchoscope occupies only 10–15% of the cross-sectional area of the trachea. Conversely, if a 5.7 mm outer diameter fiberoptic bronchoscope is introduced in a 9 mm. tracheal tube, the occupied cross section rises to 40% and, in the case of a 7 mm. tube, it even rises to 66% [26]. It is now evident how a fiberoptic bronchoscopy performed during invasive mechanical ventilation can determine inadequate ventilation, but also: a significant reduction in air flows, an increase in airway resistance, an increase in peak and plateau pressure, an auto-PEEP, and an air-trapping risk [27]. All this, in consideration of the small caliber of the trachea and the relative endotracheal tubes to be used, is decidedly more evident when bronchoscopy is performed in children, even if thin bronchoscopes are used [28].

Another use of FBO during NPV is to facilitate tracheal intubation, using the endoscopic instrument as a flexible guide spindle to aid in the proper placement of the OT tube.

In the case of negative pressure ventilation, the upper airways and trachea are completely free and the use of a fiberoptic bronchoscope, even of a larger caliber, can be used with greater confidence without the risk of inadequate ventilation.

Without having to resort to an initial orotracheal intubation, which can sometimes be difficult, before performing a percutaneous dilated tracheostomy, NPV could be used. Reported cases are, however, only sporadic. With this method, the introduction of a fiberoptic bronchoscope would find the trachea free from other tubes and could easily check the correct positioning of the dilators and then of the tracheostomy tube. The NPV would guarantee the necessary ventilatory support. In this case, for extrathoracic ventilation, the preference should be given to the "poncho" in which the grid has been positioned lower down, so as to leave more space on the neck for the doctor in charge of the operation, or a "cuirass," modified in its upper part, such as those used to ventilate patients already wearing a tracheostomy tube.

15.4 Conclusion

About a century has passed since the birth of bronchoscopy (1897) and negative external mechanical ventilation (1929). Over the years, both techniques have undergone many innovations and application developments, often being used in conjunction with each other.

Interventional rigid bronchoscopy (IRB) consists of a long metal tube with a large working channel that allows for better access to the patient's airway and the insertion of larger instruments or devices (scopes, forceps, brushes, probes, suction tubes, laser fiber optics, instruments for electrosurgery, bronchoplasty therapy, and endobronchial coagulation). Although it is equipped with a connector for connection to an anesthesia ventilator, operators using the IRB often prefer to avoid positive pressure mechanical ventilation and resort to BCV. This allows for reduced patient sedation, easier operation, fewer positive airway pressures, and thus less risk of barotrauma. It also reduces the bubbling of bronchial secretions, especially bloody secretions, which obstruct vision.

IRB is used for the removal of foreign bodies, the aspiration of very thick secretions, airway management in patients requiring clear airway obstructions and/or recalibration of the tracheobronchial axis. Furthermore, IRB is used and preferred for the placement of stents, for the treatment of tracheobronchial lesions, to better target laser therapy, to perform large-caliber biopsies, for topical treatment and control of bleeding, including the placement of tubes equipped with a hemostatic balloon.

The technological innovations that have accompanied the evolution of bronchology, in large part, can be exploited with the IRB during external negative pressure ventilation, although the latter is limited almost exclusively to the use of ventilators such as the "poncho" or "cuirass" and, as the field of intervention, the trachea and large airways.

Fiberoptic bronchoscopy (FBO), on the other hand, thanks to its highly flexible probe, easier to use, and smaller outer diameter, can be used with all types of external negative pressure ventilators, including the iron-lung (IL), and allows for very deep exploration of the bronchial tree, thus offering a significantly wider field of investigation.

This has been particularly true with the use of the most recent bronchoscopes, which have reached an external diameter of only 1.8 mm. BCV is certainly preferred to invasive positive pressure ventilation, especially when, with the latter, the internal diameter of the tracheal tube is small. With negative external ventilation during FBO, improved ventilation is ensured, reducing the risk of hypoxemia, the elevated airway pressure, and, therefore, the barotrauma. This is particularly evident in pediatrics.

Of course, all technological innovations can be used with flexible bronchoscopy alone, but, especially with more critically ill patients, the ability to increase and ensure proper ventilation with BCV makes the endoscopic procedure safer and more peaceful, reducing many risks for the patient.

Furthermore, it is important to remember that BCV can also be performed on a completely awake and cooperative patient, while with positive pressure ventilation, especially if invasive, sedation is almost always mandatory.

In conclusion, just as BCV is preferable and sometimes even necessary to conduct an effective and safe bronchoscopy, the latter can be equally useful to the patient, during ventilatory treatment, to quickly clear the airways of obstructions, to make more in-depth and precise diagnoses, and to ensure targeted and more effective therapies.

References

1. Killian G. Über direkte bronchoskopie. MWW. 1898;27:844–7.
2. Jackson C. Peroral endoscopy and laryngeal surgery. Saint Louis MO Publisher; 1915.
3. Drinker P, Shaw LA. An apparatus for the prolonged administration of artificial respiration. I. A design for adults and children. J Clin Invest. 1929;7:229–47.

4. Andersen HA, Fontana RS, Harrison EG Jr. Transbronchoscopic lung biopsy in diffuse pulmonary disease. Dis Chest. 1965;48:187–92.
5. Tsuboi E, Ikeda S, Tajima M. Transbronchial biopsy smear for diagnosis of peripheral pulmonary carcinoma. Cancer. 1967;20:687–98.
6. Ikeda S, Yanai N, Ishikawa S. Flexible bronchofiberscope. Keio J Med. 1968;17:1–16.
7. Reynolds HJ, Newball HH. Analysis of proteins and respiratory cells from human lungs by bronchial lavage. J Lab Clin Med. 1974;84(559):73.
8. Wang KP, Terry PB. Transbronchial needle aspiration in the diagnosis and staging of bronchogenic carcinoma. Am Rev Respir Dis. 1983;127:344–7.
9. Dumon JF, Shapshay S, Bourcereau J, et al. Principles for safety in application of NdYAG laser in bronchoscopy. Chest. 1984;86:163–8.
10. Ryosuke O. History of bronchoscopy. In: Bronchoscopy. Practical methods and case reports by videobronchoscopy. Tokyo: Nakayama-Shoten Co. Ltd; 1994. p. 6.
11. Dumon JF. A dedicated tracheobronchial stent. Chest. 1990;97:260–1.
12. Becker HD. Endobronchialer ultraschall. Eine neue perspektive in der bronchologie. Ultraschall Med. 1996;17:106–12.
13. Toma T, Hopkinson NS, Hillier J, et al. Bronchoscopic volume reduction with valve implants in patients with severe emphysema. Lancet. 2003;361:931–3.
14. Schwarz Y, Greif J, Becker HD, et al. Real-time electromagnetic navigation bronchoscopy to peripheral lung lesions using overlaid CT images. The first human study. Chest. 2006;129:988–94.
15. Cox G, Miller JD, McWilliams A, et al. Bronchial thermoplasty for asthma. Am J Respir Crit Care Med. 2006;173:965–9.
16. Hetzel J, Maldonado F, Ravaglia C, et al. Transbronchial cryobiopsies for the diagnosis of diffuse parenchymal lung diseases: expert statement from the cryobiopsy working group on safety and utility and a call for standardization of the procedure. Respiration. 2018;95:188–200.
17. Petrella F, Borri A, Casiraghi M, Cavaliere S, et al. Operative rigid bronchoscopy: indications, basic techniques and results. Multimed Man Cardiothorac Surg. 2014;2014:mmu006.
18. Dumon JF, Cavaliere S. Manuale di Laserterapia Endotracheobronchiale. Brescia, Italy: Edizioni CLAS International. Chapter 5, p. 65.
19. Natalini G, Cavaliere S, Seramonti V, et al. Negative pressure ventilation vs external high-frequency oscillation during rigid bronchoscopy. A controlled randomized trial. Chest. 2000;118(1):18–23.
20. Natalini G, Cavaliere S, Vitacca M, Amicucci G, et al. Negative pressure ventilation vs. spontaneous assisted ventilation during rigid bronchoscopy: A controlled randomised trial. Acta Anaesthesiol Scand. 1998;42(9):1063–9.
21. Vitacca M, Natalini G, Cavaliere S, et al. Breathing pattern and arterial blood gases during Nd-YAG laser photoresection of endobronchial lesions under general anesthesia: use of negative pressure ventilation: a preliminary study. Chest. 1997;112(6):1466–73.
22. Hideaki Mori H, Shono A, Hirade R, et al. Biphasic cuirass ventilation during anesthesia for tracheobronchial stent insertion or removal by a rigid bronchoscope: a case report. A A Pract. 2018;10(8):198–200.
23. Todisco T, Eslami A, Scarcella L, et al. Flexible bronchoscopy during iron lung mechanical ventilation in nonintubated patients. J Bronchol. 1995;2(3):200–5.
24. Cormier Y, Sériès F. Effects of lung volume and positive airway pressure on collateral resistance. Respir Physiol. 1990;80(1):103–12.
25. Cormier Y, Laviolette M, Atton L, et al. Influence of lung volume on collateral resistance in normal man. Respir Physiol. 1991;83(2):179–87.
26. Du Rand A, Blaikley J, Booton R, et al. British Thoracic Society guideline for diagnostic flexible bronchoscopy in adults. Thorax. 2013;68(Suppl 1):i1–i44.
27. Kelebeyev S, Davison W, Ford BL, et al. The effects of endotracheal tube size during bronchoscopy in simulated models of intubated patients. Laryngoscope. 2023;133(1):147–53.
28. Hsia D, Di Blasi RM, Richardson P, et al. The effects of flexible bronchoscopy on mechanical ventilation in a pediatric lung model. Chest. 2009;135(1):33–40.

Biphasic Cuirass Ventilation: Use of Biphasic Cuirass Ventilation-Supported Radiation Therapy

16

Salvatore Notaro, Giuseppe La Cerra, Vincenzo Capaldo, Andrea Imparato, and Eugenio Piscitelli

16.1 Introduction

Radiotherapy is a form of physical therapy that uses high-energy radiation, such as X-rays, gamma rays, neutrons, and protons, to destroy cancer cells and reduce tumor size [1]. It's a highly precise technique, but there can be some margin of error due to movements of the lesion related to the patient's breathing. To minimize uncertainty in targeting the lesion, various movement mitigation strategies like margins, gating, and tracking are used. However, these strategies may also affect healthy tissue surrounding the lesion. Controlled breathing techniques with mechanical ventilation can help reduce the uncertainty zone and the risk of damaging healthy tissue. Mechanical ventilation may be necessary during the procedure for patients with respiratory deficits or specific clinical conditions. In addition to traditional invasive positive pressure ventilation, high-frequency ventilation (HFV) or Jet ventilation can be used. These methods involve administering very small volumes of air at higher pressure and frequency to limit tumor movement and minimize uncertainties during the procedure [2, 3]. Alongside these techniques, we find mechanically

S. Notaro (✉) · A. Imparato · E. Piscitelli
Department of Critical Care, Intensive Care Unit and ECMO, Monaldi-Colli Hospital, Naples, Italy
e-mail: salvatore.notaro@ospedalideicolli.it; andrea.imparato@ospedalideicolli.it; eugenio.piscitelli@ospedalideicolli.it

G. La Cerra
Complex Operative Unit of Interventional Pneumology, Monaldi Hospital – Colli Hospital, Naples, Italy
e-mail: giuseppe.lacerra@ospedalideicolli.it

V. Capaldo
Department of critical care, Intensive care Unite-Federico II University, Naples, Italy

O. Alibrahim et al. (eds.), *Biphasic Cuirass Noninvasive Ventilation*, Noninvasive Ventilation. The Essentials, https://doi.org/10.1007/978-3-032-20933-7_16

assisted and non-invasive ventilation (MANIV) which is a technique that doesn't require anesthesia and is performed using a face mask. It is well tolerated by the patient and has shown good results compared to other techniques [4, 5]. Biphasic Cuirass Ventilation (BCV) is a type of negative pressure non-invasive ventilation. This method utilizes a cuirass which is connected to a ventilator via a tube. The cuirass has evolved to be more comfortable and flexible over the years. It can generate continuous negative, intermittent negative, or biphasic (negative and positive) pressure modes. Specifically, it allows for the following types of ventilation settings:

- Controlled biphasic cuirass ventilation: the patient can easily take breaths between the mandatory breaths (like Intermittent Mandatory Ventilation—IMV).
- Continuous negative pressure: it works like CPAP.
- Non-invasive Synchronized Biphasic Cuirass Ventilation (BCV): cuirass triggered breaths are akin to SIMV.
- High-frequency oscillation (HFO) can be applied in frequencies up to 1200 oscillations per minute; it uses low tidal volumes, constant mean airway pressures, and high respiratory frequency to achieve valid oxygenation and reduction of carbon dioxide.
- Cardiac synchronized: A new addition to the various modes of cuirass ventilation is the ability to time the ventilatory cycle to coincide with the cardiac cycle [6].

In some areas of radiology, cuirass ventilation is already widespread due to its advantages. One example is cardiac MR imaging. Radiology department during MRI scanning takes advantage of Cardiac ECG-triggered BCV. When the cycling of ventilation falls together with every heart beat, the imaging can be more accurate and helpful in determining structural disease, especially of the coronary arteries [6, 7].

The use of BCV in radiotherapy is not well represented in the literature, but represents a new perspective, to be combined with the invasive techniques already present and the MANIV previously described. Therefore, this chapter will review the data from a recent case report, the first example of the use of BCV in radiotherapy.

16.2 Discussion

When using highly conformal radiotherapy techniques, a stabilized breathing pattern could greatly benefit the treatment of target lesions. Usually to consider the geometric uncertainties in the position of the tumor (the target lesion in radiotherapy) induced by breathing, there are movement mitigation strategies, such as margins, gating, and tracking, which address the geometric uncertainties [8]. These strategies, however, have shortcomings. Strategies such as Internal Target Volume (ITV) or MidPosition, which span the tumor trajectory, inevitably lead to unnecessary irradiation of healthy tissues close to the target. In the literature, we find studies regarding the use of mechanical ventilation as a tool to regulate breathing pattern and minimize the movements associated with breathing. Sometimes mechanical ventilation is a mandatory choice dictated by the patient's clinical conditions or respiratory complications. Some studies have described the use of high-frequency ventilation (HFOV) during the radiotherapy procedure. The high-frequency ventilation with very low volumes and high frequency can obtain the minimum possible movement of the lesion throughout the therapy. However, this kind of ventilation generally requires anesthesia and a demanding and invasive approach. Several studies have tested the use of mechanically assisted and non-invasive ventilation (MANIV) during radiotherapy treatments. Based on current clinical practice and literature insights, different ventilation strategies can be employed to improve precision during radiotherapy. Table 16.1 summarizes these techniques, highlighting their main advantages and limitations. In detail, different ventilation methods were compared (all performed in a non-invasive way and without sedation with the aid of a face mask): volume-controlled mode (VC) that imposes regular breathing, shallow-controlled mode (SH) that intends to lower amplitudes while increasing the breathing rate (VC and SH were used to treat lung and liver tumors), and slow-controlled mode (SL) that mimics end-inspiratory breath-holds (SL was used to treat breast cancer).

The results showed that volume-controlled mode significantly reduced the amplitude changes between sessions compared to spontaneous breathing. Shallow-controlled mode showed a further reduction compared to volume-controlled mode. In all cases the techniques were well tolerated by the patients [4, 5]. Based on what has been described, it is possible to consider cuirass ventilation as an alternative ventilation technique. This could be implemented as HFOV that uses low tidal volumes, constant mean airway pressures, and high respiratory frequency (as an alternative to JET ventilation) and as Biphasic Cuirass Ventilation (BCV).

The literature is quite poor about this type of mechanical ventilation associated with radiation therapy, but in this article we report the first case report about using biphasic cuirass ventilation during definitive radiation therapy. In this case a 57-year-old man on radiation therapy for oropharyngeal cancer with OSAS and an idiopathic right-sided hemi-diaphragm eventration was unable to radiation therapy treatment positioning due to breathing difficulties while lying down. He was unable to remain in a reclining position even when wearing his continuous positive airway pressure (CPAP) device. An alternative was tracheostomy but the patient wished to avoid it. The pulmonologist therefore recommended a trial of BCV ventilation. The duration of each radiotherapy session was about 30 min. The treatment setup was the following:

1. The ventilator was preset to the "continuous negative extrathoracic pressure" setting with a maximum inspiratory pressure of 35 cm H_2O. This increased functional residual capacity allowed the patient to maintain supine treatment position while also maintaining synchrony with his natural breathing cycle.
2. The home CPAP machine was connected to the wall oxygen delivery unit with Oxygen rate flow from 3 to 5 l/min and connected to the patient with CPAP nasal prongs at a pressure setting of 10 cm H_2O.

Table 16.1 Ventilation strategies during radiotherapy: advantages and disadvantages

Type of ventilation during radiotherapy	Description	Pros	Cons
Spontaneous Breathing (SB)	Patient breathes autonomously, trying to control his breathing, without the aid of external equipment	No anesthesia needed No setup needed No training needed	Uncertainties in the position of the tumor during the treatment, increased chance to hit healthy perilesional tissue
HFOV or Jet Ventilation	Uses low tidal volumes, constant mean airway pressures, and high respiratory frequency	It works by almost freezing the breath, ensuring excellent precision during radiotherapy, and saving healthy perilesional tissue	It requires invasive ventilation and general anesthesia. Oncology patients are fragile subjects and invasive ventilation puts them at risk of VAP
MANIV	mechanically assisted and non-invasive ventilation (MANIV), performed with the aid of a mask	No anesthesia needed It's not an invasive technique Outpatient procedure It significantly increases the precision during radiotherapy compared to SB, reducing the risk of hitting healthy perilesional tissue	It requires precise setup and specific training. This type of ventilation is not always sufficient to manage patients with respiratory failure
BCV	Biphasic Cuirass Ventilation is a negative pressure non-invasive ventilation	No anesthesia needed It's not an invasive technique Outpatient procedure Able to manage patient with respiratory failure by supporting classic positive pressure NIV Able with high-frequency mode (HFO) to obtain results similar to HFOV, without invasive ventilation It significantly increase the precision during radiotherapy compared to SB, reducing the risk of hitting healthy perilesional tissue	It requires precise setup and specific training. There are not yet enough studies to validate its effectiveness

3. A size 10 cuirass was placed on the patient's chest.

The treatment lasted 7 weeks during which there were no complications. At the end of treatment, the patient was still unable to lie in a supine position for more than a few seconds without BCV assistance [7]. The main advantages of BCV are that it can be delivered as an outpatient procedure, eliminating the complexity and cost of inpatient admission; furthermore, it does not require anesthesia and is generally well tolerated by the patient and is not an invasive ventilation method.

Potential disadvantages include a steep learning curve given the relative inexperience of radiation oncology departments in administering BCV [9]. In the case described, therefore, the use of two devices for non-invasive ventilation (CPAP nasal prongs and cuirass) allowed the therapy to be carried out with good results, avoiding invasive procedure (tracheostomy) associated with an invasive type of ventilation for the patient.

A side effect of cuirass ventilation, regardless of whether or not the device has biphasic capabilities, is skin lesions and irritation that can become spots for infection [10]; however, this occurs especially for long-term use, while for radiotherapy we have relatively short sessions (in the case reported we have 30 min for each session), not comparable to chronic use of the cuirass.

One limitation for the use of biphasic cuirass ventilation during the radiation therapy is given by the need to instruct radiotherapy personnel on the use of the ventilator and on cuirass setup, in addition to the need to carry out training on the patient. This limitation may slightly delay the start of radiotherapy and is also present in the classic MANIV, mechanically assisted and non-invasive ventilation. Certainly in a broader vision it is possible to classify BCV, and cuirass ventilation in general, as MANIV. In this case we could think of applying the healthy tissue saving evidences during radiotherapy, highlighted with the MANIV and previously described, to the cuirass ventilation during radiotherapy. However, in the era of evidence-based medicine, this may not be sufficient or justified. We need further studies.

16.3 Conclusion

The use of mechanical ventilation during radiotherapy has advantages for all patients who must undergo this treatment and not only for those who need it due to respiratory deficits during the procedure. In fact, the aid of mechanical ventilation allows, combined with other strategies already carried out in radiotherapy, to reduce the probability of hitting and irradiating healthy perilesional tissue. There are several studies on the effectiveness of mechanical ventilation techniques. These concern both invasive ventilation techniques such as high-frequency ventilation or JET ventilation and non-invasive techniques with positive pressure which go by the acronym mechanically assisted and non-invasive ventilation (MANIV) [2–5].

The application of BCV in radiotherapy is not well represented in the literature; in fact, the first study about it dates back to 2020. This study is very promising, having obtained results in line with those observed with other ventilation techniques performed in radiotherapy and showing a good level of tolerance for the patient. In the specific case given as an example in this chapter, the use of BCV allowed the patient to undergo radiotherapy, saving a tracheostomy surgery and an invasive ventilation technique.

Avoiding mechanical ventilation techniques in these patients is crucial. In fact, these are generally oncology patients, therefore, immunosuppressed or in any case fragile and more susceptible to developing infections, such as VAP. Although there is not much in the literature specifically about BCV applied to radiotherapy, there are articles regarding the application of non-invasive positive pressure ventilation to radiotherapy [4, 5].

In a broader vision it is possible to classify Biphasic cuirass ventilation, and cuirass ventilation in general, as non-invasive mechanical ventilation. Consequently we could apply the results obtained with MANIV in radiotherapy and described so far also to the Biphasic Cuirass Ventilation.

However, as reasonable as it may seem, in the era of evidence-based medicine this may not be sufficient or justified.

In conclusion, BCV in radiotherapy certainly represents a new promising perspective to avoid irradiation on healthy perilesional tissue connected to the patient's respiratory movements and to avoid invasive ventilation techniques, but it requires further studies to be explored in depth.

References

1. NCI Dictionary of Cancer terms. In: Comprehensive Cancer Information – NCI. https://www.cancer.gov/publications/dictionaries/cancer-terms/def/radiotherapy. Accessed 7 Aug 2024.
2. Fritz P, Kraus H-J, Mühlnickel W, Sassmann V, Hering W, Strauch K. High-frequency jet ventilation for complete target immobilization and reduction of planning target volume in stereotactic high single-dose irradiation of stage I non–small cell lung cancer and lung metastases. Int J Radiat Oncol Biol Phys. 2010;78:136–42.
3. Santiago A, Jelen U, Ammazzalorso F, Engenhart-Cabillic R, Fritz P, Mühlnickel W, Enghardt W, Baumann M, Wittig A. Reproducibility of target coverage in stereotactic spot scanning proton lung irradiation under high frequency jet ventilation. Radiother Oncol. 2013;109:45–50.
4. Van Ooteghem G, Dasnoy-Sumell D, Lambrecht M, Reychler G, Liistro G, Sterpin E, Geets X. Mechanically-assisted non-invasive ventilation: a step forward to modulate and to improve the reproducibility of breathing-related motion in radiation therapy. Radiother Oncol. 2019;133:132–9.
5. Van Ooteghem G, Dasnoy-Sumell D, Lee JA, Geets X. Mechanically-assisted and non-invasive ventilation for radiation therapy: a safe technique to regularize and modulate internal tumour motion. Radiother Oncol. 2019;141:283–91.
6. Linton DM. Cuirass ventilation: a review and update. Critic Care Resusc. 2005;7:22–8.
7. Plein S, Bulugahapitiya S, Jones TR, Bainbridge GJ, Ridgway JP, Sivananthan MU. Cardiac MR imaging with external respirator: Synchronizing cardiac and respiratory motion—feasibility study. Radiology. 2003;227:877–82.

8. Keall PJ, Mageras GS, Balter JM, et al. The management of respiratory motion in Radiation oncology report of AAPM Task Group 76. Med Phys. 2006;33:3874–900.
9. Clinkscales W, Spence M, Gleysteen J, Hayes N, Izaguirre E, Wakefield D, Schwartz D, Rhea I, Risquez C, Sharma AM. Novel use of biphasic cuirass ventilation during definitive radiation therapy: a technical report. Pract Radiat Oncol. 2021;11:e276–81. https://doi.org/10.1016/j.prro.2020.08.003.
10. Onweni C, Rashid S, Goswami R, Treece J, Shipley LC, De Souza R, O'Neill L, Simberloff T, Baumrucker SJ. Cuirass ventilation: an alternative home-based modality for chronic respiratory failure. Home Health Care Manage Pract. 2019;32:40–4.

Oscillatory Option: Mucus Clearance Between Biphasic Cuirass Ventilation—External High-Frequency Oscillation

17

Berkan Basançelebi and Antonio M. Esquinas

17.1 Introduction

External high-frequency oscillation gained prominence in the literature following a series of studies conducted by Zamir Hayek in the late twentieth century [1–8]. Various terms have been used in the literature to describe this technique, including high-frequency negative pressure oscillation, high-frequency chest wall compression, Hayek oscillator, and high-frequency chest wall oscillation. Robert Chatburn has clarified that this technique is best described as high-frequency chest wall oscillation (HFCWO) and distinguishes it from high-frequency chest wall compression (HFCWC) [9]. In this chapter, the focus will be exclusively on high-frequency chest wall oscillation, as it pertains to EHFO. To understand the utility of this technique, a brief review of normal mucus physiology and its dysfunction is essential.

Airway mucus is a fluid secreted by mucus-producing cells, including the goblet cells of the pseudostratified columnar surface layer and the mucus cells of the submucosal glands. The fluid has a complicated, viscoelastic structure that is made up of glycoproteins, proteins, and lipids in an aqueous matrix [10]. Mucus along with serous fluid makes the airway surface fluid that is the most suitable environment for the airways. This fluid is indispensable for the maintenance of normal ciliary function and general airway hygiene. Duncan Rogers emphasized its physiological importance by the statement "getting airway secretions right: not too runny, not too thick; not too wet, not too dry" [11–13]. The production of about 10 mL of mucus per day is the main defense that protects the lower respiratory tract. Any interference with secretion or mucociliary clearance may cause the accumulation of mucus,

B. Basançelebi (✉)
Department of Electroneurophysiology, Vocational School, Istanbul Medipol University, Istanbul, Turkey

A. M. Esquinas
Intensive Care Unit, Hospital General Universitario Morales Meseguer, Murcia, Spain

O. Alibrahim et al. (eds.), *Biphasic Cuirass Noninvasive Ventilation*, Noninvasive Ventilation. The Essentials, https://doi.org/10.1007/978-3-032-20933-7_17

which, in turn, can depress lung function, reduce lung defenses, and increase the risk of infections and, potentially, neoplasia [10, 12]. Mucus production and clearance are like yin and yang, and they have to be in balance. If the balance is disturbed, whether as a cause of or a result of the disease, there is often a necessity to use airway clearance techniques.

17.2 Airway Clearance Techniques

Conventional chest physiotherapy is one of the oldest methods that has been used in the past to improve the clearance of the airways. It essentially represents a set of procedures, e.g., postural drainage, vibration, shaking, percussion, autogenic drainage, the active cycle of breathing technique, forced exhalation techniques, huffing, coughing maneuvers, and their mixtures [12]. Basançelebi referred to these methods as a single group of manual techniques and exercises [14]. Van der Schans et al., in their systematic review, noted that the scientific evidence supporting manual airway clearance techniques for cystic fibrosis patients is not robust. They suggested that the limited evidence might be attributed to inadequate frequency and amplitude of percussion and oscillations [12, 15]. A meta-analysis also found no significant difference between manual techniques, such as conventional chest physiotherapy, positive airway pressure, forced exhalation, and autogenic drainage [16]. These uncertainties have led to the development and definition of assistive devices and mechanical techniques aimed at providing more effective airway clearance.

Mechanical airway clearance techniques, such as intermittent positive pressure breathing, intrapulmonary percussive ventilation, mechanical insufflation-exsufflation, non-invasive ventilation, oscillatory positive expiratory pressure, temporary positive expiratory pressure, high-frequency chest wall compression, and high-frequency chest wall oscillation (referred to as EHFO in this chapter), operate through several potential mechanisms. These mechanisms include air-liquid shear forces (which create multiple mini-coughs), the Scherer model, radial displacement of the airway, mechanical rheological effects, and possibly an increase in ciliary beat [9, 12]. While these mechanical techniques are thought to offer potential advantages over conventional chest physiotherapy, guidelines from the American College of Chest Physicians consider them as alternatives to traditional methods for cystic fibrosis management [12, 17].

17.3 Mechanisms of Action for Mucus Clearance via EHFO

Mucus clearance from the airways is an important biological function that supports overall respiratory health by getting rid of inhaled particles, pathogens, and surplus mucus. The main mechanisms put into effect for this aim are mucociliary transport, the cough reflex, and the utilization of mechanical devices such as Hayek RTX Oscillator (EHFO).

Mucociliary transport is the fundamental mechanism, which refers to the concerted work of cilia and mucus. The respiratory epithelium consists of ciliated cells which are responsible for the movement of mucus in an upward direction by their coordinated beating from the pharynx, where it is to be discharged. This process is called the mucociliary escalator. EHFO helps mucociliary transport by producing quick oscillatory pressures that resonate the airway walls. Such vibrations free mucus from the airway surface and facilitate its transport to the central airways (see Fig. 17.1). By creating turbulence in the airways, the action of EHFO is further enhanced to bring about more mucus clearance [10, 11, 18].

A cough is one of the body's protective reflexes, whose purpose is to rid the lower airways of mucus. The cough reflex is induced when mucus or irritants come in contact with the sensory receptors; thus the respiratory muscles reflexively contract and air is forcefully exhaled. EHFO can be this supply for the reflex by dislodging mucus, thus allowing the patient to effectively get rid of it through coughing. Through loosening of mucus, EHFO makes the cough reflex more efficient; thereby it becomes easier to clear the lungs [10, 19].

A wide range of different mechanical devices and methods are employed to help with the clearance of mucus. External high-frequency oscillation (EHFO) is an example of a technique that employs a rapidly inflating and deflating cuirass to create oscillations. These changes in pressure aid in loosening and mobilizing mucus, which can be very helpful for patients with, for example, cystic fibrosis, as in these cases normally used methods of mucus clearance may not bring results [15, 16, 20]. EHFO produces oscillations that cause mechanical vibrations in the entire airways and the generation of the shear forces at the mucus airway wall interface resulting

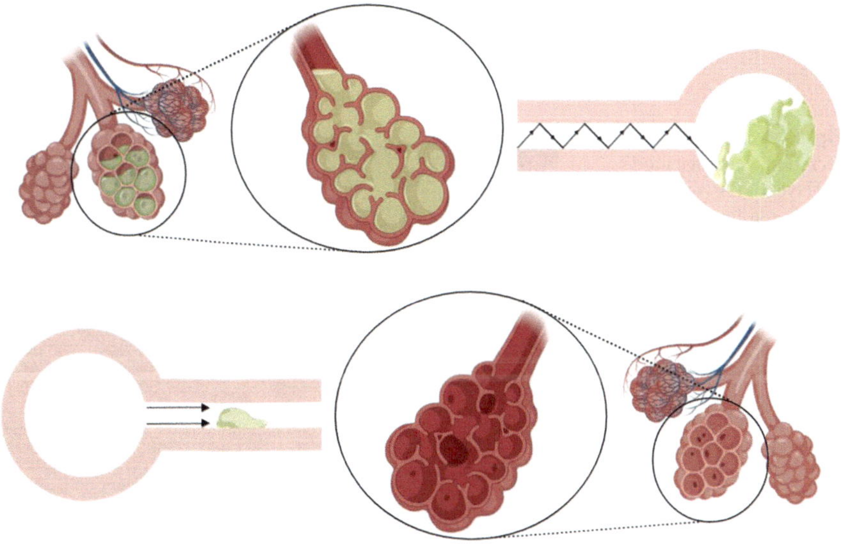

Fig. 17.1 Mechanisms of action for mucus clearance

in the breaking of the adhesive and cohesive forces that bind the mucus to the wall. By loosening the mucus, EHFO helps its transport to the central airways that can be more easily cleared by coughing or suctioning. This method is particularly suitable for people with thick, narrow mucus [3, 21, 22]. By reducing the mucus viscosity and elasticity, EHFO makes it easier to transport. This rheology alteration facilitates its flow, aiding in its clearance from the airways [10, 23]. EHFO also promotes airflow by allowing air to bypass mucus obstructions and plugs, promoting the movement of mucus toward larger airways where it can be more easily thrown out. Additionally, by increasing ciliary beat frequency, EHFO promotes the mucociliary escalator, which naturally transports mucus toward the mouth. This is an important role to the body's natural defense mechanisms. Patients with weak cough, EHFO promote mobilize mucus from distal to the central airways and oscillative flow produces rapid air pressure shifts (see Figs. 17.2 and 17.3) [21].

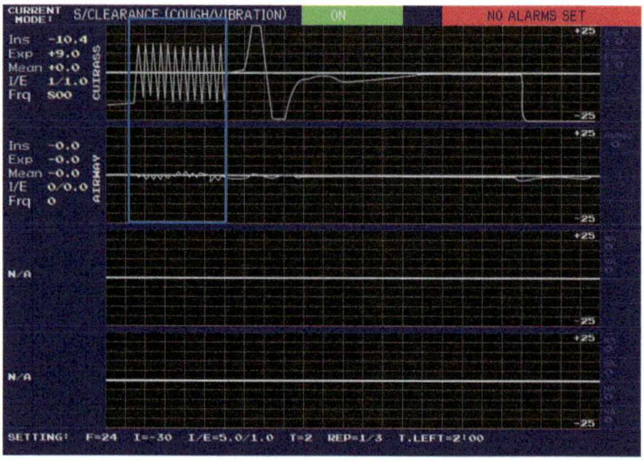

Fig. 17.2 Vibration option of secretion clearance mode in Hayek RTX (with permission from [25]

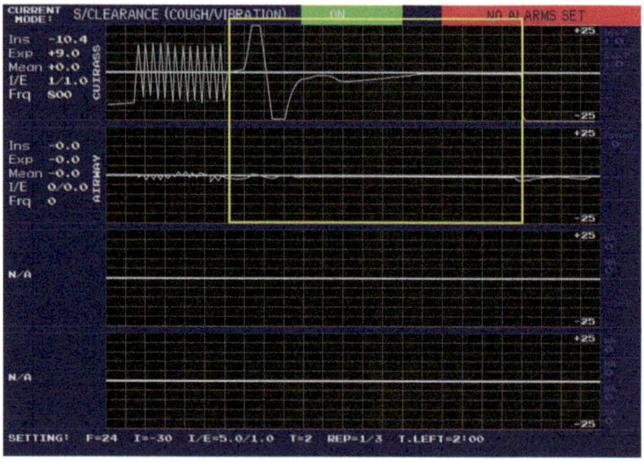

Fig. 17.3 Cough option of secretion clearance mode in Hayek RTX (with permission from [25])

17.4 Indications, Contraindications, and Key Precautions of EHFO

Vibration mode is normally used when the clinical objective is to loosen and mobilize retained secretions and/or recruit atelectatic regions without the use of an invasive airway. Manufacturer guidance and clinical reviews cite retained secretion states such as atelectasis, postoperative sputum retention, pneumonia with mucus plugging, chronic obstructive pulmonary disease (COPD) or asthma/bronchiolitis exacerbations, bronchiectasis and cystic fibrosis, and neuromuscular weakness with an ineffective cough, as the most common examples of usage of the device [9, 24, 25]. Cough (assisted cough) mode is an indication to be used after vibration when secretions have been moved toward central airways and a high-flow expiratory "cough surrogate" is required to remove them; in particular, it is very effective in neuromuscular disease, spinal cord injury, tracheostomized/intubated patients requiring non-invasive airway clearance, and the condition in which peak cough flow is insufficient [9, 24, 26–28]. In reality, clinicians accomplish the sequential use of both modes within a single airway clearance session, and depending on the burden and response, they may be repeated several times per treatment block.

Absolute/strong contraindications for the use a Hayek cuirass for EHFO/assisted cough involve mainly safety and interface issues: skin that has been burned or wounds that are actively draining under the shell/seal, chest anatomy that does not allow a hermetic seal, lack of a viable airway (natural or artificial), cardiopulmonary arrest, body weight that is above the system's safe seal/fit limit (~180 kg), and any indwelling line/tube/drain whose skin entry point is located directly under the seal (lines may go through the cuirass if the entry points are outside the seal) [25]. One important physiologic precaution is the case of unstable or collapsible upper airway obstruction (e.g., obstructive sleep apnea, bulky soft tissue obstruction): the negative pressure phases can increase the degree of collapse, and thus patients must have a patent airway or be "stented" with CPAP or airway adjuncts if necessary. Since vibration/cough can rapidly move large volumes of secretions into the upper airway, the treatment should be done before meals/bolus feeds, continuous feeding may need to be stopped, and oral or tracheal suction must be readily available in patients with impaired airway protection [25]. Moreover, there are also relative contraindications that can be inferred from chest physiotherapy/HFCWO literature such as recent or active significant hemoptysis, recent rib/vertebral fractures, severe osteoporosis, or markedly increased bleeding risk, wherein the vigorous oscillation or expulsive cycles may cause the injury or bleeding to get aggravated; therefore, in such situations, EHFO should either be completely avoided or given only with very gentle settings and close monitoring [14, 29, 30].

17.5 Complications and Side Effects of EHFO

Generally, EHFO is seen as a low barotrauma method in comparison with positive pressure ventilation; however, it is not devoid of side effects. The complications that have been reported and expected are skin pressure injury or breakdown at seal contact points, in particular if the device is used for a longer period or the seals are worn; discomfort/pain due to oscillation, in some cases limiting the achievable pressures; and hypothermia/heat loss resulting from the large chest area being exposed under the cuirass in smaller children or during long sessions [25, 26]. Aspiration or airway obstruction by mobilized secretions is a very significant risk from the clinical point of view in case suctioning or expectoration are not facilitated, especially in a situation of weak cough, bulbar dysfunction, or reduced consciousness. Consequently, there is a strong focus on airway protection and timed suctioning during the final seconds of the cough cycles in artificial airways [25]. Transient desaturation during heavy secretion mobilization, gastric distension or reflux in susceptible patients, and therapy failure/delay of escalation if EHFO is used when invasive ventilation is obviously required are some of the less common but recognized potential issues [9, 26]. When patients have preexisting air-leak syndromes (e.g., pneumothorax), BCV is sometimes the option to avoid high airway pressures; however, it still needs careful monitoring and an individualized risk benefit assessment instead of being considered universally safe [31].

17.6 Vibration Option of Secretion Clearance Mode in Hayek RTX

The Hayek RTX vibration mode is, in essence, an external high-frequency oscillation (EHFO) that is very rapidly and with a very small amplitude delivered to the chest of the patient: in other words, the device produces quick small upward/downward pressure changes on the chest which physically deliver the oscillatory mechanical energy to the chest wall and lungs and thus oscillatory airflow is generated in the lung which helps to loosen mucus from the lung wall and also enhance peripheral-to-central secretion transport and, additionally, gas exchange at very small tidal volumes can be facilitated. Clinically it is used as the first phase of Secretion Clearance Mode (see Fig. 17.2), and usually it is switched on with assisted-cough cycles to imitate the airway clearance "mobilize then expel" [24, 32, 33].

The manufacturer instructions indicate that practical starting values should be first used, and these values should then be adjusted according to the patient's tolerance and visible chest wall movement: vibration with 600–800 cycles/min and approximately −20 to −40 cmH_2O for 3–5 min per bout in adults; in children, 700–1000 cycles/min at −15 to −30 cmH_2O for 2–5 min and in infants, 800–1200 cycles/min at −5 to −20 cmH_2O for 2–4 min (see Table 17.1) [25].

The clinician attempts to create an airtight and comfortable seal between the cuirass and the patient, and then make sure the airway is patent (open and clear) at the bedside. The operator tests recommended settings after starting the device

Table 17.1 Starting parameters and settings for EHFO

Mode	Settings	Adult	Pediatric	Infant
Vibration	CPM	600–800	700–1000	800–1200
	Pressure, cmH_2O	−20 to −40	−15 to −30	−5 to −20
	Duration, min	3–5	2–5	2–4
Cough	Inspiratory pressure, cmH_2O	−20 to −40	−15 to −30	−10 to −20
	Expiratory pressure, cmH_2O	+20 to +40	+15 to +30	+5 to +20
	CPM	12–24	24–36	36–60
	I:E	4:1 to 6:1	5:1 to 6:1	5:1 to 6:1
	Duration, min	2	1–2	1–2
	Session	3–6	4–6	5–6

The table was created based on manufacturer's recommendations [5, 25]

while adjusting frequency and pressure according to observed clinical outcomes which include audible or auscultatory movement of secretions and comfortably increased ventilation and facilitated expectoration. Usually, clinician runs short vibration intervals followed by cough mode (commonly ~3–4 min vibration and ~2 min cough, repeated as necessary) and, at the same time, they prepare to suction or assist expectoration as secretions reach the upper airway and they time therapy before meals or pause continuous feeds when it is appropriate. Continuous monitoring of oxygenation, ventilation, hemodynamics, and skin/seal condition is also recommended during the whole period [25, 34].

17.7 Cough Option of Hayek RTX

The Hayek RTX cough mode (see Fig. 17.3) is a single integrated cuirass-delivered profile that happens after the device's vibration/oscillation phase in the Secretion Clearance Mode. Its objective is to perform a high-flow expiratory "huff-cough" directly from the mobilized secretions without changing the interfaces. From a mechanical point of view, the RTX first goes for a relatively long, comfortable negative pressure inspiratory "loading" phase to open the chest and increase lung volume, then it quickly changes to a very brief, higher positive pressure expulsive phase thus creating a very sharp inspiratory-to-expiratory transition as well as very high-peak expiratory flows that detach the mucus from the central airways and push it proximally for expectoration or suctioning; at the same time, the lung inflation between the cycles is preserved [24, 25, 35].

The manufacturer initially recommends the parameters to be changed in accordance with the chest wall movement, secretion response, and tolerance: for adult patients, the inspiratory pressure is approximately −20 to −40 cmH_2O with the following expiratory pressure +20 to +40 cmH_2O at 12–24 cycles/min, with the I:E ratio being about 4:1 to 6:1, the duration of the short periods being approximately 2 min; for children, the pressures are −15 to −30/+15 to +30 cmH_2O, the number of cycles is 24–36 per minute with the I:E ratio varying between 5:1 and 6:1, and the length of the time is 1–2 min; and for infants, the values are −10 to −20/+5 to

+20 cmH_2O at 36–60 cycles/min, and the I:E ratio that targets the same duration is 1–2 min (see Table 17.1) [5, 25].

At the patient side, healthcare providers make a secure airtight and comfortable cuirass seal and check for an open upper airway; they start from the lower end of these ranges and then change the inspiratory depth, expulsive pressure, and cycle rate depending on the non-distressing but effective cough surrogate that they have achieved (thoracoabdominal rise visible, secretion movement audible, auscultation improved, and expectoration facilitated); usually, they are mixing intervals of short vibration with intervals of short episodic cough and also getting ready to suction as secretions arrive at the pharynx. They are advised to also keep a continuous monitor on SpO_2/CO_2 trend, hemodynamics, skin condition, and the performance of the seal, and pain, air-leak syndromes, or poor tolerance; they lessen the cough pressures or stop them altogether [25, 35].

17.8 Future Directions: Mucus Clearance Between Biphasic Cuirass Ventilation

Biphasic cuirass ventilation (BCV) secretion clearance mode pairing EHFO with an assisted-cough cycle through a single cuirass already has a quite convincing mechanistic role in disorders dominated by tenacious or bulky airway/alveolar material, but the subsequent stage is to delineate the extent to which it can actually alter the standards of care as opposed to simply being an adjunct option [24]. In pulmonary alveolar proteinosis (PAP), whole lung lavage (WLL) is still the standard treatment for advanced disease, and it generally involves manual chest percussion to mobilize the proteinaceous surfactant during lavage [36–38]. The major proof of concept example demonstrated that the use of BCV intra-operatively as "automated percussion" during WLL not only promoted the removal of the lavage fluid but also resulted in a positive bilateral clinical recovery without any complications, thus supporting the notion that BCV can effectively deliver the oscillatory energy even under one lung ventilation and can potentially replace the laborious manual methods [39]. As a result, the next segment of research on PAP should, first, conduct prospective comparative trials of BCV-assisted WLL versus conventional WLL with manual percussion, measuring lavage efficiency (effluent clarity/volume), peri procedural oxygenation, and complication rates; second, determine the oscillation "dose" (frequency, pressure span, bout duration, sequencing with ventilator settings) for various PAP phenotypes and body sizes in order to achieve the greatest surfactant mobilization while keeping derecruitment at a minimum; third, evaluate the use of BCV as a clearance device either before or after the lavage to extend the interval between WLL sessions and help patients who have an incomplete response to granulocyte-macrophage colony-stimulating factor-based therapies [37, 40].

Besides PAP, the most dramatic scenarios are to be severe clinical situations in which secretion retention leads to exacerbations or intubation risk. In cystic fibrosis and non-CF bronchiectasis, BCV is a respirator-free option which not only can ventilate but also can clear secretions; however, most of the evidence is still in the form of the observations and reports of the particular devices; hence the field requires the performance of the HFCWO versus HFCWC trials, intrapulmonary percussive ventilation, and mechanical insufflation-exsufflation through endpoints such as exacerbation rate, forced expiration volume in one second (FEV_1) slope, antibiotic days, and quality-of-life score changes to name a few [9, 25, 28]. In neuromuscular disease and spinal cord injury, BCV's incorporated vibration plus cough pattern can be the designation as a home-based hybrid for those patients who are not able to produce effective peak cough flows or are averse to positive pressure interfaces; upcoming protocols must associate BCV parameters with objective cough flow goals and remote monitoring to lower infection-related hospitalizations [24, 27, 28]. In acute care postoperative lobar atelectasis, pneumonia with mucus plugging, COPD/asthma exacerbations, and pediatric secretion retentive respiratory failure future moves may be centered around timely, protocolized BCV secretion clearance mode as an "intubation avoidance" bundle and as a post-extubation strategy for re-collapse prevention, especially in airway surgery or difficult weaning high-risk groups [24, 41].

The focus of the relevant technology and future clinical trials is on identifying different indications as well as targeting a new generation of BCV that includes personalized, optimal, and intelligent treatment. This target may include next-generation BCV secretion clearance targets that integrate real-time indicators such as chest wall tightness/permeability, chest wall displacement, oscillatory flow, SpO_2/CO_2 trends, and even localize secretion movement via bedside acoustic markers so that the machine can automatically adjust the vibration and cough force to a specific physiological "clearance dose". There will be a strong need for multi-center registries and pragmatic trials to outline the safety envelopes (fragile chest wall, severe airflow obstruction, air-leak syndromes) and standardize the outcome reporting thus making BCV a well-documented airway clearance technique which can be applied not only in rare diseases such as PAP but also in those which are characterized by high-burden chronic/acute secretion retentive disorders.

17.9 Summary

External high-frequency oscillation (EHFO) is a non-invasive airway clearance method specifically aimed at facilitating the expulsion of mucus in the case of chronic respiratory diseases. EHFO achieves the effect of the rapid oscillations through the use of a cuirass, shell, or poncho. The vibrations resulting from the oscillations loosen the mucus that is sticking to the airway walls, thus enabling the operator to clear it more easily. Usually, the device is operated at frequencies from 8 to 1200 cycles per minute, which not only increases the mobility of the mucus but also reduces its viscosity. To date, several clinical trials have demonstrated the capability of EHFO to raise lung function parameters and the overall quality of life of patients suffering from mucus retention problems.

It works to free the airways of cystic fibrosis patients and thereby improve lung functions. Likewise, in patients with bronchiectasis and neuromuscular disorders,

EHFO lowers the frequency of exacerbations and consequent hospital admissions. To sum up, EHFO is acknowledged as a safe and efficacious treatment, barely causing a mild discomfort type side effect if any. It is an important tool in chronic lung disease management, thereby giving the patient a choice of different or combined airway clearance techniques.

References

1. Petros A, Fernando S, Shenoy V, Al-Saady N. The Hayek Oscillator Nomograms for tidal volume and minute ventilation using external high frequency oscillation. Anaesthesia. 1995;50:601–6.
2. Hardinge FM, Stradling JR. Effects of short term high frequency negative pressure ventilation on gas exchange using the Hayek oscillator in normal subjects. Thorax. 1995;50:44–9.
3. Hayek Z. External high-frequency oscillation. In: Rügheimer E, editor. Respiratorische Therapie nach operativen Eingriffen. Berlin/Heidelberg: Springer; 1995.
4. Hayek Z, Ryan CA, Peliowski A, et al. High frequency external oscillation without intubation. Pediatr Res. 1985;19:406.
5. United Hayek Industries. Hayek RTX respirator operator's manual. London: United Hayek Industries; 2020.
6. Eyal FG, Hayek Z, Armengol J, Jones RL. Comparison of high-frequency negative-pressure oscillation with conventional mechanical ventilation in normal and saline-lavaged cats. Crit Care Med. 1986;14:724–9.
7. Penny DJ, Hayek Z, Rawle P, et al. Ventilation with external high frequency oscillation around a negative baseline increases pulmonary blood flow after the Fontan operation. Cardiol Young. 1992;2:277–80.
8. Hayek Z, Ryan CA, Eyal F, et al. Comparison of high-frequency chest wall compression with conventional mechanical ventilation in cats. Crit Care Med. 1987;15:676–81.
9. Chatburn RL. High-frequency assisted airway clearance. Respir Care. 2007;52:1224–35.
10. King M. Physiology of mucus clearance. Paediatr Respir Rev. 2006;7:212–4.
11. Rogers DF. Airway clearance: physiology, pharmacology, techniques, and practice. Respir Care. 2007;9:1134–49.
12. Hess DR. Airway clearance: physiology, pharmacology, techniques, and practice. Respir Care. 2007;52:1392–6.
13. Button BM, Button B. Structure and function of the mucus clearance system of the lung. Cold Spring Harb Perspect Med. 2013;3:a009720.
14. Basançelebi B. Non invasive mechanical ventilation and respiratory physiotherapy and pulmonary rehabilitation. In: Esquinas AM, Alahmari M, editors. Respiratory care in non invasive mechanical ventilatory support: principles and practice. 1st ed. New York: Nova Science Publishers Inc.; 2021. p. 407–15.
15. van der Schans CP, Prasad A, Main E. Chest physiotherapy compared to no chest physiotherapy for cystic fibrosis. Cochrane Database Syst Rev. 2000.
16. Thomas J, Cook DJ, Brooks D. Chest physical therapy management of patients with cystic fibrosis: a meta-analysis. Am J Respir Crit Care Med. 1995;151:846–50.
17. Dennis Mccool F, Rosen MJ. Nonpharmacologic airway clearance therapies ACCP evidence-based clinical practice guidelines. Chest. 2006;129:250S–9S.
18. Fahy JV, Dickey BF. Airway mucus function and dysfunction. N Engl J Med. 2010;363:2233–47.
19. Gibson PG, Simpson JL, Ryan NM, Vertigan AE. Mechanisms of cough. Curr Opin Allergy Clin Immunol. 2014;14:55–61.
20. Scherer TA, Barandun J, Martinez E, et al. Effect of high-frequency oral airway and chest wall oscillation and conventional chest physical therapy on expectoration in patients with stable cystic fibrosis. Chest. 1998;113:1019–27.

21. Morrison L, Agnew J. Oscillating devices for airway clearance in people with cystic fibrosis. Cochrane Database Syst Rev. 2014.
22. Linton DM. Cuirass ventilation: a review and update. Critic Care Resusc. 2005;7:22–8.
23. Hansen LG, Warwick WJ, Hansen KL. Mucus transport mechanisms in relation to the effect of high frequency chest compression (HFCC) on mucus clearance. Pediatr Pulmonol. 1994;17:113–8.
24. DeRusso M, Miller AG, Caccamise M, Alibrahim O. Negative-pressure ventilation in the pediatric ICU. Respir Care. 2024;69:354–65.
25. United Hayek Industries. Application of the Hayek RTX. London: United Hayek Industries; 2020.
26. Hassinger AB, Breuer RK, Nutty K, et al. Negative-pressure ventilation in pediatric acute respiratory failure. Respir Care. 2017;62:1540–9.
27. Gipsman AI, Lapinel NC, Mayer OH. Airway clearance in patients with neuromuscular disease. Paediatr Respir Rev. 2023;47:33–40.
28. Onweni C, Rashid S, Goswami R, et al. Cuirass ventilation: an alternative home-based modality for chronic respiratory failure. Home Health Care Manag Pract. 2020;32:40–4.
29. Flume PA, Mogayzel PJ, Robinson KA, et al. Cystic fibrosis pulmonary guidelines. Am J Respir Crit Care Med. 2012;182:298–306.
30. Tripathi AK, Sankari A. Postural drainage and vibration. StatPearls; 2024.
31. Hino H, Suzuki Y, Ishii E, Fukuda M. Biphasic cuirass ventilation for treatment of an air leak after pneumothorax in a patient with nemaline myopathy: a case report. J Anesth. 2016;30(6):1087–90.
32. Kato K, Sato N, Takeda S, et al. Marked improvement of extensive atelectasis by unilateral application of the RTX respirator in elderly patients. Intern Med. 2009;48:1419–23.
33. Al-Saady NM, Fernando SSD, Petros AJ, et al. External high frequency oscillation in normal subjects and in patients with acute respiratory failure. Anaesthesia. 1995;50:1031–5.
34. United Hayek Industries. Frequently asked questions. London: United Hayek Industries; 2020.
35. Mefford G, Fernandez D. Biphasic cuirass ventilation for pulmonary compromise due to neuro-muscular illness or injury. J Pulm Tech. 2010;10:28–33.
36. Awab A, Khan MS, Youness HA. Whole lung lavage-technical details, challenges and management of complications. J Thorac Dis. 2017;9:1697–706.
37. Campo I, Luisetti M, Griese M, et al. Whole lung lavage therapy for pulmonary alveolar proteinosis: a global survey of current practices and procedures. Orphanet J Rare Dis. 2016;11:115.
38. Shrestha D, Dhooria S, Munirathinam GK, et al. How We Do It: Whole Lung Lavage. Sarcoidosis Vasc Diffuse Lung Dis. 2022;39:e2022017.
39. Nakamura K, Omura S, Kajiura K, Ishigaki M. Removal of lung lavage fluid during whole-lung lavage using biphasic cuirass ventilation chest percussion in a patient with autoimmune pulmonary alveolar proteinosis. Lung India. 2019;36:540–2.
40. Wołoszczak J, Wrześniewska M, Hrapkowicz A, et al. A comprehensive outlook on pulmonary alveolar proteinosis—a review. Int J Mol Sci. 2024;25:7092.
41. Bodhey A, Bodhey M, Shallik NA, et al. Biphasic cuirass ventilation for airway surgeries: a comprehensive review. Cureus. 2024;16:757–77.

Biphasic Cuirass Ventilation in Pulmonary Rehabilitation

18

Inês Filipa Silva

18.1 Respiratory Rehabilitation

Respiratory Rehabilitation as a multidisciplinary approach to lung disease management is defined by the European Respiratory Society and the American Thoracic Society (ATS) as "a comprehensive intervention based on a thorough patient assessment followed by patient-tailored therapies, which include, but are not limited to, exercise training, education, and behaviour change, designed to improve the physical and psychological condition of people with chronic respiratory disease and to promote the long-term adherence of health-enhancing behaviours" [1].

It stands as an undeniable asset in the multidisciplinary management of patients with chronic respiratory diseases. Its benefits are widely recognized, with robust evidence demonstrating significant improvements in exercise capacity, dyspnea, quality of life, and reduction in hospitalizations. Additionally, it enhances treatment adherence, empowers patients to self-manage their condition, and reduces the long-term functional impact of the disease. While rehabilitation may be tailored to a specific disease or symptom, it encompasses a wide range of therapeutic strategies in both acute and chronic settings, aiming to relieve symptoms, reduce complications, and improve functional outcomes. For example, exercise training constitutes a central key of pulmonary rehabilitation, aiming for improved aerobic capacity, skeletal muscle strength, and symptom relief in the long-term management of chronic illness. However, in such physiological deterioration conditions, medical devices are often used for therapeutic support [2].

Among these devices, high-frequency chest wall oscillation (HFCWO) and high-frequency chest wall compression (HFCWC) are airway clearance techniques that utilize high-frequency pressure variations to assist lung function. These methods work by altering transrespiratory pressure—either increasing it to enhance

I. F. Silva (✉)
Unidade Local de Saúde de Trás-os-Montes e Alto Douro, Vila Real, Portugal

O. Alibrahim et al. (eds.), *Biphasic Cuirass Noninvasive Ventilation*, Noninvasive Ventilation. The Essentials, https://doi.org/10.1007/978-3-032-20933-7_18

inspiratory flow or decreasing it to promote greater expiratory flow. In contrast, non-assisted techniques depend on the natural force of passive exhalation to produce oscillations in the chest wall, as seen with devices like the Flutter and Acapella.

The Cough Assist (mechanical insufflator-exsufflator) is the most commonly used method. It is a device that simulates an effective cough, promoting secretion clearance in patients with an ineffective natural cough. It works through a rapid alternation between positive pressure (insufflation) and negative pressure (exsufflation), mobilizing secretions from the lower airways to the upper airways.

Biphasic Cuirass Ventilation (BCV) is a more recent method that provides non-invasive ventilatory support by applying alternating negative and positive pressures via a rigid shell (cuirass) fitted to the thorax. This technique supports both inspiration and expiration, mimicking natural respiratory cycles and facilitating ventilation without requiring an invasive interface. In addition to aiding gas exchange, BCV may contribute to airway clearance by generating thoracic oscillations and promoting mucus mobilization, as it is discussed in this chapter.

18.2 Cuirass Ventilation

Ventilation machines have long been updated since their most infamous external machine in history—the iron lung, during the Polio epidemic in the twentieth century, as a therapeutic weapon for respiratory failure and loss of respiratory drive due bulbospinal affectation in poliomyelitis [3].

In current ages, positive pressure machines such as biphasic positive airway pressure (BiPAP) or continuous positive airway pressure (CPAP) are the gold-standard for a myriad of pulmonary and respiratory illnesses. However, negative pressure ventilation is not a completely obsolete practice; it has been demonstrated that it provides more homogeneous lung inflation, more favourable pressure–volume curves, reduced energy loss and work of breathing, resulting in less hysteresis and more homogeneous alveolar expansion [4].

The cuirass is a plastic barrel-shaped device that interfaces the thoracic cavity and upper abdomen all around and applies alternating positive and negative pressure, mimicking the natural motion of the diaphragm during breathing. Expiration is facilitated by the positive pressure, whereas inspiration occurs as negative pressure expands the chest cavity [5].

The vast abilities and modes in a single machine plan to work intertwined to assist and promote ventilation in a non-invasive manner closer to the physiological ventilation, through pendulous differential pressures through the chest cavity, instead of mask delivery.

The cuirass apparatus contains five different types of ventilation modes: Continuous Negative Pressure, Controlled Biphasic Cuirass Ventilation (BCV), Non-Invasive Synchronized BCV, High-Frequency Chest Wall Oscillation (HFCWO), and Cardiac Synchronization.

- Controlled BCV corresponds to a mode in which the entire ventilatory cycle is determined by the ventilator, with pre-set respiratory rate, inspiratory and expiratory pressures, and timing. It is typically employed in situations of absent or severely impaired respiratory drive, where ventilation is entirely machine-dependent. In contrast, non-invasive synchronized (assisted) BCV requires an intact patient drive, as the ventilator detects the patient's inspiratory effort and delivers the pre-set pressure support in synchrony, thereby ensuring effective ventilation.
- High-frequency oscillation, as high as 1200 oscillations per minute, alternating between positive and negative pressure, has demonstrated benefits in gas exchange and secretion clearance. This specific setting of the BCV machine plays a crucial role in pulmonary rehabilitation, as described forward [6].

Nonetheless, the cuirass shows promising prowess as a ventilation alternative in situations where traditional methods impose as a challenge: oral and airway surgery. Although small, the sample size demonstrated the cuirass as a success as a standalone ventilation mechanism (without tracheal intubation), offering stable ventilation as gas exchange, without complications [7].

18.3 BCV in Rehabilitation

According to Mefford [8], secretion clearance consists of a spectrum of physiological processes aiming to secretion exteriorization, where in each step therapeutic targets present themselves useful in helping an otherwise healthy and functioning physiological process: cough and mucus expulsion. Such therapeutic mediators can act in secretion modification, mobilization between different airway compartments, culminating in expectoration.

- *Modification*

Amid acute pulmonary disease or chronic disease exacerbations, sputum production often increases, and its clearance can be further hindered due to intensified airway inflammation and obstruction, as well as increased secretion viscosity. Furthermore, the affected airway and its ciliary clearance may not withstand, further increasing the likelihood of complications. Thus, mucus clearance, namely its property's modification, comprises an important role in pulmonary rehabilitation [9].

Given the conditions in which bacteria thrives and further promotes inflammation in muco-obstructive diseases, hydration of airway mucus through aerosolized solutions, namely hypertonic solutions that allow ion modulation, is a direct method of thinning out secretions and promoting its clearance. Another therapeutic weapon is N-acetylcisteine, a drug that acts by diluting mucins present in mucus [10].

In line with the biophysics of mucin conglomerates in mucus viscosity, the authors state oscillatory airflow techniques aim to thin out viscosity mucous gel layers, as well as extrathoracic oscillatory compressors, thus promoting clearance and cough efficacy, that aligns with previous findings, namely mechanical insufflation-exsufflation techniques in neuromuscular disease models [11].

- *Mobilization*

Mobilizing-retained secretion is fundamental for effective airway clearance. To remove significant amounts of mucus, secretions must be actively transported from the peripheral to central airways.

A variety of therapeutic interventions is available to facilitate this mobilization, including the active cycle of breathing (ACB), autogenic drainage (AD), forced expiratory techniques (FET), strategic positioning, chest percussion, oscillatory therapies, and intermittent positive pressure breathing (IPPB).

Conventional chest physiotherapy methods, such as postural drainage combined with manual percussion, typically require the support of trained personnel. However, these approaches can be physically demanding and may pose risks, especially when specific drainage positions lead to clinical instability. This risk depends on factors such as the patient's overall condition, the location of retained secretions, and the extent of ventilation-perfusion mismatch.

Oscillatory techniques contribute significantly to mucus mobilization by generating bursts of airflow that help lift and move the mucus layer upward. Devices such as oscillatory vests or air bladder systems work by rapidly compressing and releasing the chest wall, resulting in high-frequency chest wall compression (HFCWC) [12].

Alternatively, the Hayek biphasic cuirass delivers true high-frequency chest wall oscillation (HFCWO) by alternating positive and negative pressures within a rigid shell. This dynamic pressure system closely replicates natural breathing mechanics, promoting airway patency and minimizing the obstruction that can sometimes occur with positive airway pressure (PAP) devices.

Nonetheless, regardless of the technique employed, an effective cough—spontaneous or assisted—remains essential to achieving complete airway clearance.

- *Expectoration*

Once pulmonary secretions that have been retained are adjusted to a viscosity that allows normal flow and are moved toward the larger airways, effective airway clearance requires that these secretions be expelled from the respiratory tract. The natural cough serves as the primary and most effective mechanism for expectoration. However, when the cough is weak or ineffective, various support techniques can be applied. If the cough function is compromised, the overall secretion clearance process is likely impaired. The aforementioned positive pressure devices (CoughAssist, etc.) promote airway expansion, then cough is promoted by negative pressure for secretion mobilization. This is especially useful in acute settings, such as pneumonia or tracheobronchitis where bronchorrhea is predominant, or chronic illnesses such as COPD and neuromuscular disease, where both the airway structure and the neuromuscular component, both playing a crucial role in secretion mobilization, are damaged.

Therefore, BCV machine plans on intervening in multiple modalities, as its HFCWO and ventilation modes work by amplifying natural cough processes coupled with its built-in cough assist function. By amplifying cough mechanisms, it holds potential to assist in each step of the secretion exteriorization spectrum as discussed earlier, making it a valuable asset able to act in multiple physiological processes in a single machine, contrasting the need for multiple devices and/or therapies with various purposes in order to achieve mucus clearance.

According to the manufacturer, BCV modalities for pulmonary rehabilitation include two main functions: vibration mode, which delivers HFCWO by quickly shifting pressure between two levels (ranging from −50 to +50 cm H_2O) at rates up to 20 times per second; the cough simulator, which gives a long, deep breath followed by a sharp, fast exhale, pushing mucus up through the airways to be expelled more easily. In addition, the BCV actively supports lung expansion through its continuous negative pressure and non-invasive ventilation (NIV) modes. Thus, it improves chest wall motion and airway opening, making it especially useful for patients with impaired respiratory function.

Additionally, the lack of need for facial masks or other invasive systems lowers the risk of infection and other complications such as barotrauma, facial trauma, and upper airway iatrogeny. The Hayek device shows great promise circumventing some of the shortcomings of positive pressure mask-type devices, whether for ventilation or rehabilitation purposes. However, preliminary research comparing multiple devices designed for airway clearance show no difference between the BCV device and other cough assist devices or other therapeutic weapons, namely in Cystic Fibrosis [13, 14].

Moreover, cuirass-type devices raises the question of its feasibility in the frail patient, often with weak and ankylosed thoracic cavities, that might not endure external pressure without some musculoskeletal trauma. In an acute setting, patients with invasive tubes or catheters also raise the question of its safety. The lack of wide clinical trials using BCV discerningly in different pulmonary diseases and settings makes it all the more difficult to standardize its use in a medical practice setting; thus more research is warranted before implementing.

References

1. Spruit MA, Singh SJ, Garvey C, ZuWallack R, Nici L, Rochester C, et al. An official American Thoracic Society/European Respiratory Society statement: key concepts and advances in pulmonary rehabilitation. Am J Respir Crit Care Med. 2013;188(8):e13–64.
2. Troosters T, Janssens W, Demeyer H, Rabinovich RA. Pulmonary rehabilitation and physical interventions. Eur Respir Rev. 2023;32(168).
3. Eichel T, Dreux ML. Negative or positive? The iron lung and poliomyelitis-Zurich, 1951. Anaesth Intensive Care. 2017;45(7):13–20.

4. Katira BH, Cereda M. Negative pressure is the positive way to breathe! Am J Respir Crit Care Med. 2023;207(5):505–6.
5. Annunziata A, Calabrese C, Simioli F, Coppola A, Flora M, Marotta A, et al. Negative-pressure ventilation in neuromuscular diseases in the acute setting. J Clin Med. 2022;11(9).
6. Linton DM. Cuirass ventilation: a review and update. Crit Care Resusc. 2005;7(1):22–8.
7. Bodhey A, Bodhey M, Shallik NA, Al Nadhari M, Griess HF, Al Ani O, et al. Biphasic cuirass ventilation for airway surgeries: a comprehensive review. Cureus. 2024;16(12):e75477.
8. Mefford GW. Biphasic cuirass ventilation for airway secretions. In: Esquinas AM, editor. Humidification in the intensive care unit: the essentials. Cham: Springer; 2023. p. 313–21.
9. Placidi G, Cornacchia M, Polese G, Zanolla L, Assael BM, Braggion C. Chest physiotherapy with positive airway pressure: a pilot study of short-term effects on sputum clearance in patients with cystic fibrosis and severe airway obstruction. Respir Care. 2006;51(10):1145–53.
10. Hill DB, Button B, Rubinstein M, Boucher RC. Physiology and pathophysiology of human airway mucus. Physiol Rev. 2022;102(4):1757–836.
11. Ren S, Li W, Wang L, Shi Y, Cai M, Hao L, et al. Numerical analysis of airway mucus clearance effectiveness using assisted coughing techniques. Sci Rep. 2020;10(1):2030.
12. Chatburn RL. High-frequency assisted airway clearance. Respir Care. 2007;52(9):1224–35; discussion 35–7.
13. Trimble A, Zeman K, Wu J, Ceppe A, Bennett W, Donaldson S. Effect of airway clearance therapies on mucociliary clearance in adults with cystic fibrosis: a randomized controlled trial. PLoS One. 2022;17(5):e0268622.
14. Miyagawa T, Ichiba T. Comparison of mucus clearance between biphasic cuirass ventilation device and mechanical cough assist device on the differences of rheological property and lung mechanics. Respir Care. 2018;63(Suppl_10):3023606.

Part IV

Critical Care Anesthesiology

Byphasic Cuirass Ventilation-Nasal High-Flow Oxygen

19

Elisa Salsano, Oriana Rossi, and Cecilia Rispoli

19.1 Introduction

Biphasic cuirass ventilation (BCV) technology applies uniform pressure across the thorax, facilitating even lung expansion and homogeneous ventilation to address various forms of acute and chronic respiratory failure [1]. Biphasic cuirass ventilation (BCV) assists spontaneous breathing and supports ventilation through a biphasic pressure application. During inspiration, negative pressure actively moves the diaphragm caudally, while positive pressure during expiration enhances air expulsion from the lungs. This expiratory positive pressure is particularly effective in facilitating carbon dioxide clearance, weaning patients from mechanical ventilation, increasing cardiac output, and promoting alveolar recruitment. Consequently, BCV may also contribute to reducing complications associated with invasive mechanical ventilation, such as ventilator-associated pneumonia, laryngeal injury, and respiratory muscle atrophy, potentially improving patient quality of life [2, 3].

Furthermore, a significant advantage of BCV is its compatibility with various noninvasive positive pressure ventilation interfaces, including CPAP and HFNO. In patients already receiving NIV, the application of BCV can reduce the required pressure support and inspired oxygen fraction, while simultaneously increasing tidal volumes and enhancing carbon dioxide removal [4].

E. Salsano (✉)
Geriatric and Intensive Geriatric Care Unit, San Giuseppe Moscati Hospital, Avellino, Italy
e-mail: elisa.salsano@aornmoscati.it

O. Rossi
Medical Department, University Aldo Moro, Bari, Italy

C. Rispoli
Emergency Department, Antonio Cardarelli Hospital, Naples, Italy

O. Alibrahim et al. (eds.), *Biphasic Cuirass Noninvasive Ventilation*, Noninvasive Ventilation. The Essentials, https://doi.org/10.1007/978-3-032-20933-7_19

19.2 The Rationale for the Use of BCV for the De-escalation Therapy

Contemporary cuirass ventilation devices offer a therapeutic approach to significant challenges in chronic lung disease, specifically secretion clearance, carbon dioxide retention, and respiratory muscle fatigue. Noninvasive Synchronized Biphasic Cuirass Ventilation, when applied periodically, can offer some relief for each of these problems, similarly to the benefits observed with intermittent noninvasive positive pressure ventilation.

The application of cuirass ventilation has demonstrated benefits in intubated patients receiving positive pressure ventilation [5, 6]. The imposition of biphasic extra-thoracic pressures facilitates a reduction in pressure support requirements and is associated with physiological improvements in oxygenation and cardiac output [7]. Particularly with adaptive positive pressure ventilatory modes, a progressive and rapid decrease in required inspired pressure support is observable. Biphasic cuirass ventilation effectively enables rapid weaning from positive pressure support, leading to increased spontaneously generated tidal volumes, enhanced CO_2 removal, and reduced inspired oxygen requirements [4].

The prolonged use of NIV in critically ill, ventilator-dependent patients remains controversial due to its association with a significant risk of NIV failure. These patients frequently develop mask intolerance and exhibit increased mortality. In routine intensive care unit (ICU) practice, this represents a complex and unresolved challenge necessitating the development of alternatives to prolonged NIV. Moreover, this underscores the importance of re-evaluating NIV-dependent de-escalation strategies to facilitate liberation from conventional mask-based NIV.

HFNO is often a useful alternative tool in the de-escalation phase in patients with low or middle muscular weakness, who are not hypercapnic and have not developed the physiological effects of respiratory muscular weakness and other ventilatory effects of prolonged NIV.

However, HFNO alone is insufficient in cases of severe respiratory muscle fatigue, as it cannot deliver the necessary supportive pressures to achieve adequate tidal volumes and overall respiratory volumes. In such instances, negative pressure ventilation may offer a valuable alternative by facilitating lung recruitment and providing sufficient respiratory support, thereby alleviating muscle fatigue.

In an interesting clinical case, Borges and Esquinas described the successful de-escalation of respiratory support in a 58-year-old woman with ARDS post-COVID-19 and secondary pulmonary fibrosis who exhibited respiratory fatigue and orofacial mask intolerance. The combined use of high-flow nasal cannula and negative pressure ventilation enabled a progressive weaning from NIV [8].

19.3 Conclusion

Although not widely employed, negative pressure ventilation offers a potentially beneficial noninvasive ventilation method for select clinical conditions. Patients with anatomical orofacial abnormalities or intolerance to conventional noninvasive ventilation could particularly benefit from this approach. While current literature describes few cases, the SARS-CoV-2 pandemic has underscored the necessity for developing novel noninvasive ventilation methods to ensure comprehensive therapeutic strategies across diverse patient populations.

References

1. Bauer AR. Mechanical respirator for newborn infants and other patients: preliminary report. JAMA. 1956;161(8):723–5. https://doi.org/10.1001/jama.1956.62970080003016a.
2. Linton DM. Cuirass ventilation: a review and update. Crit Care Resusc. 2005;7(1):22–8.
3. Onweni C, Rashid S, Goswami R, et al. Cuirass ventilation: an alternative home-based modality for chronic respiratory failure. Home Health Care Manag Pract. 2020;32:40. https://doi.org/10.1177/1084822319875111.
4. Takeda S, Nakanishi K, Takano T, et al. The combination of external high-frequency oscillation and pressure support ventilation in acute respiratory failure. Acta Anaesthesiol Scand. 1997;41:670–4. https://doi.org/10.1111/j.1399-6576.1997.tb04765.x.
5. Gaitini, Krimerman, Smorgik, Gruber, Varzberger. External high frequency ventilation for weaning from mechanical ventilation. Recent advances in anaesthesia, pain, intensive care and emergency 1990;5:137–8.
6. Bennett MR, Blair KE, Fiehler PC, Kline LR. Chest wall oscillation in acute resp failure utilizing the Hayek oscillator. Am Rev Resp Dis. 1993;147(Supplement 4):A983.
7. Sideno B, Vaage J. Ventilation by external highfrequency oscillations improves cardiac function after coronary artery bypass grafting. Eur J Cardiothorac Surg. 1997;11:248–57. https://doi.org/10.1016/s1010-7940(96)01042-1.
8. Borges J, Esquinas A. Biphasic cuirass ventilation in the escalation of non-invasive ventilation in COVID-19: Case report. https://doi.org/10.4081/monaldi.2023.2510.

Biphasic Cuirass Ventilation in Hypoxemic Respiratory Failure

20

Munir Mohamed Mimun

20.1 Introduction

Biphasic cuirass ventilation (BCV) represents a noninvasive ventilatory support modality that has experienced a notable resurgence in recent decades, particularly in the management of patients with hypoxemic respiratory failure. This condition, defined by an arterial oxygen partial pressure (PaO_2) below 60 mmHg while breathing room air at sea level, or a PaO_2/FiO_2 ratio less than 300 mmHg according to the Berlin criteria for acute respiratory distress syndrome [1], constitutes a significant clinical challenge requiring effective and, when possible, less invasive therapeutic interventions.

The concept of external negative pressure ventilation is not new to respiratory medicine. Indeed, the "iron lungs" used during poliomyelitis epidemics in the first half of the twentieth century operated under similar principles [2]. However, modern BCV technology represents a significant evolution from those primitive devices, offering precise control of applied pressures, greater patient comfort, and the ability to provide both negative and positive pressure in a biphasic manner [3].

The clinical relevance of BCV in the current context is based on its unique capacity to provide ventilatory support while preserving, and even improving, physiological aspects that may be compromised with conventional positive pressure ventilation. As Shekerdemian and Bohn note in their review on cardiovascular effects of mechanical ventilation [4], positive pressure ventilation can have significant adverse

M. Mohamed Mimun (✉)
Department of Internal Medicine, Consorci Sanitari de Terrassa – Hospital Universitari, Terrassa, Spain
e-mail: 26106@cst.cat

O. Alibrahim et al. (eds.), *Biphasic Cuirass Noninvasive Ventilation*, Noninvasive Ventilation. The Essentials, https://doi.org/10.1007/978-3-032-20933-7_20

hemodynamic effects, particularly in patients with cardiovascular compromise or right ventricular dysfunction. BCV, by operating through external pressure, avoids many of these complications while providing effective ventilatory support [5].

20.2 Pathophysiology of Hypoxemic Respiratory Failure

20.2.1 Definition and Diagnostic Criteria

Hypoxemic respiratory failure is a condition in which blood oxygen levels are insufficient to meet the body's oxygen demands, defined by a significant decrease in arterial oxygen pressure (PaO_2) despite adequate ventilation in the patient. Clinical and radiological criteria are used to determine its severity, including the PaO_2/FiO_2 ratio and the presence of bilateral infiltrates on chest radiography [6].

Under normal conditions, oxygen passes from the alveoli to the blood through the alveolar-capillary membrane. In hypoxemic respiratory failure, whether due to diffusion problems, ventilation-perfusion mismatch, or airway closure, this process is compromised. The result is decreased systemic oxygenation, forcing the body to activate compensatory mechanisms (such as increased respiratory rate and cardiac output).

20.2.2 Underlying Mechanisms

Pathophysiological mechanisms include:

- *Ventilation/Perfusion (V/Q) Mismatch*: V/Q mismatch occurs when there is an imbalance between the amount of air reaching the alveoli (ventilation) and the amount of blood flowing through the surrounding capillaries (perfusion). For example, in conditions such as pneumonia, pulmonary edema, or alveolar collapse, certain lung segments may receive little air due to obstruction or filling of the alveoli. However, perfusion in these areas may remain nearly normal. This means that blood passing through these capillaries is not adequately oxygenated, as the available oxygen in the alveoli is insufficient.
- *Alveolar Damage*: Inflammatory or infectious processes that alter the integrity of the alveolar-capillary membrane. Alveolar damage affects the lungs' ability to perform optimal gas exchange and can induce hypoxemia through several mechanisms [7, 8]:
  - Alveolar-Capillary Membrane Alteration: When direct damage to the alveoli occurs (for example, in severe inflammatory processes such as acute respiratory distress syndrome [ARDS]), the structure of the alveolar-capillary membrane is compromised. This increases the thickness of the diffusion barrier, hindering oxygen passage into the blood and delaying gas exchange.

- Alveolar Edema and Fluid Accumulation: Damage to the alveoli can cause fluid leakage into the alveolar space. This edema reduces the surface area available for gas exchange and acts as an additional barrier to oxygen, reducing its diffusion into the capillaries.
- Alveolar Collapse (Atelectasis): Destruction or damage to the alveolar structure can lead to partial or complete collapse of some alveoli. By reducing the number of functional units for ventilation, the amount of oxygen that can be absorbed decreases, contributing to hypoxemia.

• *Intrapulmonary Shunt*: Caused by lung areas that do not participate in gas exchange [9]. Deoxygenated blood circulating through these poorly ventilated areas mixes with blood that has been oxygenated in other lung zones. This mixing effect decreases the overall oxygen concentration in arterial blood, leading to hypoxemia.

20.3 Physiological Foundations and Mechanism of Action of BCV

20.3.1 Basic Operating Principles

The biphasic cuirass ventilation system operates through physiological principles that more naturally reproduce the normal respiratory process. According to the detailed description by Bodhey et al. [3], the device consists of a rigid or semi-rigid cuirass that adapts to the patient's thoracic contour, creating an airtight chamber around the chest. This cuirass is connected to a control unit that generates and regulates the pressures applied during the respiratory cycle.

During the inspiratory phase, the system generates negative pressure within the thoracic chamber. This negative pressure, typically configured between −15 and −25 cm H_2O according to available studies, causes chest wall expansion similar to what would occur with respiratory muscle contraction during spontaneous breathing. Yamashita et al. [10] reported successful use of negative pressures of −21 cmH_2O in their series of critically ill patients, demonstrating significant improvements in ventilatory parameters.

The externally applied negative pressure creates a transpulmonary pressure gradient that facilitates airflow into the alveoli without the need to directly pressurize the airway.

In the expiratory phase, the system applies external positive pressure, typically between +5 and +10 cmH_2O, which actively assists air exit from the lungs. This biphasic characteristic distinguishes modern BCV systems from old negative pressure ventilators that relied solely on passive elastic chest recoil for expiration. Yamashita et al. [10] used expiratory pressures of +7 cmH_2O, observing improvement in CO_2 elimination and overall ventilatory mechanics. In several studies [3, 10], the I:E ratio was 1:1 (Fig. 20.1).

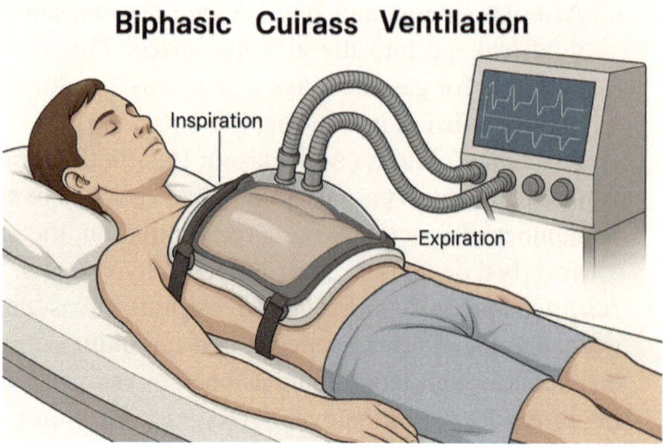

Fig. 20.1 Graphic illustration of the biphasic cuirass ventilation. (Mohamed Mimun M.)

20.3.2 Cardiovascular Physiological Effects

The interaction between ventilation and the cardiovascular system has been extensively studied, and BCV presents unique advantages in this aspect. During conventional positive pressure ventilation, increased intrathoracic pressure reduces the pressure gradient for venous return, which can decrease right ventricular preload and, consequently, cardiac output [4]. This effect is particularly pronounced in hypovolemic patients or those with right ventricular dysfunction.

Furthermore, Sato et al. [11] investigated the effects of extrathoracic mechanical ventilation in patients with pulmonary hypertension secondary to lung disease. Their findings suggest that BCV can reduce mean pulmonary artery pressure, possibly through several mechanisms: improvement of alveolar oxygenation with reduction of hypoxic pulmonary vasoconstriction and decrease in mean intrathoracic pressure that reduces right ventricular afterload.

20.3.3 Effects on Respiratory Muscle Function

A fundamental aspect of BCV is its capacity to maintain or even improve respiratory muscle function. Cropp and DiMarco [12] conducted a controlled study in eight patients with severe chronic obstructive pulmonary disease (COPD), applying intermittent negative pressure ventilation for 3–6 hours daily for three consecutive days. Results showed significant increases in maximal inspiratory pressure (PImax) of 14% and maximal expiratory pressure (PEmax) of 12%, in addition to an average reduction of 8 mmHg in $PaCO_2$, compared to the control group that received no intervention.

Montserrat et al. [13] corroborated these findings in a similar study during acute COPD exacerbations. They observed that negative pressure ventilation not only improved arterial gases acutely but also preserved respiratory muscle strength measured by maximal respiratory pressures. The authors suggest this is because BCV assists ventilation without completely suppressing patient respiratory work, allowing some degree of muscle activity that prevents disuse atrophy.

20.3.4 Effects on Ventilation and Perfusion Distribution

Corrado and Gorini [2], in their comprehensive review on negative pressure ventilation, describe how BCV can improve ventilation distribution by promoting expansion of all lung regions in a more physiological manner. This is particularly relevant in patients with atelectasis or basal consolidations, where positive pressure ventilation may be less effective in recruiting these areas.

20.4 Clinical Applications in Hypoxemic Respiratory Failure

20.4.1 Acute Respiratory Failure

The application of BCV in acute respiratory failure has been documented in several observational studies. Yamashita et al. [10] reported a series of 18 critically ill patients with acute respiratory failure treated with BCV in the intensive care unit. Of these patients, 15 were intubated and receiving conventional mechanical ventilation when BCV was added as adjuvant therapy. Results showed significant improvements in tidal volume, PaO_2/FiO_2 ratio, and shunt fraction ($p < 0.05$).

20.4.2 Acute Respiratory Distress Syndrome (ARDS)

Although specific evidence in ARDS is limited, the physiological basis for BCV use in this condition includes several favorable aspects. First, external negative pressure can promote more homogeneous alveolar recruitment without the risks associated with high airway pressures. Second, preservation of cardiac output may be particularly beneficial in these patients who frequently present hemodynamic instability. Third, the ability to apply continuous negative pressure between breaths (analogous to PEEP but with negative pressure) may help maintain alveolar recruitment [14], although the cited studies were performed in animals and there is no solid evidence in humans.

20.4.3 Weaning from Mechanical Ventilation

One of the most promising applications of BCV is in the process of weaning from mechanical ventilation, particularly in patients with difficult or prolonged weaning. Onweni et al. [5] describe successful use of BCV as a bridge between invasive ventilation and spontaneous breathing in patients with post-ICU respiratory muscle weakness. The authors suggest that BCV offers advantages in this context by providing partial ventilatory support while allowing the patient to maintain control of their breathing pattern and continue exercising their respiratory muscles.

Almeida Borges and Esquinas [15] reported an illustrative case of a COVID-19 patient with prolonged dependence on noninvasive positive pressure ventilation

(NIV). After several weeks of continuous NIV with progressive mask intolerance, BCV was implemented along with HFNO as a de-escalation strategy, proving to be a ventilation alternative.

20.5 Configuration and Clinical Management

20.5.1 Patient Evaluation and Selection

Appropriate patient selection is crucial for BCV success. Based on available evidence and reported clinical experience, ideal candidates include patients with hypoxemic respiratory failure of reversible cause, mild to moderate respiratory acidosis, neuromuscular disease, bilateral diaphragmatic paralysis/paresis, chronic alveolar hypoventilation, atelectasis or difficulty clearing or expectorating secretions and pediatric patients in whom difficulty maintaining facial seal compromises efficacy, especially those who do not tolerate or present incompatibility with facial mask use [2, 5, 15, 16, 17].

Absolute contraindications, according to Corrado and Gorini's review [2], include sleep apnea syndrome, severe obesity, severe kyphoscoliosis, claustrophobia, rib fractures, and recent abdominal surgery.

20.5.2 Configuration Parameters

Initial BCV configuration should be based on parameters reported in available literature, although specific evidence on titration protocols is limited. Yamashita et al. [10] used inspiratory negative pressures of −21 cmH_2O and expiratory positive pressures of +7 cmH_2O with good results. Cropp and DiMarco [12] employed similar ranges, between −20 and −25 cmH_2O for negative pressure.

Initial respiratory rate is generally configured to match the patient's spontaneous rate, typically between 12 and 20 breaths per minute in adults. The inspiration:expiration (I:E) ratio is adjusted according to underlying pathology, although no studies have systematically evaluated different configurations. Clinical practice suggests using 1:1 ratios as a starting point, with adjustments based on patient response [10, 12].

An important aspect is the possibility of applying continuous negative pressure between breaths, analogous to the concept of PEEP in positive pressure ventilation. Although specific evidence is limited, some authors suggest that continuous negative pressures of −2 to −5 cmH_2O may help maintain alveolar recruitment and improve functional residual capacity [18].

20.5.3 Monitoring and Adjustments

Monitoring during BCV treatment should be comprehensive and continuous. Essential parameters include continuous pulse oximetry, baseline and follow-up arterial blood gases, vital signs including heart rate and blood pressure, respiratory pattern and apparent respiratory work, and patient comfort level.

Performing arterial blood gases before BCV initiation and subsequently after implementation allows parameter adjustments and response evaluation. There is no established time for performing controls, but sessions in various clinical series were around 30 minutes and 2 hours of treatment.

20.5.4 Complications and Management

BCV complications are generally minor compared to invasive ventilation but require appropriate recognition and management. In these studies, the most common side effects were poor adherence, upper airway obstruction, and musculoskeletal pain. All negative pressure ventilators restrict movement and back pain is a common problem [2, 19]. BCV has been associated with rib fractures and pneumothorax in a low percentage, but it is a possible complication [20].

Skin pressure injuries at cuirass contact points are the most frequent, reported in 5–10% of cases in long series [19]. Prevention includes adequate padding of cuirass edges, regular skin inspection, and position changes when possible.

Device intolerance, manifested as claustrophobia or anxiety, occurs in approximately 5–10% of patients according to different series [19]. Strategies to improve tolerance include detailed explanation of the procedure before starting, gradual initiation with low pressures, judicious use of anxiolytics if not contraindicated, and presence of trained personnel to reassure the patient.

20.6 Scientific Evidence and Clinical Outcomes

20.6.1 Literature Review

Scientific evidence on biphasic cuirass ventilation in hypoxemic respiratory failure is limited and comes mainly from observational studies and case series. Yamashita et al. [10] documented BCV use in 18 critically ill patients with acute respiratory failure, reporting significant improvements in ventilatory parameters ($p < 0.05$). However, most of these patients were receiving conventional mechanical ventilation simultaneously, limiting conclusions about BCV efficacy as a single modality.

In COPD patients, controlled studies by Cropp and DiMarco [12] and Montserrat et al. [13] demonstrated improvements in respiratory muscle function and blood gas parameters, although with small samples. Corrado and Gorini's review [2] constitutes the most complete available analysis but explicitly acknowledges the absence of large-scale randomized clinical trials.

During the COVID-19 pandemic, reports such as that by Almeida Borges and Esquinas [15] documented BCV use in SARS-CoV-2 pneumonia, suggesting viability in this context when combined with other respiratory support modalities.

20.6.2 Comparison with Other Modalities

Direct comparison between BCV and other noninvasive ventilation modalities is limited by the scarcity of comparative studies. Main identified differences include:

Hemodynamic effects: Unlike positive pressure ventilation which can reduce venous return, BCV facilitates venous return during inspiration [4].

Tolerance and complications: BCV avoids facial masks, benefiting patients with facial injuries or facial pressure intolerance. However, it can cause its own limitations including movement restriction and skin injuries at contact points [2, 19].

Specific populations: Evidence suggests potential utility in mechanical ventilation weaning in patients with muscle weakness [5] and in pediatric patients with difficulties tolerating facial interfaces [17], although these observations require validation in more rigorous studies.

20.6.3 Areas of Controversy and Future Research

Main areas of controversy include:

Lack of standardized protocols: There is no consensus on optimal parameters. Studies have used different pressures (Yamashita: −21/+7 cmH_2O; Cropp and DiMarco: −20 to −25 cmH_2O) without unified criteria for titration [10, 12].

Patient selection criteria: Although absolute contraindications are established (undrained pneumothorax, rib fractures), criteria to identify patients who will benefit remain poorly defined.

Role in ARDS: Evidence in humans is practically non-existent, limited to animal model studies [14].

Future research priorities:

- Randomized clinical trials comparing BCV with standard noninvasive ventilation
- Development of evidence-based configuration and titration protocols
- Identification of clinical predictors of favorable response
- Cost-effectiveness studies considering equipment and potential savings
- Research in specific populations (pediatric, neuromuscular)

20.7 Conclusions

Biphasic cuirass ventilation represents a noninvasive respiratory support modality that, based on fundamental physiological principles of natural breathing, offers a valuable therapeutic alternative in the management of hypoxemic respiratory failure. Through controlled application of external negative and positive pressures, BCV provides unique advantages that distinguish it from conventional positive pressure ventilation modalities, particularly in terms of cardiovascular function preservation, respiratory muscle activity maintenance, and ventilation/perfusion distribution optimization.

The reviewed scientific evidence, although limited in scope and methodological quality, suggests that BCV may be especially beneficial in specific clinical contexts. Patients with chronic obstructive pulmonary disease, those in the process of mechanical ventilation weaning with respiratory muscle weakness, pediatric populations with difficulties tolerating facial interfaces, and patients with contraindications to positive pressure ventilation emerge as groups that could obtain the greatest benefits from this technology. Experience accumulated during the COVID-19 pandemic has renewed interest in this modality, highlighting additional advantages such as reduced aerosolization risk and preservation of critical healthcare resources.

However, it is essential to recognize the significant limitations currently facing BCV clinical implementation. The absence of large-scale randomized clinical trials, lack of standardized configuration and titration protocols, and limited equipment availability constitute important barriers to its wider adoption. These limitations underscore the urgent need for rigorous research to definitively establish BCV's place in the modern therapeutic algorithm of respiratory failure.

In conclusion, biphasic cuirass ventilation reminds us that innovation in respiratory medicine does not always require completely new technologies, but also the revision and refinement of established concepts through the application of modern knowledge. In an era where personalized medicine and less invasive interventions are increasingly valued, BCV offers a therapeutic option that, with the generation of more robust scientific evidence and development of evidence-based protocols, has the potential to occupy an important place in the comprehensive management of selected patients with hypoxemic respiratory failure. The challenge for the medical community is now to generate the necessary evidence to precisely define when, how, and in whom to use this promising therapeutic modality.

References

1. Force ADT, Ranieri VM, Rubenfeld GD, Thompson BT, Ferguson ND, Caldwell E, et al. Acute respiratory distress syndrome: the Berlin definition. JAMA. 2012;307(23):2526–33.
2. Corrado A, Gorini M. Negative-pressure ventilation: is there still a role? Eur Respir J. 2002;20(1):187–97.
3. Bodhey A, Bodhey M, Shallik NA, Al Nadhari M, Griess HF, Al Ani O, Sainuddin S, Thomas KP, ElHanfi O, Jose S, Nair A. Biphasic cuirass ventilation for airway surgeries: a comprehensive review. Cureus. 2024;16(12):e75477.
4. Shekerdemian LS, Bohn D. Cardiovascular effects of mechanical ventilation. Arch Dis Child. 1999;80(5):475–80.
5. Onweni C, Rashid S, Goswami R, Treece J, Shipley LC, De Souza R, et al. Cuirass ventilation: an alternative home-based modality for chronic respiratory failure. Home Healthc Manag Pract. 2020;37(4):253–9.
6. Frat JP, Thille AW, Mercat A, et al. High-flow oxygen through nasal cannula in acute hypoxemic respiratory failure. N Engl J Med. 2015;372(23):2185–96.
7. West JB. Respiratory physiology: the essentials. 9th ed. Philadelphia, PA: Lippincott Williams & Wilkins; 2012.
8. Tobin MJ. Principles and practice of mechanical ventilation. 3rd ed. New York: McGraw-Hill; 2013.

9. Hilbert G, et al. Noninvasive ventilation in immunocompromised patients with pulmonary infiltrates, fever, and acute respiratory failure. N Engl J Med. 2001;344(7):481–7.
10. Yamashita T, Taniwaki Y, Takayama H, Sato H, Hino M, Okuda K, et al. Efficacy of biphasic cuirass ventilation in the critical care department. Crit Care. 2012;16(Suppl 1):P132.
11. Sato Y, Saeki N, Asakura T, Aoshiba K, Kotani T. Effects of extrathoracic mechanical ventilation on pulmonary hypertension secondary to lung disease. J Anesth. 2016;30(4):663–70.
12. Cropp A, DiMarco AF. Effects of intermittent negative pressure ventilation on respiratory muscle function in patients with severe chronic obstructive pulmonary disease. Am Rev Respir Dis. 1987;135(5):1056–61.
13. Montserrat JM, Martos JA, Alarcon A, Celis R, Plaza V, Picado C. Effect of negative pressure ventilation on arterial blood gas pressures and inspiratory muscle strength during an exacerbation of chronic obstructive lung disease. Thorax. 1991;46(1):6–8.
14. Skaburskis M, Helal R, Zidulka A. Hemodynamic effects of external continuous negative pressure ventilation compared with those of continuous positive pressure ventilation in dogs with acute lung injury. Am Rev Respir Dis. 1987;136(4):886–91.
15. Almeida Borges J, Esquinas AM. Biphasic cuirass ventilation in the escalation of non-invasive ventilation in COVID-19: case report and review. Monaldi Arch Chest Dis. 2023;93(4):2510.
16. Driver AG, Blackburn BB, Marcuard SP, Austin EH Jr. Bilateral diaphragm paralysis treated with cuirass ventilation. Chest. 1987;92(4):683–5.
17. Shekerdemian LS, Schulze-Neick I, Redington AN, Bush A, Penny DJ. Negative pressure ventilation as haemodynamic rescue following surgery for congenital heart disease. Intensive Care Med. 2000;26:93–6.
18. Gorini M, Corrado A, Villella G, Ginanni R, Augustynen A, Tozzi D. Physiologic effects of negative pressure ventilation in acute exacerbation of chronic obstructive pulmonary disease. Am J Respir Crit Care Med. 2001;163(7):1614–8.
19. Corrado A, Confalonieri M, Marchese S, Mollica C, Villella G, Gorini M, et al. Iron lung vs mask ventilation in the treatment of acute on chronic respiratory failure in COPD patients: a multicenter study. Chest. 2002;121(1):189–95.
20. Zibrak JD, Hill NS, Federman EC, Kwa SL, O'Donnell C. Evaluation of intermittent long-term negative-pressure ventilation in patients with severe chronic obstructive pulmonary disease. Am Rev Respir Dis. 1988;138(6):1515–8.

21 Clinical Applications of Biphasic Cuirass Ventilation in Pulmonary and Critical Care: Pneumonia, Pneumothorax, Barotrauma, and Air Leak Syndromes

Salvatore Notaro, Giuseppe La Cerra, Vincenzo Capaldo, Andrea Imparato, and Eugenio Piscitelli

21.1 Introduction

An "iron lung" historically provided negative pressure ventilation in patients with severe poliomyelitis [1]. With negative pressure ventilation, after positioning the patient inside a special container, a negative pressure is generated outside the chest and, with the iron lung, also in the abdomen. Pathophysiologically, this extrathoracic negative pressure causes a lifting of the thorax and an enlargement of the internal volume with a consequent reduction of the pleural pressure (Ppl) and, thus, of the alveolar pressure (PA). The difference between the negative pressure which is present at the alveolar level (PA) and the one present at the level of the upper airways (Pawo), in close contact and, there fore, equal to that of the ambient air, will determine the inspiratory act which will consists in an aspiration of air from the external environment towards the alveoli. This mechanism emulates exactly natural breathing and, therefore, respects normal respiratory physiology. The negative pressure will also involve the abdomen. The lifting of this part of the human body causes a lowering of the diaphragm, which, associated with the lifting of the chest, increases the negativity inside the chest and, therefore, increases the volume and flows of the inspired air [2].

S. Notaro (✉) · A. Imparato · E. Piscitelli
Department of Critical Care, Intensive Care Unit and ECMO, Monaldi-Colli Hospital, Naples, Italy

G. La Cerra
Complex Operative Unit of Interventional Pneumology, Monaldi Hospital – Colli Hospital, Naples, Italy

V. Capaldo
Department of Critical Care, Intensive Care Unite-Federico II University, Naples, Italy

O. Alibrahim et al. (eds.), *Biphasic Cuirass Noninvasive Ventilation*, Noninvasive Ventilation. The Essentials, https://doi.org/10.1007/978-3-032-20933-7_21

Biphasic cuirass ventilation (BCV), an emerging technology using a negative pressure ventilation (NPV) method, has spread into clinical practice. It only requires fitting an external cuirass to the body to generate negative pressure, compared with positive pressure ventilation, which requires intubation or a mask. BCV could assist in spontaneous breathing and support ventilation by enabling negative pressure in the inspiratory phase to move the diaphragm downward and positive pressure in the expiratory phase to push air back out of the lungs. BCV has been reported to improve lung function, oxygenation, and cardiac output and reduce the risk of barotrauma [3].

The Cuirass Ventilation can be applied using a noninvasive chest wall cuirass in as many different patterns as routine positive pressure ventilation and can be set in different modes:

- Controlled biphasic cuirass ventilation resembles intermittent mandatory ventilation (IMV); the patient can breathe whenever desired between the mandatory breaths.
- Continuous negative pressure equals CPAP and can be set at any pressure around the baseline to increase the functional residual capacity.
- Noninvasive Synchronized Biphasic Cuirass Ventilation (BCV): Cuirass-triggered breaths are akin to the spontaneous breaths in the synchronized ventilation (SIMV).
- High-frequency oscillation (HFO) can be applied in frequencies up to 1200 oscillations per minute, for the achievement of oxygenation and reduction of carbon dioxide.
- A significant benefit of externally applied cyclical negative and positive (biphasic) pressure is the ability to assist in coughing and secretion clearance from the airways.
- Cardiac synchronized: A new addition to the various modes of cuirass ventilation is the ability to time the ventilatory cycle to coincide with the cardiac cycle. This is done by sensing the electrocardiograph signals to drive the negative pressure ventilator rate and timing. This mode of noninvasive cardiac synchronized biphasic cuirass ventilation has been reported to have benefits in specific cardiac diseases, enhancing cardiac output. It could also be used in the radiology department during MRI scanning. In highly sensitive magnetic resonance scanning of the heart and thorax, cardiac and ventilatory interaction often interferes with precise imaging [3].

Noninvasive ventilation (NIV) effectively reduces the need for endotracheal intubation [4] and is associated with a decreased risk of respiratory infections, including nosocomial pneumonia, in patients with acute respiratory failure [5]. In literature reports, the application of the device for negative mechanical ventilation (NPV) has been widely used in important pathological conditions like acute respiratory failure in COPD [6, 7] and neuromuscular patients [8], in various clinical fields such as neonatology [9, 10], pediatrics [11], rehabilitation [12], and endoscopic or surgical treatments of the airways [13, 14].

Positive pressure ventilation, especially during invasive mechanical ventilation and in prolonged periods of ventilatory support, is related to reduced possibility of clearance of the airways, the insufficiency of the cough mechanism, and it is also linked to the reduced participation of the patient in ventilatory mechanics, especially if sedated. This may lead to the obstruction of the airways caused by bronchial secretions, bronchial obstruction phenomena, an increased onset of pneumonia, increases in airway pressure, and even barotrauma [15, 16]; it can cause pneumothorax, pneumomediastinum, and subcutaneous emphysema.

This chapter will be discussed using cuirass ventilation in pneumonia, barotrauma, pneumothorax, and air leak syndrome.

21.2 Pneumonia

Pneumonia is a form of acute respiratory infection most commonly caused by viruses or bacteria [17]. The literature describes the use of Cuirass Ventilation in acute respiratory failure due to pneumonia, with some case reports. The following relevant cases are cited.

The first one describes a case of a 71-year-old man who was admitted to the ICU with acute exacerbation of chronic obstructive pulmonary disease (COPD) due to pneumonia and pneumococcal sepsis. He was intubated due to worsening of the exchanges, initially ventilated in a controlled manner, subsequently with support ventilation, which ended with self-extubation after almost 2 weeks of invasive ventilation; at this point, it was decided to support the respiratory activity with external ventilation via the Hayek Oscillator. It was used with an initial frequency of 120 cycles/min, gradually reduced to 25 cycles/min, an I/E ratio of 1 1, an inspiratory pressure of −22 cmH_2O, and an expiratory pressure of 10 cmH_2O. This ventilation allowed for a significant improvement in the patient's clinical state and a gradual improvement in arterial blood gases (ABG). The patient expected a large amount of sputum. He was discharged 13 days after extubation [18].

The second case describes a case of a 39-year-old paraplegic man suffering from poliomyelitis contracted in childhood who was admitted to the ICU with acute respiratory failure due to pneumonia. He was intubated and ventilated with CMV and IMV for 14 days. It was impossible to wean the patient from the ventilator with conventional methods (SIMV, pressure support); therefore, cuirass ventilation was started and implemented for 7 h, starting with a frequency of 120 cycles/min, gradually decreasing to 30 cycles/min, an I/E ratio of 1:1, an inspiratory pressure of −25 cmH_2O, and an expiratory pressure of −8 cmH_2O. The patient expelled a large amount of mucus through the endotracheal tube. After 4 days, he could breathe spontaneously, ventilation was discontinued, and extubation was performed. The authors of this case report conclude that External Ventilation with cuirass was successfully applied in other patients. Reventilation was achieved within seconds, and the hazards of reintubation were eliminated. Cuirass Ventilation is an additional mode of mechanical ventilation in patients with respiratory failure; it is virtually free from complications [18].

A third case report described a case of COVID-19 pneumonia admitted to the ICU and treated with NIV.

This patient, after a few weeks of prolonged use of NIV, began to develop tachypnea hypercarbia and intolerance to the interface mask. She also began to develop muscular weakness and residual lung fibrosis, which resulted in secondary ventilatory dependency. However, prolonged endotracheal intubation in COVID-19 patients has been shown to have poor outcomes. Therefore, the patient was treated by combining HFNC and BCV to avoid orotracheal intubation. HFNC is a valuable alternative tool in the de-escalation phase in patients with low or middle muscular weakness with hypercapnia. BCV technology was applied during the 30 min of discontinuation of NIV.

BCV device assists spontaneous breathing and supports ventilation by enabling negative pressure in the inspiratory phase to move the diaphragm downward actively and positive pressure in the expiratory phase to push air back out of the lung. This technique allowed prolonged NIV weaning with de-escalation and physiotherapy and avoidance of orotracheal intubation [19].

21.3 Barotrauma-Pneumothoraces

Barotrauma is physical damage to body tissues caused by a difference in pressure between a gas space inside or in contact with the body and the surrounding fluid. Several case reports suggest that Biphasic Cuirass Ventilation (BCV), compared to noninvasive positive pressure ventilation (NPPV), may be associated with lower airway pressures and improved patient compliance, potentially reducing the risk of barotrauma. In clinical practice, BCV has been used successfully in patients with pneumothorax or air leak syndromes, particularly when NPPV was insufficient or contraindicated due to elevated airway pressures. Moreover, BCV has been employed as an alternative or in combination with low-intensity NPPV, enabling adequate ventilation while minimizing pressure-related complications [20–22].

The literature further supports these observations through several case reports documenting the effective use of cuirass ventilation in the management of pneumothorax and barotrauma. The most relevant examples are outlined below.

The first case is an 82-year-old woman with spinal tuberculosis and pulmonary fibrosis with hypoventilation who was admitted to hospital due to sudden dyspnea due to pneumodiastinum, initially treated with NPPV IPAP/EPAP 15/4 cmH_2O, RR 33braths/min, and subsequent occurrence evolution into pneumothorax and hypercapnia. Therefore, BCV started in control mode, inspiratory/expiratory pressure −24/+8 cmH_2O, RR 25/min, 2 h × 2 sets/d, while NPPV was restarted at low-intensity spontaneous mode IPAP/EPAP 9/4 cmH_2O. This resulted in an increased tidal volume and decreased PCO_2; subsequently, BCV was interrupted, and IPAP increased until rehabilitation [21].

In the second case, a 79-year-old man with idiopathic pulmonary fibrosis developed a pneumothorax followed by nosocomial pneumonia. Arterial blood gas analysis revealed respiratory acidosis. Respiratory support consisted of non-invasive positive pressure ventilation (NPPV), initiated at low pressure, combined with biphasic cuirass ventilation (BCV) in synchronized mode, with inspiratory/expiratory pressures of −21/+7 cmH2O for two 2-hour sessions per day. Over the following 5 days, tidal volume increased during the combined use of BCV and NPPV compared with NPPV alone, accompanied by a gradual reduction in PaCO2 levels and clinical improvement. Thereafter, he was weaned from BCV support, and pulmonary rehabilitation was resumed [21].

The third case is subcutaneous and mediastinal emphysema in a 39-year-old woman with late-onset Pompe disease who was undergoing noninvasive positive pressure ventilation (NPPV). Even if the patient had a history of pneumothorax, she did not present it at the time of admission. She had not undergone adequate respiratory rehabilitation, which resulted in decreased respiratory compliance. They have theorized that the emphysema had been caused by a gain in airway pressure due to NPPV. A decrease in inspiratory pressure of NPPV from 14 cmH_2O to 9 cmH_2O made the patient dyspneic and hypoxic. They first tried with cuirass ventilation alone, but the result was dyspnea and hypoxia. Combining cuirass ventilation (control mode) and NPPV (assist control mode) could decrease the inspiratory pressure to 7 cmH_2O. After 26 days of treatment, the patient recovered from subcutaneous and mediastinal emphysema. After the treatment, her maximum inspiratory capacity was expanded from 400 to 600 ml, which indicates improved thoracic compliance. Thus, a combination of cuirass ventilation and NPPV is beneficial in managing barotrauma that may occur during NPPV in a respirator-dependent patient [22].

21.4 Leaks Syndrome

Pulmonary air leak syndromes involve the dissection of air out of the normal pulmonary airspaces and include pulmonary interstitial emphysema, pneumothorax, pneumomediastinum, pneumopericardium, pneumoperitoneum, subcutaneous emphysema, and systemic air embolism [23].

The literature describes the use of Cuirass Ventilation in pulmonary air leak syndromes with some case reports. The following relevant case is cited: an 11-year-old child who comes to the emergency room for dyspnea, suffering from a neuromuscular disease. Nemaline disease is a congenital disorder that affects skeletal muscles. On admission, the patient had chest pain, worsening dyspnea, tachycardia (140 beats/min), and hypotension. An X-ray showed the right pneumothorax with the mediastinum shifted to the left. A tension pneumothorax was diagnosed and treated with immediate chest tube placement. Although the pneumothorax improved, hypercapnia and hypoxemia persisted; therefore, non-invasive positive pressure ventilation (NPPV) was initiated, leading to improved gas exchange. The inspiratory and expiratory pressures were modified to avoid barotrauma. Unfortunately, even if NPPV gradually improved hypercapnia and oxygenation up to the normal ranges, the air leak continued, and chemical pleurodesis was performed. At this point, it was hypothesized that the persistent air leak was due to increased positive airway pressure induced by NPPV and, therefore, the respiratory therapy from

NPPV to BCV, which supported the patient's respiration by a cuirass fitted around the chest; the patient wore the cuirass in the respiratory-triggered mode while sleeping; the respiratory rate was set at 20 breaths/ min, inspiratory: expiratory ratio at 2.5:1.0, inspiratory pressure at −14 cmH_2O, and positive pressure during the active expiratory phase at +3 cmH_2O. BCV maintained the adequate respiratory status. The air leak gradually resolved during the next few days [20].

21.5 Discussion

Biphasic cuirass ventilation (BCV) is a NPV method. It could be considered an advanced model of the iron lung. It consists of a cuirass and a pressure source capable of providing both positive and negative pressure, which supports spontaneous breathing more physiologically than positive pressure ventilation. While with the iron lung, patients may experience a certain sense of claustrophobia, as the entire body except the head is inside the ventilator; the newer cuirass is more versatile and comfortable. Contemporary BCV models are available in different measures from neonatal to adult, allowing for a better fit and easy adjustment [24]. Another advantage of modern NPV devices is that patients have heads completely free so that they can talk, drink, eat, blow their nose, expectorate, and, in the case of the cuirass and the "poncho," they also can free their arms and lower limbs [2]. A further strength of curtain ventilation is improved patient-ventilator interaction and the development of more portable devices with comfortable flexibility. The latest generation of devices can apply many ventilation models obtainable with positive pressure devices. Furthermore, they can provide normal to high respiratory rates and swinging and expiratory assistance (coughing). Among the NPV methods, it is worth mentioning high-frequency oscillation (HFO), which, with frequencies of up to 1200 oscillations per minute, allows the achievement of better oxygenation, the reduction of carbon dioxide, and the mobilization of secretions from the periphery of the lung as occurs with the thorax physiotherapy [3]. Double Positive + Negative Synchronized Ventilation (DPNSV) is also worth mentioning. In this case, a ventilator acting directly on the airways with the release of positive pressure operates simultaneously with another ventilator acting externally to the chest with negative pressure, and both are perfectly electronically synchronized with each other. The transpulmonary pressure (PL) or the total pressure of the respiratory system (Prs) is doubled. Therefore, an improvement in ventilation is obtained. However, we have seen that the characteristic of this double synchronized ventilation is that the pressures inside the thorax, particularly at the alveolar level, are counterbalanced and, therefore, eliminated [2, 25].

The literature about BCV is based on case reports, but it looks very promising. It could be helpful in acute respiratory failure due to pneumonia. In fact, with the help of a Pulmo Vista® system, an increase in the areas ventilated with DPNSV instead of positive pressure ventilation has been seen in favor of the posterior areas of the thorax. These areas are difficult to ventilate in a non-prone patient. This has also resulted in increased alveolar recruitment [2].

The use of external high-frequency oscillation (EHFO) combined with pressure support ventilation (PSV) was evaluated in patients with acute respiratory failure.

By applying alternating negative and positive pressures via a cuirass device, the authors observed early improvements in oxygenation and a rapid decrease in $PaCO_2$. The technique also facilitated secretion clearance and improved cardiac output without adverse hemodynamic effects. EHFO proved to be a valuable supportive strategy to enhance ventilation and airway hygiene in the acute care setting [26].

The increase in sputum seems to be one of the main advantages of using BCV, and it is also thanks to the cough support function. As can be seen from the case reports in the introduction, the association of BCV with positive pressure ventilation simultaneously (DPNSV) or for a phase (BCV and then IPPV or NPPV) is very effective. In the case of pneumothorax, where positive ventilation may be ineffective or worsen the clinical outcome, BCV finds space. In this case, the patient's outcome can be improved by using BCV or the NPPV + BCV combination in the acute phase [21, 22]. Cuirass ventilators are designed to apply equal pressure throughout the thorax, allowing for even lung expansion and uniform ventilation [24]. However, although biphasic cuirass ventilation (BCV) avoids positive airway pressure, pneumothorax has been reported as a potential complication. In one study, a patient with severe COPD developed a pneumothorax shortly after using a negative pressure ventilation device (poncho wrap), despite the absence of invasive ventilation or airway pressure [27].

As seen for the treatment of pneumothorax, a similar argument can be applied to the treatment of leak syndrome, where positive pressure ventilation is often ineffective, promoting the persistence of the air leak; BCV, using negative pressure instead of positive pressure, could resolve it.

Finally, a relevant comparative study assessed the efficacy of negative pressure ventilation (NPV) versus conventional mechanical ventilation (CMV) in patients with COPD and acute respiratory failure. The results showed similar mortality rates between the two groups, but significantly shorter ventilation times in patients treated with NPV. Moreover, NPV proved to be effective in preventing endotracheal intubation in a substantial proportion of cases. However, no significant difference was observed in hospital stay duration [28].

A common complication of cuirass ventilation, regardless of whether or not the device has biphasic capabilities, is skin lesions and irritation that can become spots for infection [24]. Cuirass ventilation is contraindicated for patients who are deformed or burned such that the cuirass cannot be applied and for patients with absolute upper airway obstruction [29].

21.6 Conclusion

As can be seen from the studies carried out to date and partly reported in this article, it emerges that BCV is a clinically valid tool to treat respiratory failure due to pneumonia, barotrauma, and pulmonary air leak syndrome as a support to positive pressure ventilation or as a replacement where positive pressure ventilation is ineffective or may worsen the patient's clinical condition. BCV helps treat conditions of hypoxemia and hypercapnia, reduce and resolve dyspnea, and work on respiratory mechanics. Interesting uses are given by the high-frequency oscillation (HFO) to increase sputum and improve alveolar exchanges and by noninvasive cardiac synchronized biphasic cuirass ventilation, which is very helpful in specific cardiac diseases, enhancing cardiac output. It could also be used in the radiology department during MRI scanning, where ventilatory interaction often interferes with precise imaging. However, case reports on BCV are almost exclusively available in the literature. Therefore, further studies are needed to prove the efficacy and correct use of BCV alone or in association with positive pressure ventilation techniques.

References

1. Drinker PA. The iron lung. JAMA. 1986;255:1476.
2. Vincenzi U. A new mode of mechanical ventilation: positive + negative synchronized ventilation. Multidiscip Respir Med. 2021; https://doi.org/10.4081/mrm.2021.788.
3. Linton DM. Cuirass ventilation: a review and update. Crit Care Resusc. 2005;7:22–8.
4. Mehta S, Hill NS. Noninvasive ventilation. Am J Respir Crit Care Med. 2001;163:540–77.
5. American Thoracic Society. Guidelines for the management of adults with hospital-acquired, ventilator-associated, and healthcare-associated pneumonia. Am J Respir Crit Care Med. 2005;171:388–416.
6. Corrado A, Gorini M, De Paola E, Bruscoli G, Tozzi D, Augustynen A, Nutini S, Ginanni R. Iron lung treatment of acute on chronic respiratory failure: 16 yrs of experience. Monaldi Arch Chest Dis. 1994;49(6):552–5.
7. Corrado A, Gorini M, Villella G, Augustynen A, Tozzi D, De Paola E. Negative pressure ventilation in COPD patients with acute on chronic respiratory failure. Monaldi Arch Chest Dis. 1997;52(1):60–3.
8. Annunziata A, Calabrese C, Simioli F, Coppola A, Flora M, Marotta A, Di Spirito V, Didonna F, Cicalese M, Fiorentino G. Negative-pressure ventilation in neuromuscular diseases in the acute setting. J Clin Med. 2022;11(9):2589. https://doi.org/10.3390/jcm11092589. PMID: 35566729; PMCID: PMC9101364.
9. Cvetnic WG, Waffarn F, Martin JM. Continuous negative pressure and intermittent mandatory ventilation in the management of pulmonary interstitial emphysema: a preliminary study. J Perinatol. 1989;9(1):26–32.
10. Sills JH, Cvetnic WG, Pietz J. Continuous negative pressure in the treatment of infants with pulmonary hypertension and respiratory failure. J Perinatol. 1989;9(1):43–8.
11. Samuels MP, Southall DP. Negative extrathoracic pressure in treatment of respiratory failure in infants and young children. BMJ. 1989;299:1253–7.
12. Huang H-Y, Chou P-C, Joa W-C, et al. Pulmonary rehabilitation coupled with negative pressure ventilation decreases decline in lung function, hospitalizations, and medical cost in COPD. Medicine. 2016; https://doi.org/10.1097/MD.0000000000005119.
13. Vitacca M, Natalini G, Cavaliere S, Clini E, Foccoli P, Candiani A, Ambrosino N. Breathing pattern and arterial blood gases during Nd-YAG laser photoresection of endobronchial lesions under general anesthesia: use of negative pressure ventilation: a preliminary study. Chest. 1997;112(6):1466–73. https://doi.org/10.1378/chest.112.6.1466. PMID: 9404740.
14. Petrella F, Borri A, Casiraghi M, et al. Operative rigid bronchoscopy: indications, basic techniques and results. Multimed Man Cardiothorac Surg. 2014;2014(mmu006) https://doi.org/10.1093/mmcts/mmu006.
15. Anzueto A, Frutos-Vivar F, Esteban A, et al. Incidence, risk factors and outcome of barotrauma in mechanically ventilated patients. Intensive Care Med. 2004;30:612–9.
16. Ioannidis G, Lazaridis G, Baka S, et al. Barotrauma and pneumothorax. J Thorac Dis. 2015;7(Suppl 1):S38–43.

17. World Health Organization. Pneumonia. https://www.who.int/health-topics/pneumonia. 2024.
18. Gaitini L, Vaida S, Krimerman S, et al. External high-frequency ventilation in patients with respiratory failure (external ventilation). Intensive Care Med. 1995;21:191.
19. Almeida Borges J, Esquinas AM. Biphasic cuirass ventilation in the escalation of non-invasive ventilation in COVID-19: case report and review. Monaldi Arch Chest Dis. 2023. https://doi.org/10.4081/monaldi.2023.2510.
20. Hino H, Suzuki Y, Ishii E, Fukuda M. Biphasic cuirass ventilation for treatment of an air leak after pneumothorax in a patient with nemaline myopathy: a case report. J Anesth. 2016;30:1087–90.
21. Tada M, Kadowaki T, Tsubouchi Y, et al. Concurrent use of biphasic cuirass ventilation and low-intensity noninvasive positive pressure ventilation. Clin Pulm Med. 2020;27:26–9.
22. Furusawa Y, Yamamoto T, Oya Y, et al. Treatment of subcutaneous and mediastinal emphysema with cuirass ventilation in a patient with Pompe disease undergoing non-invasive positive pressure ventilation. Rinsho Shinkeigaku. 2010;50:306–10.
23. El Ouali I, Habib Chorfa S, El Hamzaoui H, et al. Pulmonary air leak syndrome in rheumatoid arthritis patient. SAGE Open Med Case Rep. 2022;10:2050313X221125361. https://doi.org/10.1177/2050313X221125361.
24. Onweni C, Rashid S, Goswami R, et al. Cuirass ventilation: an alternative home-based modality for chronic respiratory failure. Home Health Care Manag Pract. 2019;32:40–4.
25. Carpagnano GE, Sabato R, Lacedonia D, Di Gioia R, Saliani R, Vincenzi U, Foschino Barbaro MP. New non-invasive ventilator strategy applied to COPD patients in acute ventilator failure. Pulm Pharmacol Ther. 2017;46:64–8.
26. Takeda S, Nakanishi K, Takano T, et al. The combination of external high-frequency oscillation and pressure support ventilation in acute respiratory failure. Acta Anaesthesiol Scand. 1997;41:670–4.
27. Zibrak JD, Hill NS, Federman EC, Kwa SL, O'Donnell C. Evaluation of intermittent long-term negative-pressure ventilation in patients with severe chronic obstructive pulmonary disease. Am Rev Respir Dis. 1988;138:1515–8.
28. Corrado A, Gorini M, Ginanni R, et al. Negative pressure ventilation versus conventional mechanical ventilation in the treatment of acute respiratory failure in COPD patients. Eur Respir J. 1998;12:519–25.
29. Mori H, Shono A, Hirade R, Nikai T, Saito Y. Biphasic cuirass ventilation during anesthesia for tracheobronchial stent insertion or removal by a rigid bronchoscope: a case report. A&A Pract. 2018;10:198–200.

Biphasic Cuirass Ventilation in Trauma: Chest, Head, and Spinal Injuries

22

Akiva Nachshon and Peter Vernon van Heerden

22.1 Introduction

Biphasic cuirass ventilation (BCV) has a role to play in the management of trauma patients for specific indications, where it either adds to, or in some cases is superior to, intermittent positive pressure ventilation (IPPV) via either an endotracheal or tracheostomy tube. This chapter will discuss some of the instances where BCV is useful in trauma patients.

22.2 Mass Casualties

Due to the simplicity (of use of devices used to deliver BCV), BCV is ideal for ventilatory support of patients where the number of injured patients requiring support overwhelms the medical staff available or where the skill set of the medical staff is such that they are unable to provide IPPV. Even if patient numbers are not overwhelming and staff skills are adequate, then BCV could still be considered for trauma patients requiring ventilatory support initially, particularly where airway protective reflexes and level of consciousness (LOC) do not preclude BVC in favor of IPPV.

An example of mass trauma where BCV would be very useful as a modality of ventilatory support would be for the treatment of people exposed to "poison gas" as a weapon of mass destruction. Respiratory distress is a hallmark of poisoning with both mustard gas-type poisons [1, 2] as well as with organophosphate-based poisons [3, 4]. BCV could be applied in the field or in casualty reception areas by

A. Nachshon · P. V. van Heerden (✉)
Department of General Intensive Care, Department of Anesthesiology, Critical Care and Pain Medicine, Hadassah University Hospital, Jerusalem, Israel
e-mail: Akivan@Hadassah.org.il; Vernon@Hadassah.org.il

O. Alibrahim et al. (eds.), *Biphasic Cuirass Noninvasive Ventilation*, Noninvasive Ventilation. The Essentials, https://doi.org/10.1007/978-3-032-20933-7_22

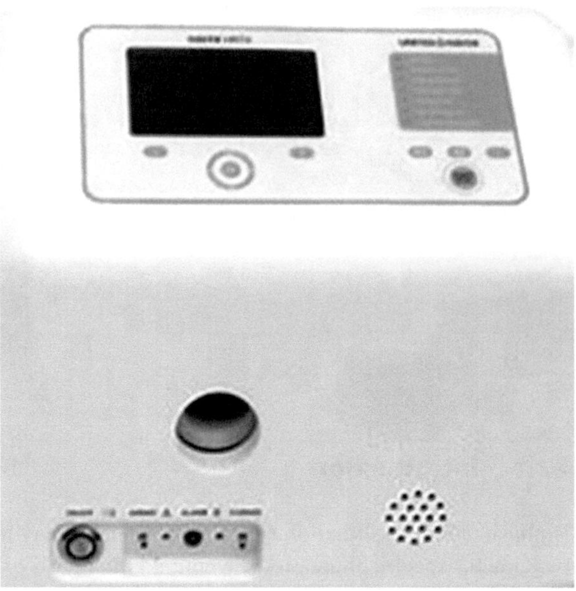

Fig. 22.1 Example of a portable BCV

medical personnel with minimal training, such as army medics or ambulance personnel. Small battery-operated BCV devices have been developed for exactly this purpose. An example is the military grade Hayek HRTX BVC ventilator (Hayek Medical, London, UK), which is able to operate for up to 6 hours off an on-board battery or via 12 V or 24 V power input (e.g., from a car battery)—see Fig. 22.1. The advantages of BCV in this setting are that it can be rapidly applied by staff with little training, and there is no need for intubation of the trachea (with the associated need for medications such as sedatives and muscle relaxants). Patients can receive ventilatory support while awake and able to interact with caregivers.

Another example of mass casualty event where BCV would be useful is in the management of multiple patients with crush injuries to the chest as may occur during an earthquake (see management of flail chest below). Early stabilization of the chest wall and ventilatory support could potentially save lives, as well as prevent complications such as nosocomial pneumonia in such patients.

22.3 Chest Injury

Blunt chest injury, with fracture/dislocation of one or more ribs and/or the sternum, carries significant morbidity and risk of mortality [5, 6], even for a single fractured rib [7]. The main causes of early morbidity and mortality in this setting are as follows:

Disruption of the mechanics of the chest wall, with reduced minute ventilation and functional residual capacity (FRC) and thus impaired ability to cough. This effect is especially seen with flail chest where a segment of the chest wall moves paradoxically during the respiratory cycle, due to disruption of continuity of several ribs at two points along their course.

Damage to underlying lung tissue, such as pulmonary contusion, which affects lung compliance and gas exchange.

Collection of fluid, air, or blood in the pleural space, interfering with lung expansion.

Disruption of elements of the tracheobronchial tree.

Pain, which can greatly impair deep inspiration and cough. This in turn impairs clearance of secretions, lung atelectasis, and the development of nosocomial chest infections. Of note, there is sometimes reluctance to apply a cuirass because of fear of causing pain to the patient. However, patients almost always report a reduction in pain once the cuirass is in place and continuous negative pressure (CNEP) is activated.

BCV has a number of important roles in preventing morbidity and mortality in the setting of blunt chest trauma as follows:

Early application of the cuirass and institution of CNEP causes expansion of the chest and lungs (improving FRC) and also stabilizes the chest wall, reducing paradoxical chest wall movement. This maneuver also significantly reduces pain in the chest wall as the ends of fractured ribs are distracted from each other. Less strong analgesics allows the patient to more effectively take part with their own rehabilitation, as well as avoiding common side-effects, such as sedation and constipation. Supplemental oxygen therapy can be given via nasal cannulae, facemask, or high-flow nasal cannulae (HFNC) as necessary.

A relative contra-indication to BCV in this setting is if the patient has undergone associated urgent laparotomy due to difficulties in applying the cuirass or if the patient has an associated head injury, with depressed LOC and poor airway protection. Aspiration of oro-pharyngeal and/or gastric contents will then be an ongoing risk.

With adequate analgesia and patient co-operation, oscillation and cough simulation may be added to aid clearance of chest secretions (sputum clearance mode).

If minute ventilation is inadequate, due to impaired lung or chest wall compliance, then intermittent or mandatory ventilation may be added to the CNEP and sputum clearance modes to add ventilatory support.

The alternative to this external splinting of the chest wall, ventilatory support, and sputum clearance is of course tracheal intubation and IPPV, so-called "internal splinting" of the chest. Because of the complexity and complications of this approach (use of sedatives and possibly muscle relaxants, blocking some of the natural defense mechanisms of the respiratory system such as coughing and sputum clearance, nosocomial chest infection), IPPV may be withheld until there is no choice but to intubate the patient—this may delay effective chest wall splinting, ventilatory support, and sputum clearance and increase the associated morbidity and mortality. The fact that such "splinting" is required for long periods of time also results in reluctance to initiate IPPV until late in the course of the episode.

It should be noted that there is a recent trend to surgical correction of the unstable chest wall after trauma [8], but that this approach is not without complications [9]. The authors contend that early use of a BCV device, together with adequate analgesia (with emphasis on regional chest blocks) and chest physiotherapy, is effective in most blunt chest injuries.

BCV use is relatively contra-indicated in the presence of a ruptured diaphragm and undrained pleural collections of air, fluid, and blood.

22.4 Head Injury

BCV has very little utility in the early management of head injury where there is a depressed LOC and impaired upper airway reflexes or where very precise control of PCO_2 is needed for the management of intracranial hypertension. However, after the acute phase, when the patient is recovering and entering the rehabilitation phase, then BCV may play a large part:

If there is *disordered central control of ventilation* due to the head injury involving the brainstem then a mode of ventilation using a BCV device which guarantees a minimum minute ventilation may be crucial to safely managing the patient in the long term.

A BCV device may be useful to aid *secretion clearance* and avoidance of nosocomial chest infection.

Night-time ventilatory support for when the patient is asleep and supine may also be provided by BCV if the FRC is marginal.

BCV allows for the management of the patient without use of sedative medications (such as may be needed to tolerate an endotracheal tube and IPPV), allowing the patient to eat, drink, and talk while receiving respiratory support and allowing the caregivers to assess the neurologic status of the patient. Such support can also be safely provided in a rehabilitation facility or at home by caregivers with a minimum amount of training.

22.5 Spinal Injury

In much the same way as in head injury, BCV has a limited role to play in the management of acute spinal injury. BCV may be a very useful treatment modality in such patients when they enter the rehabilitation phase of their injury.

Spinal injury affects respiration depending on the level of the injury. High cervical injury may result in phrenic nerve impairment, together with tetraplegia. This will affect function of the diaphragm as well as intercostal muscles and require full ventilatory support. If the phrenic nerves are preserved, but some/all of the intercostal nerves are affected then the patient may require variable levels of ventilatory support. The final level of injury does not reveal itself until months after the initial insult, with some recovery of function possible until years later. The better the initial resuscitation and early fixation of the spinal injury, the better the long-term outlook. During the initial phase the patient is usually managed with IPPV.

Later on, when the functional spinal level is more defined, then the degree of ventilatory support required can be better assessed. Such support provided by BCV allows the patient to eat, drink, and talk, unlike management via tracheostomy (where these are all much more difficult). BCV can also be used during weaning from IPPV, such that the patient may be on BCV for increasing lengths of time until free of IPPV. He/she may then progress to increasing period off BCV until free of ventilation during the day and only require BCV at night as a safety measure. In other words BCV may be used as a weaning tool.

There are more invasive means of dealing with complete phrenic nerve paralysis, such as diaphragmatic pacing, but this is expensive and has associated complications [10].

22.6 Conclusion

BCV has a very useful and defined role to play in the management of trauma patients.

References

1. Taghaddosinejad F, Fayyaz AF, Behnoush B. Pulmonary complications of mustard gas exposure: a study on cadavers. Acta Med Iran. 2011;49(4):233–6. PMID: 21713733.
2. Geraci MJ. Mustard gas: imminent danger or eminent threat? Ann Pharmacother. 2008;42(2):237–46. https://doi.org/10.1345/aph.1K445. Epub 2008 Jan 22. PMID: 18212254.
3. Eason MP. Sarin exposure: a simulation case scenario. South Med J. 2013;106(1):55–62. https://doi.org/10.1097/SMJ.0b013e31827cd12d. PMID: 23263315.
4. Lee EC. Clinical manifestations of sarin nerve gas exposure. JAMA. 2003;290(5):659–62. https://doi.org/10.1001/jama.290.5.659. PMID: 12902371.
5. Dogrul BN, Kiliccalan I, Asci ES, Peker SC. Blunt trauma related chest wall and pulmonary injuries: an overview. Chin J Traumatol. 2020;23(3):125–38. https://doi.org/10.1016/j.cjtee.2020.04.003. Epub 2020 Apr 20. PMID: 32417043; PMCID: PMC7296362.
6. Majercik S, Pieracci FM. Chest Wall trauma. Thorac Surg Clin. 2017;27(2):113–21. https://doi.org/10.1016/j.thorsurg.2017.01.004.
7. Kishawi SK, Ho VP, Bachman KC, Alvarado CE, Worrell SG, Argote-Greene LM, Linden PA, Towe CW. Are we underestimating the morbidity of single rib fractures? J Surg Res. 2021;268:174–80. https://doi.org/10.1016/j.jss.2021.06.048. Epub 2021 Jul 27. PMID: 34329822; PMCID: PMC8678162.
8. Slobogean GP, Kim H, Russell JP, Stockton DJ, Hsieh AH, O'Toole RV. Rib fracture fixation restores inspiratory volume and peak flow in a full thorax human cadaveric breathing model. Arch Trauma Res. 2015;4(4):e28018. https://doi.org/10.5812/atr.28018. PMID: 26848471; PMCID: PMC4733518.
9. Thiels CA, Aho JM, Naik ND, Zielinski MD, Schiller HJ, Morris DS, Kim BD. Infected hardware after surgical stabilization of rib fractures: outcomes and management experience. J Trauma Acute Care Surg. 2016;80(5):819–23. https://doi.org/10.1097/TA.0000000000001005. PMID: 26891160; PMCID: PMC4840052.
10. Monden KR, Coker J, Charlifue S, Bennett SJ, Draganich C, Coons D, Marino RJ, Berliner J. Long-term follow-up of patients with ventilator-dependent high tetraplegia managed with diaphragmatic pacing systems. Arch Phys Med Rehabil. 2022;103(4):773–8. https://doi.org/10.1016/j.apmr.2021.03.005. Epub 2021 Mar 22. PMID: 33766556.

Biphasic Cuirass Ventilation During Emergency Tracheal Intubation

23

Tony Zitek

23.1 Introduction

Although advances in the approach to airway management including the widespread use of video laryngoscopy [1] have increased the safety of rapid sequence intubation (RSI), a study from 2016 by Bodily et al. demonstrated that approximately 1 in 3 patients undergoing RSI experience oxygen desaturation [2]. Additionally, post-intubation cardiac arrest has been reported to occur in as many as 1 in 25 emergency intubations [3]. While recent data suggests that delayed sequence intubation (DSI) may offer a means to improve preoxygenation as compared to standard RSI [4], the act of paralyzing a patient to allow for the passage of an endotracheal tube, nonetheless, ceases the patient's respiration and puts them at risk for hypoxemia and worsening acidosis. Therefore, additional safety measures are warranted.

Biphasic cuirass ventilation (BCV) with the BCV device (Hayek Medical, London, United Kingdom) has been most extensively studied with regards to its use in treating respiratory failure from neuromuscular disorders [5–8]. However, the BCV device can and has been used to avoid intubation in patients with respiratory failure due to a variety of other conditions, including bronchiolitis [9, 10], pneumonia [9, 10], asthma [9, 10], congenital heart disease [11], and cystic fibrosis [12]. That being said, should a patient still require tracheal intubation despite a trial of BCV or should a patient not be a good candidate for a trial of BCV before intubation, the BCV device can still be used during emergency tracheal intubation to increase the safety of the procedure. Unfortunately, at this time, the published data to support this strategy are limited to a single case report [13].

This chapter will describe how the use of BCV during emergency tracheal intubation may be useful to prevent worsening hypoxemia and acidosis. This chapter

T. Zitek (✉)
Department of Emergency Medicine, The Permanente Medical Group, Modesto, CA, USA

O. Alibrahim et al. (eds.), *Biphasic Cuirass Noninvasive Ventilation*, Noninvasive Ventilation. The Essentials, https://doi.org/10.1007/978-3-032-20933-7_23

will also explain how to use the BCV device during emergency airway management and will discuss barriers to implementation.

23.2 Hypoxemic Respiratory Failure

A common indication for emergency tracheal intubation is hypoxemic respiratory failure. In general, patients who are intubated for hypoxemic respiratory failure have already been trialed on supplemental oxygen through a face mask (such as a non-rebreather), noninvasive positive pressure ventilation, high-flow nasal cannula, or BCV. These patients may be hypoxemic despite these noninvasive means of providing supplemental oxygen or they may be normoxemic with supplemental oxygen but expected to deteriorate. In either case, patients who are intubated for hypoxemic respiratory failure have an increased risk of developing worsening hypoxemia during RSI. In particular, one study reported that about 25% of patients undergoing RSI for hypoxemic respiratory failure develop an oxygen saturation of 83% or less during RSI [14]. Delayed sequence intubation (DSI) may reduce the incidence of hypoxemia during endotracheal intubation attempts by improving preoxygenation [4], but it does not provide more oxygen to patients after paralysis as compared to RSI.

One strategy that has been suggested to prevent desaturation during RSI is "apneic oxygenation," which is the administration of supplemental oxygen via nasal cannula during the apneic period of RSI [15]. While paralyzed and apneic, the patient can be given supplemental oxygen at 15 L/minute by a standard nasal cannula or up to 40 L/minute using a high-flow nasal cannula. Systematic reviews have reported that the use of apneic oxygenation during emergency intubation reduces the incidence of hypoxemia in both adults and children [16–18].

While apneic oxygenation is a useful tool to help prevent hypoxemia during emergency tracheal intubation, data also suggest that apneic oxygenation may not reduce the incidence of hypoxemia when a patient requires intubation specifically for respiratory failure [19]. In other words, apneic oxygenation seems to reduce the incidence of hypoxemia during emergency intubations for non-respiratory conditions, but it is not clear that apneic oxygenation provides a meaningful benefit to patients being intubated for respiratory failure. Perhaps the amount of oxygen transferred to the alveoli through apneic oxygenation is too small to be clinically significant if the patient is already having trouble oxygenating. Therefore, a new strategy to prevent hypoxemia during intubation of patients with respiratory failure is warranted.

The use of BCV during RSI may provide a solution to this problem. A BCV device in biphasic mode will use negative inspiratory pressure and positive expiratory pressure so that a patient's chest will rise and fall even while they are paralyzed. In addition to the BCV device, the patient can be placed on a nasal cannula (either standard or high flow). Functionally, the patient will then be receiving oxygen as they would for apneic oxygenation, but they would also be ventilated by the BCV device. This would likely prolong the time to desaturation substantially more than standard apneic oxygenation. However, there is, unfortunately, a lack of published data to support this strategy. The author of this chapter has used this strategy on several patients with success and has published one case report using this strategy [13]. Otherwise, no published data are available.

23.3 Severe Acidosis

Standard RSI is dangerous in patients who have severe acidosis because the apneic period of RSI could lead to worsening acidosis which may result in hemodynamic collapse or cardiac arrhythmia [20]. In fact, some sources specifically recommend avoiding intubation in patients with severe metabolic acidosis [21]. When intubation is necessary, some physicians may choose to avoid paralysis in patients with severe acidosis, which may help reduce the risk of worsening acidosis by allowing the patient to continue breathing during the intubation attempt. However, the use of sedatives without paralysis is associated with a substantially lower first-pass success rate as compared to RSI with paralytics [22], making this strategy less than ideal. Another strategy that has been suggested during the intubation attempt for patients with severe acidosis is to sedate and paralyze them (as is typical for RSI), but to also provide bag-valve mask ventilation during the apneic period, which appears to be safe [21, 23]. However, this strategy is limited by the fact that a patient cannot receive bag-valve mask ventilation while a laryngoscope is in their pharynx, so some worsening acidosis is still expected.

Therefore, new strategies for intubating severely acidotic patients are needed, and one such strategy is using BCV during the intubation attempt. If the BCV device is attached to the patient and turned on to the biphasic mode, the patient can be ventilated while they are paralyzed. To the author's knowledge, BCV use during intubation is the only strategy that can ventilate a paralyzed patient while the clinician is actively trying to intubate the patient with a laryngoscope in the patient's pharynx. The patient can potentially have the benefit of allowing the clinician a higher chance of first-pass success (through paralysis) while minimizing the drop in pH (through continued ventilation). Unfortunately, as mentioned before, only one case report has been published describing the use of BCV during tracheal intubation [13], so the benefits of BCV in this regard are largely theoretical at this point.

23.4 Other Difficult Intubations

While hypoxemic respiratory failure and severe acidosis were specifically mentioned as indications for use of the BCV device during tracheal intubation, BCV could be used to assist with nearly all intubations, both expected easy and expected difficult. The ability of the BCV device plus a nasal cannula to both oxygenate and ventilate a paralyzed patient should theoretically make almost all intubations safer. For example, currently, apneic oxygenation might be used to avoid hypoxemia in a patient being intubated for a depressed mental status due to an intracranial hemorrhage. While the data discussed above suggest that the use of apneic oxygenation in such a patient reduces the chances of hypoxemia during the intubation attempt, it is likely that the use of the BCV device plus a nasal cannula would further reduce the chances of hypoxemia.

The only case report that has been published about the use of the BCV device during intubation described a patient for whom a reliable pulse oximetry could not be obtained [13]. Tracheal intubation without a pulse oximeter is very dangerous, as a patient could be critically hypoxemic and the clinicians may not know. By providing oxygenation through the combination of the BCV device and a nasal cannula, the team caring for the patient described in the case report felt they made a dangerous situation safer.

23.5 How to Use BCV During Emergency Intubation

The use of the BCV device during emergency tracheal intubation is straightforward. First, place the patient on a nasal cannula (standard or high flow) during the preoxygenation period. It is likely that a high-flow nasal cannula will provide the best oxygenation for this procedure, so consider using that, if available. If a standard nasal cannula is used, the patient should also be preoxygenated with another device, such as a non-rebreather face mask or noninvasive positive pressure ventilation. For teenagers and adults, turn the flow rate on the nasal cannula to 15 L/minute (standard) or 40 L/minute (high flow). For a young child this can be reduced to 5–10 L/minute.

Next, place the BCV device (if not already on) over the patient's chest and connect the tubing to the respirator. Make sure to choose the correct shell size (12 different sizes are available). The appropriate setup of the BCV device for a patient with a standard nasal cannula is shown in Fig. 23.1. After the shell is on the patient, set the respirator to the negative pressure mode at −20 cm H_2O, which ensures the shell has a tight seal on the chest wall. Once a tight seal has been confirmed, strap

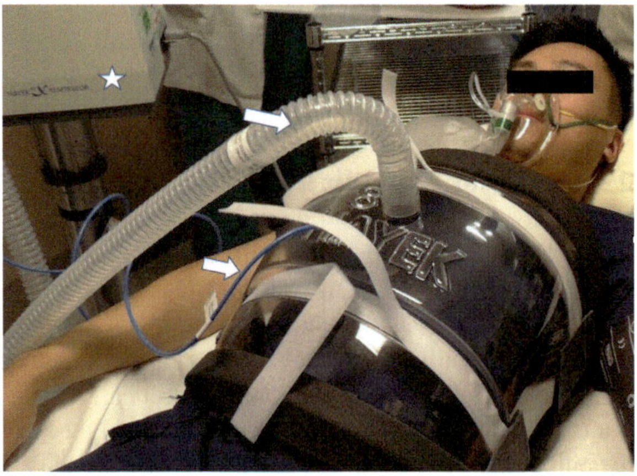

Fig. 23.1 A patient with a non-rebreather face mask over a standard nasal cannula with an end-tidal CO_2 detector. The plastic shell for the BCV device is placed over the patient's chest. The shell is connected to the respirator (star) by two tubes (arrows)—the clear wide bore tube and the blue cuirass sensor tube

the shell in place. Then, switch the BCV device to the biphasic ("control") mode. The settings for optimal ventilation will vary, but a reasonable starting point is an inspiratory pressure of −25 cc H_2O, an expiratory pressure of +5 cm H_2O, and a respiratory rate of 20.

The BCV device and a nasal cannula should be left in place throughout the entirety of the intubation and can be discontinued once the correct location of the endotracheal tube has been confirmed.

23.6 Barriers to Implementation

Currently, the primary barrier to the use of BCV to assist with tracheal intubation is the lack of availability of the BCV device in most hospitals. Secondly, most emergency medicine and critical care physicians do not know how to use the BCV device, but, as described above, the application of the device is simple. In a hospital that the author of this chapter worked at that had access to a BCV device; an additional barrier to use of the BCV device during intubation was the perceived length of time it would take to set up the device. However, the time required to set up the BCV device is expected to be only a few minutes.

If a patient is in cardiac arrest, the BCV device should not be used since the shell will impede chest compressions. Otherwise, there are no known absolute contraindications to the use of BCV during tracheal intubation, but the BCV device will inhibit clinicians from accessing the chest wall. Therefore, if a procedure requiring access to the chest wall is imminent (such as chest tube placement, pericardiocentesis, and electrical cardioversion), then it may be best not to use the BCV device during emergency airway management.

23.7 Conclusion

The BCV device can be used during emergency tracheal intubation to improve oxygenation and ventilation of the patient while they are paralyzed. Although this technique shows promise, currently, no research studies and only one case report have been published about this technique so far.

References

1. Lewis SR, Butler AR, Parker J, Cook TM, Smith AF. Videolaryngoscopy versus direct laryngoscopy for adult patients requiring tracheal intubation. Cochrane Database Syst Rev. 2016;11(11):CD011136. https://doi.org/10.1002/14651858.CD011136.pub2.
2. Bodily J, Webb H, Weiss S, Braude D. Incidence and duration of continuously measured oxygen desaturation during emergency department intubation. Ann Emerg Med. 2016;67:389–95.
3. Heffner AC, Swords DS, Neale MN, Jones AE. Incidence and factors associated with cardiac arrest complicating emergency airway management. Resuscitation. 2013;84:1500–4.

4. Bandyopadhyay A, Kumar P, Jafra A, Thakur H, Yaddanapudi LN, Jain K. Peri-intubation hypoxia after delayed versus rapid sequence intubation in critically injured patients on arrival to trauma triage: a randomized controlled trial. Anesth Analg. 2023;136(5):913–9.
5. Almeda M, Puranik S, Felker M, Daftary AS. Biphasic cuirass ventilation in a patient with congenital myotonic dystrophy. Am J Respir Crit Care Med. 2020;201:15–20.
6. Braun SR, Sufit RL, Giovannoni R, O'Connor M, Peters H. Intermittent negative pressure ventilation in the treatment of respiratory failure in progressive neuromuscular disease. Neurology. 1987;37:1874.
7. Corrado A, Gorini M, De Paola E. Alternative techniques for managing acute neuromuscular respiratory failure. Skull Base. 1995;15:84–9.
8. Imitazione P, Annunziata A, Lanza M, Fiorentino G. Combined high flow nasal cannula and negative pressure ventilation as a novel respiratory approach in a patient with acute respiratory failure and limb-girdle muscular dystrophy. Acta Myol. 2021;40:101–4.
9. Nunez CA, Hassinger AB. Predictors of negative pressure ventilation response in pediatric acute respiratory failure. Respir Care. 2020;65(1):91–8. https://doi.org/10.4187/respcare.07020.
10. Hasinger AB, Breuer RK, Nutty K, Ma CX, Al Ibrahim OS. Negative-pressure ventilation in pediatric acute respiratory failure. Respir Care. 2017;62(12):1540–9. https://doi.org/10.4187/respcare.05531.
11. Shime N, Toida C, Itoi T, Hashimoto S. Continuous negative extrathoracic pressure in children after congenital heart surgery. Crit Care Resusc. 2006;8(4):297–301.
12. Onweni C, Rashid S, Goswami R, Treece J, Shipley LC, et al. Cuirass ventilation: an alternative home-based modality for chronic respiratory failure. Home Health Care Manag Pract. 2020;32(1):40–4.
13. Zitek T, Berkeley RP, Hodnick R, Davis K, Dado N, Slattery DE. A novel technique to intubate patients without reliable pulse oximetry. Am J Emerg Med. 2018;36(11):2131.e1–2.
14. McKown AC, Casey JD, Russell DW, Joffe AM, Janz DR, Rice TW, Semler MW. Risk factors for and prediction of hypoxemia during tracheal intubation of critically ill adults. Ann Am Thorac Soc. 2018;15(11):1320–7. https://doi.org/10.1513/AnnalsATS.201802-118OC.
15. Weingart SD, Levitan RM. Preoxygenation and prevention of desaturation during emergency airway management. Ann Emerg Med. 2012;59(3):165–75.e1.
16. Pavlov I, Medrano S, Weingart S. Apneic oxygenation reduces the incidence of hypoxemia during emergency intubation: a systematic review and meta-analysis. Am J Emerg Med. 2017;35(8):1184–9. https://doi.org/10.1016/j.ajem.2017.06.029.
17. Binks MJ, et al. Apnoeic oxygenation during intubation in the intensive care unit: a systematic review and meta-analysis. Heart Lung. 2017;46(6):452–7. https://doi.org/10.1016/j.hrtlng.2017.08.001.
18. George S, Wilson M, Humphreys S, Gibbons K, Long E, Schibler A. Apnoeic oxygenation during paediatric intubation: a systematic review. Front Pediatr. 2022;10:918148. https://doi.org/10.3389/fped.2022.918148. eCollection 2022.
19. White LD, Melhuish TM, White LK, et al. Apnoeic oxygenation during intubation: a systematic review and meta-analysis. Anaesth Intensive Care. 2017;45(1):21–7.
20. Manthous CA. Avoiding circulatory complications during endotra- cheal intubation and initiation of positive pressure ventilation. J Emerg Med. 2010;38:622–31.
21. Lentz S, Grossman A, Koyfman A, Long B. High-risk airway management in the emergency department. Part I: diseases and approaches. J Emerg Med. 2020;59(1):84–95. https://doi.org/10.1016/j.jemermed.2020.05.008.
22. Brown CA, Bair AE, Pallin DJ, Walls RM. Techniques, success, and adverse events of emergency department adult intubations. Ann Emerg Med. 2015;65:363–3701.
23. Casey JD, Janz DR, Russell DW, et al. Bag-mask ventilation during tracheal intubation of critically ill adults. N Engl J Med. 2019;380:811–21.

BCV: Ventilation During Anesthesia in Ear Nose and Throat (ENT) Procedures

24

Abhijit S. Nair and Ashok Lal

24.1 Introduction

Biphasic Cuirass Ventilation (BCV) is a non-invasive ventilation technique that uses a cuirass, or shell-like device, to facilitate ventilation. The approach differs from more traditional methods of positive pressure ventilation, which usually requires airway adjuncts and intubation. BCV utilizes the negative pressure ventilation method used in the iron lung ventilation that was used during the polio pandemic. However, unlike iron lung ventilation, BCV offers better control of both the inspiration and expiration [1, 2]. As the gases are not forced into the lungs by positive pressure, the chances of barotrauma and volutrauma are less with BCV. Also, as airway adjuncts like the endotracheal tube are not required, various airway injuries and ventilator-associated pneumonia are lesser [3–5].

Patients with impeded respiratory function may benefit from preoperative BCV use. It is a beneficial modality for improving lung function before surgery, particularly for people who have obesity, neuromuscular disorders, or chronic obstructive pulmonary disease (COPD). Because BCV is non-invasive, patients can comply with treatment more easily and feel more comfortable, which makes it a useful choice for preoperative respiratory support and optimization. BCV can also facilitate weaning when used postoperatively after cardiothoracic surgeries and in patients who have barotrauma and positive pressure ventilation is not feasible [6, 7].

A. S. Nair (✉) · A. Lal
Department of Anesthesiology, Ibra Hospital, Ibra, Sultanate of Oman
e-mail: ashock.lal@moh.om

O. Alibrahim et al. (eds.), *Biphasic Cuirass Noninvasive Ventilation*, Noninvasive Ventilation. The Essentials, https://doi.org/10.1007/978-3-032-20933-7_24

24.2 BCV in the Ear, Nose, Throat (ENT), and Airway Surgeries

The nature of the surgical field makes ventilation a major challenge for ENT and airway surgeries. The anesthesiologists need to share the airway with the surgeons. The airway may become obstructed or compromised by procedures involving the larynx, trachea, or nasal cavity, which may make conventional positive pressure ventilation challenging. Endotracheal tubes and other airway devices are more challenging to use for these surgeries because continuous access to the airway is frequently required [8–10]. Due to its unconventional ventilatory characteristics, BCV is particularly beneficial in various surgeries like micro-laryngeal surgeries and tracheal surgeries.

24.3 Initial Use of BCV for Airway Surgeries (Hayek Oscillator)

Dr. Zamir Hayek developed the non-invasive, high-frequency Hayek Oscillator chest ventilator. It is particularly useful for paticnts with chronic respiratory failure, during anesthesia for various airway surgeries, and in critical care areas because it regulates both respiratory cycle phases. To preserve functional residual capacity and enhance gas exchange, the device oscillates around a baseline of negative pressure. This strategy eliminates the need for endotracheal intubation, making it useful in various clinical settings, including micro-laryngeal surgery. Earlier, the entire machinery was bulky and cumbersome to use. However, the present equipment is portable and less space-occupying [11, 12].

Twenty-five patients (nine women and sixteen men), between the ages of 25 and 75, weighing 52 and 105 kg, all requiring an upper airway endoscopy, were recruited in the study by Dilkes et al. [13]. BCV was administered during the procedure. After suxamethonium and propofol were used to induce anesthesia, a nasal airway was placed, and a baseline $ETCO_2$ was recorded. After the procedure was completed, the ensuing $ETCO_2$ was obtained. The various indications for which endoscopy was performed were different vocal cord pathologies like polyps, nodules, edema, suspected malignancy, and hemangiomas. The authors used the following settings for BCV: frequency of 30–300 CPM, cuirass inspiratory pressures of −15 to −30 cm H_2O, cuirass expiratory pressures of +5 to +12 cm H_2O, and inspiratory-expiratory ratio 1:1 to 1:3. All the procedures were uneventful with the only complication being epistaxis which was due to insertion of the nasal airway.

Monks et al. (1995) also successfully used a Hayek oscillator in 41 patients undergoing micro-laryngeal surgery, without using an endotracheal tube [14]. The settings used by the authors were as follows. The initial settings were a rate of 90 cycles/min, an inspiratory pressure of −24 cm of water, an expiratory pressure of +10 cm of water, and an I: E ratio of 1:1, and a change in the respiratory rate as necessary. The airway was managed with mask ventilation till the scope was introduced by the surgeons for the micro-laryngeal surgery. Broomhead et al. described using the Hayek oscillator in a patient with a difficult airway, whose airway management was even impossible with a fiberoptic bronchoscope, based on the nasal endoscopy findings of a large mass at the epiglottis that occluded the airway [15]. General anesthesia was induced with propofol and atracurium, and lungs were ventilated manually till the Hayek oscillator was initiated. The 40-minute surgery involving debulking of the tumor was uneventful.

24.4 The Present BCV Equipment

Over the years, the machines providing BCV have improved significantly in terms of portability and various features, thus facilitating its use in various acute and chronic conditions, including airway surgeries. The present BCV machines are easy to operate, fully computerized, and easy to set up. The various modes available are continuous negative, mandatory controlled ventilation, ventilatory synchronized, and secretion clearance. Currently, four adult-sized and seven pediatric cuirass are available for BCV [16].

24.5 Anesthesia Management Using a BCV

The method by which cuirass ventilation operates is by covering the upper abdomen and anterior chest with an airtight seal using a cuirass. Applying alternately positive and negative pressure inside the cuirass allows for ventilation. Thus, ventilation can occur without the need for a jet ventilation device in the airway, a supraglottic airway, or a tracheal tube. The ability to perform surgery on the larynx and trachea without time constraints or the risk of developing hypercapnia from apneic techniques is a significant benefit of cuirass ventilation. The patient selection for BCV in airway surgery is very important. A few indications are narrow tracheal lumens due to disease and securing the airway is impossible, prolonged surgery, history of previous airway surgeries in which there was a need for repeated intubations to facilitate surgery. After connecting essential monitors like non-invasive blood pressure monitoring cuff, electrocardiography, and pulse-oximeter, anesthesia is induced with an opioid like fentanyl/sufentanil, an induction agent like propofol, and neuromuscular blockade is achieved with either suxamethonium initially followed by a long-acting non-depolarizing neuromuscular blocker like atracurium, cisatracurium, or rocuronium. Oxygen insufflation is done using a facemask or by using a high-flow nasal oxygenation (HFNO) and simultaneously the BCV is initiated. General anesthesia needs to be maintained with a propofol target-controlled infusion with Bispectral Index (BIS) monitoring, targeted to a BIS ranging 50–60. A target-controlled infusion (TCI) of remifentanil also can be used or boluses of fentanyl can be administered, at the discretion of the attending anesthesiologist. The airway is kept open with a suspension laryngoscope for the duration of the proposed surgery. This provides uninterrupted access to the surgeon for the airway surgery. At the end of the surgery, BCV is terminated, neuromuscular blockade is reversed, and, thereafter, the patient breathes spontaneously. Monitoring carbon dioxide (CO_2) is challenging as end-tidal carbon dioxide ($ETCO_2$) monitoring, which is considered a standard of care for general anesthesia, is not possible. In such situations, the use of transcutaneous CO_2 monitoring is ideal and recommended. The other option is serial arterial blood gas (ABG) analysis which needs an arterial line. It is not only cumbersome, but also costly, and does not provide the results immediately. Postoperatively, the patients need to be monitored either in a high-dependency unit or an intensive care unit (ICU) for vital parameters, especially respiratory events like desaturation, stridor, or any cardiovascular event [17, 18].

When BCV is used for surgeries like biopsies and minimal resections, a tracheostomy can be avoided, which otherwise is a requirement either because the airway cannot be secured with a definitive airway, or might be necessary postoperatively due to edema as a result of airway instrumentation, thereby causing respiratory distress and hypoxemia.

Kristensen et al. reported their experience of 14 airway surgeries which were performed using BCV [18]. They selected the cases based on the nature of the airway when securing it with a definitive airway was impossible. The patients also were the ones who had previous airway surgeries, and an endotracheal tube was placed and was subjected to repeated extubation and intubations, intraoperatively, causing morbidity. Another criterion was when the expected surgical time was supposed to be long. Based on the report, all the cases were successfully managed with meticulous selection, planning, and perioperative management.

24.6 Case Series

Mori et al. used BCV in a series of 3 patients undergoing tracheobronchial stenting [19]. BCV was useful for assisting spontaneous breathing during tracheobronchial stenting procedures, where positive pressure ventilation was not possible. In all three cases, the authors did not experience severe respiratory acidosis or hypoxemia. The operations were completed without requiring ECMO during the interventions.

Nishiyama et al. reported successful use of BCV in an infant requiring ventilation for persistent atelectasis [20]. Initially, a nasal NIV was initiated but was unsuccessful due to a poorly fitting mask and also subsequent skin ulceration due to the nasal mask. The authors used BCV using a Respiratory Therapy External (RTX; Medivent, London, UK) device. With the initial use of BCV, the infant improved. However, after 4 weeks, positive pressure ventilation using an airway pressure release ventilation mode was initiated due to bronchiolitis. Subsequently, BCV was reinitiated and the child was nursed over BCV over 6 weeks, after which the infant was successfully weaned and discharged.

To treat a COVID-19 pneumonia patient who needed prolonged NIV and developed face mask intolerance, ventilator dependency due to residual lung fibrosis, and respiratory muscular weakness, Borges and Esquinas reported a case combining BCV with HFNO [21]. The authors suggested that BCV is a safe and effective non-invasive technique for weaning from prolonged NIV support.

Clinkscales et al. reported the use of BCV in a patient with head and neck malignancy who required radiotherapy [22]. After the first 5 treatment sessions of radiation, the patient was not able to lie supine. After a multidisciplinary approach, it was decided to use BCV for all his subsequent radiation sessions. The authors mentioned that although the entire process of setting up the BCV was time-consuming, it was still worth doing it as it helped the patient receive the necessary treatment for the underlying malignancy.

24.7 Limitations of Using BCV in Airway Surgeries

The combination of cuirass ventilation and airway surgery has certain limitations. Since it is impossible to measure the ventilatory minute volume directly during surgery, transcutaneous CO_2 measurement or frequent arterial blood gas samples must be used. Before inserting the suspension laryngoscope, a baseline measurement of the minute volume of cuirass ventilation can be made using a face mask or a supraglottic airway device. Every open-airway technique has a monitoring ventilation challenge. Placing the suspension laryngoscope requires special preparation due to the cuirass's position above the front surface of the thorax. The function of cuirass ventilation in conjunction with airway surgery in patients who are morbidly obese has not been explored to date. Not every patient undergoing airway surgery is a good fit for BCV. The safety and effectiveness of this ventilation technique depend on the careful selection of patients. Patients who require high levels of positive end-expiratory pressure (PEEP), have open wounds, or have severe chest wall deformities might not be the most suitable candidates for BCV. BCV use necessitates specific tools and learning. The surgical team must collaborate closely together to ensure smooth integration with the surgical procedure, and anesthesia providers need to be conversant about the monitoring and operation of BCV systems. Widespread adoption of BCV equipment may be hampered by the limited availability of the equipment in some healthcare settings.

24.8 Conclusions

For ENT and airway surgeries, BCV provides a useful substitute for conventional ventilation techniques. The ability to deliver non-invasive ventilation while preserving an open surgical field improves surgical results, lowers complications after surgery, and increases patient safety. However, careful patient selection, specialized training, and close teamwork within the surgical team are necessary for the successful implementation of BCV in these surgical contexts. The use of transcutaneous CO_2 monitoring is recommended with the use of BCV for airway surgeries. With new opportunities to enhance patient care and surgical results, BCV is expected to become increasingly important in the management of complex airway surgeries.

References

1. Meyer JA. A practical mechanical respirator, 1929: the "iron lung". Ann Thorac Surg. 1990;50(3):490–3. https://doi.org/10.1016/0003-4975(90)90508-4.
2. Braun NMT. Negative pressure noninvasive ventilation (NPNIV): history, rationale, and application. Nocturnal Non-Invasive Ventilation. 2015:27–71. Published 2015 Oct 1. https://doi.org/10.1007/978-1-4899-7624-6_2.
3. Yamashita T, Taniwaki Y, Takayama H, Sakamoto Y. Efficacy of biphasic cuirass ventilation in the critical care department. Crit Care. 2012;16(Suppl 1):P132. https://doi.org/10.1186/cc10739.
4. Linton DM. Cuirass ventilation: a review and update. Crit Care Resusc. 2005;7(1):22–8.
5. Onweni C, Rashid S, Goswami R, Treece J, Shipley LC, De Souza R, et al. Cuirass ventilation: an alternative home-based modality for chronic respiratory failure. Home Health Care Manag Pract. 2020;32(1):40–4.
6. McBride WT, Ranaldi G, Dougherty MJ, et al. The hemodynamic and respiratory effects of continuous negative and control mode cuirass ventilation in recently extubated cardiac surgery patients: part 2. J Cardiothorac Vasc Anesth. 2012;26:873–7.
7. Hino H, Suzuki Y, Ishii E, Fukuda M. Biphasic cuirass ventilation for treatment of an air leak after pneumothorax in a patient with nemaline myopathy: a case report. J Anesth. 2016;30:1087–90.
8. Li LT, Chitilian HV, Alfille PH, Bao X. Airway management and anesthesia for airway surgery: a narrative review. Transl Lung Cancer Res. 2021;10(12):4631–42. https://doi.org/10.21037/tlcr-21-917.
9. Prust RS, Calkins JM. Considerations for managing the airway in the ENT patient. Contemp Anesth Pract. 1987;9:49–72.
10. Patel A. The shared airway. Curr Anaesth Crit Care. 2001;12(4):213–7.
11. Hardinge FM, Davies RJ, Stradling JR. Effects of short term high frequency negative pressure ventilation on gas exchange using the Hayek oscillator in normal subjects. Thorax. 1995;50(1):44–9. https://doi.org/10.1136/thx.50.1.44.
12. Eyal FG, Gur I, O'Donnell KT, Hamm CR. Efficacy of noninvasive biphasic cuirass ventilation in neonates: comparison with invasive positive pressure ventilation. Chest. 2008;134(4):7S.
13. Dilkes MG, McNeill JM, Hill AC, Monks PS, McKelvie P, Hollamby RG. The Hayek oscillator: a new method of ventilation in microlaryngeal surgery. Ann Otol Rhinol Laryngol. 1993;102(6):455–8. https://doi.org/10.1177/000348949310200609.
14. Monks PS, Broomhead CJ, Dilkes MG, McKelvie P. The use of the Hayek oscillator during microlaryngeal surgery. Anaesthesia. 1995;50(10):865–9. https://doi.org/10.1111/j.1365-2044.1995.tb05853.x.
15. Broomhead CJ, Dilkes MG, Monks PS. Use of the Hayek oscillator in a case of failed fibreoptic intubation. Br J Anaesth. 1995;74:720–1.
16. Available from: https://www.hayekmedical.com/oldsite8322/archives/product/hayek-rtx. Last accessed on 31st Aug 2024.
17. Kristensen MS, Hesselfeldt R, Schmidt JF. Improvements in cuirass ventilation for airway surgery: origins in Copenhagen on the 70th anniversary of the first intensive care unit. Br J Anaesth. 2023;131(4):644–8. https://doi.org/10.1016/j.bja.2023.07.021.
18. Kristensen MS, Hesselfeldt R, Schmidt JF. Modern cuirass ventilation for airway surgery: unlimited access to the larynx and trachea in anaesthetised patients. Br J Anaesth. 2023;131:e106e9.
19. Mori H, Shono A, Hirade R, Nikai T, Saito Y. Biphasic cuirass ventilation during anesthesia for tracheobronchial stent insertion or removal by a rigid bronchoscope: a case report. A A Pract. 2018;10(8):198–200. https://doi.org/10.1213/XAA.0000000000000660.
20. Nishiyama K, Komori M, Sato T, Kondo I, Suzuki Y, Kominami H, Tsukamoto K, Kawamata M. Biphasic cuirass ventilation in an infant with severe respiratory failure. J Anesth. 2009;23(1):166–7. https://doi.org/10.1007/s00540-008-0675-6.

21. Almeida Borges J, Esquinas AM. Biphasic cuirass ventilation in the escalation of non-invasive ventilation in COVID-19: case report and review. Monaldi Arch Chest Dis. 2023;93(4) https://doi.org/10.4081/monaldi.2023.2510.
22. Clinkscales W, Spence M, Gleysteen J, Hayes N, Izaguirre E, Wakefield D, et al. Novel use of biphasic cuirass ventilation during definitive radiation therapy: a technical report. Pract Radiat Oncol. 2021;11(3):e276–81. https://doi.org/10.1016/j.prro.2020.08.003.

Biphasic Cuirass Non-invasive Ventilation (BCV) Outside ENT Anaesthesia

25

Preethi Thomas, Praburam Selvaraj, Marzooq Aslam, Anas N. Shallik, and Nabil A. Shallik

25.1 Introduction

Biphasic Cuirass Ventilation (BCV) is an artificial ventilation technique that uses negative pressure to the thorax and upper abdomen with a tight-fitting device referred to as a cuirass. This creates negative intrathoracic and alveolar pressure, allowing the patient to spontaneously aspirate air from the upper respiratory airways, which facilitates oxygenation and carbon dioxide removal.

BCV is the modern application of the iron lung, which provided artificial ventilation for many patients in the polio epidemic. It is a physiological form of artificial ventilation with some benefits for long-term patient ventilation in that it does not require sedation, upper airway manipulation, or paralysis of the muscles. Once the patient is on BCV, he or she can be programmed in assist mode on the negative pressure ventilator to maintain respiratory muscle strength, even with prolonged ventilation (Fig. 25.1a, b).

P. Thomas · P. Selvaraj · M. Aslam
Department of Anaesthesia and Perioperative Medicine, Hamad Medical Corporation, Doha, Qatar
e-mail: pthomas@hamad.qa; PSelvaraj2@hamad.qa; Maslam@hamad.qa

A. N. Shallik
Royal College of Surgeons in Ireland Medical University of Bahrain, Manamah, Bahrain

N. A. Shallik (✉)
Department of Anaesthesia and Perioperative Medicine, Hamad Medical Corporation, Doha, Qatar

Clinical Anaesthesiology Department, Weill Cornell Medical College in Qatar, Doha, Qatar

Clinical Anaesthesiology Department, College of Medicine, Qatar University, Doha, Qatar
e-mail: nshallik@hamad.qa

O. Alibrahim et al. (eds.), *Biphasic Cuirass Noninvasive Ventilation*, Noninvasive Ventilation. The Essentials, https://doi.org/10.1007/978-3-032-20933-7_25

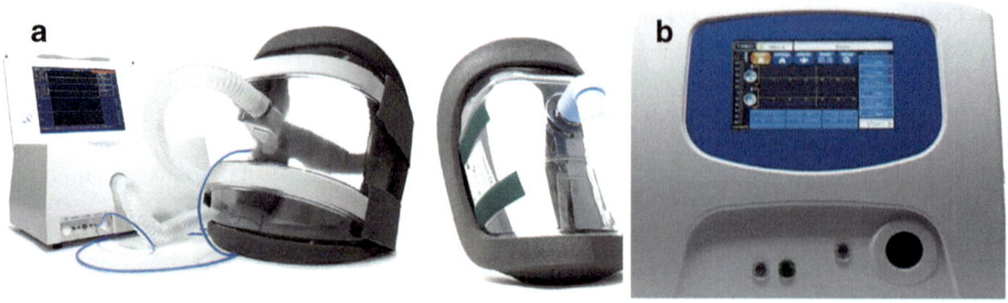

Fig. 25.1 (**a**, **b**) Biphasic Cuirass Ventilator machines from two Different Companies. BCV is gaining popularity as a technique for tubeless anaesthesia in upper airway tumour resection surgery instead of using endotracheal intubation. This gives the surgeon an entire and unobstructed view of the supraglottic, glottic, and laryngeal areas and enables them to perform tumour resection and provide proper haemostasis of the area [1]

25.1.1 Physiology

BCV comes with an external, transparent plastic shell, having cushioned edges, that provides a tongue-like seal over the chest. It has a wide-bore port for attaching tubing that connects to the cuirass ventilator. The device generates negative pressure assistance for a naturally aspirated tidal volume, alternating with minimal preset positive pressure to aid physiological elastic recoil during expiration. Thus, BCV can replicate respiration perfectly with control of both respiratory phases. BCV is an effective and non-invasive mode of ventilation in patients with neuromuscular disorders and difficult airways. BCV offers a physiological negative pressure mode of ventilation, creating the competent tidal volumes necessary for effective ventilation and adequate respiratory rates. BCV encourages respiratory muscle strength and cardiac output, and, hence, is successful in weaning from artificial ventilation dependence. Since there are complications and effects of the invasive nature of positive pressure ventilation, BCV offers a safe and effective mode of ventilation for long-term artificial ventilation.

There is no requirement for airway intervention equipment, unless aspiration is present, in which oxygenation may be provided by supplemental oxygen through a face mask, high-flow nasal oxygen, or other suitable means. Monitoring should be done routinely as per the American Society of Anaesthesiologists (ASA) requirements, and transcutaneous CO_2 monitoring should be done to ensure proper CO_2 washout.

25.1.2 General Considerations

Although BCV is primarily indicated for critical care, it is being performed off the ventilator for anaesthetic ventilation. The ventilation with BCV is close to normal, with evidence on record of adequate gas exchange without external airway intervention, particularly for airway surgeries that do not require intubation and/or airway devices. The potential for such a ventilation method provides a lot of safety, and the oxygenation and ventilation aspect does not require gas or volume monitoring, allowing for transcutaneous CO_2 measurement to assess the adequacy of ventilation.

When BCV is a mode of artificial ventilation during anaesthesia for non-airway surgery, there are specific considerations as follows.

Type of Anaesthesia: BCV needs no airway intervention, since gas exchange is through an open upper airway. In the absence of a good seal, gas anaesthesia usage is also compromised. Therefore, total intravenous anaesthesia (TIVA) is the ideal technique, with depth of anaesthesia monitoring, along with standard ASA monitoring and transcutaneous CO_2 measurement.

Type of Surgery: BCV can safely be performed in the context of extremity surgery, endoscopic urology, and GI endoscopies, among others [1].

Airway Equipment: BCV will not necessitate the use of airway equipment, but if the level of anaesthesia is sufficient, supraglottic airway devices may be utilized. This allows for the administration of an anaesthetic workstation and taking further volume counts utilizing gas anaesthesia to a certain extent.

Space Requirements: BCV will require adequate space for the cuirass shell and the implementation of the ventilatory assist device.

Noise Pollution and Chest Movement: Operation of the BCV devices will generate some noise and cause heightened chest movement, which may be a concern in specific operating room settings.

Microsurgery: BCV can be safely used in microsurgery when minimal airway manipulation is indicated.

Intraoperative Fluoroscopy: BCV does not interfere with intraoperative fluoroscopy. The handle of the BCV device does not interfere with fluoroscopy.

Patient Positioning: Adequate patient positioning is mandatory for the achievement of effective ventilation with BCV and patient comfort.

25.2 Using BCV in Non-ENT Anaesthesia

25.2.1 BCV Paediatric Use

BCV has been used almost exclusively within a paediatric population. It should be noted that Dr. Hayek's first case series involved only the paediatric age group, and the plastic shell is available in all sizes to accommodate children and adults. No airway intervention is required, which helps avoid airway complications in paediatric patients undergoing general anaesthesia procedures. BCV permits natural physiological ventilation even with a deeper plane of sedation during procedures in a state of sedation [2].

25.2.2 Radiotherapy

BCV was effectively and safely utilized in repeated radiotherapeutic interventions for a patient who needed radiation therapy for oropharyngeal malignancy and experienced significant intolerance to the supine position caused by comorbid OSA and idiopathic hemi-diaphragmatic eventration. The setup at treatment on a daily basis is challenging, but may be one of the options in the management of patients intolerant to treatment positioning during radiation therapy and tracheostomy alternatives [3].

25.2.3 Resuscitation

A recent article highlighted the need to have cuirass ventilation devices on hand to deliver emergency respiratory assistance by first responder teams that are not trained to provide immediate medical intervention, even if they are in full protective anti-chemical suits. This type of ventilation assistance is valuable during a mass casualty situation, like a nerve agent attack, where time is of the essence and resources will most probably be scarce.

During an emergency, the goal is to save a life by providing respiratory support as soon as possible, thereby enabling the individual to obtain sufficient oxygen. Most practices would require advanced, prompt airway management interventions, starting with laryngoscopy, intubation, and positive pressure ventilation for reversing muscle paralysis. However, the practical usefulness of the procedures will be influenced by the turbulent environment, multiple patient requirements, and the level of inadequate training and practice.

This cuirass ventilation method provides a new option that does not require additional advanced airway procedures, such as intubation, but ventilates for you and clears secretions—a very useful feature of airway management in victims of nerve agent exposure.

With the simplicity of training and use, it is a practical addition to the first responders' arsenal. If done early in the most severe emergencies, it could improve the outcome of such patients and assist in reaching the goal of greater pre-treatment survival [4].

25.2.4 Emergency Department (ED)

BCV has been applied effectively in the emergency department from the time of patient arrival, during the course of preoxygenation in rapid sequence induction, and can be finished without pause to allow intubation. In patients who are expected to have a difficult intubation, if not possible to perform awake fiberscopic intubation, adequate oxygenation is still possible by breathing through a bag-valve-mask (BVM) device.

As soon as a patient is totally paralyzed with neuromuscular blocking drugs (NMBDs), the support can be switched from passive BCV when the patient remains awake to complete active BCV after the NMBD takes effect.

Patients will also desaturate during anaesthetic intubation if they have unrecognized underlying pulmonary pathology. This situation can be prevented by employing BCV [5].

25.2.5 Critical Care

BCV was also used in the treatment of COVID-19 patients who needed long-term non-invasive ventilation (NIV) and became dependent on neck masks with resultant mask intolerance because of severe and residual lung fibrosis and respiratory muscle weakness. The innovation of applying BCV and high-flow nasal oxygenation (HFNO) to decrease the burden of therapy non-invasively and enhance outcomes from extended NIV was a historic synergy, and it was a novel ventilation approach to reduce endotracheal tube dependence in COVID-19 patients who were ventilator-dependent [6].

Using the Hayek Oscillator in a Case of Failed Fiberoptic Intubation: A recent article describes how the Hayek Oscillator, as a form of BCV, was utilized in a challenging intubation scenario. The patient underwent LASER debulking of a pharyngeal tumour through no intubation, and BCV was effectively utilized to maintain adequate ventilation during this surgical intervention. The case demonstrates the use of BCV in airway surgery. However, it indicates the potential for BCV to be used in non-airway surgery when other methods of ventilation are not feasible [7].

25.2.6 A New Method to Intubate Patients with Unreliable Pulse Oximetry

BCV may be used during rapid sequence intubation (RSI) of a patient with unreliable pulse oximetry. BCV successfully maintained oxygenation and ventilation throughout the intubation procedure, illustrating how such procedures are facilitated in airway management in patients at high risk. This indicates a degree of functional capacity through the use of BCV in emergencies and in maintaining patients throughout airway management procedures, which can also be used in procedures that demand airway and non-airway/invasive surgical management, where ventilatory assistance is required [8].

25.2.7 Biphasic Cuirass Ventilation During Bronchoscopy: Key Considerations

Biphasic Cuirass Ventilation (BCV) has the additional advantage during bronchoscopy of delivering non-invasive ventilatory support without interfering with the airway. Unlike positive pressure ventilation, BCV allows free access to the tracheobronchial tree and is particularly useful in rigid and flexible bronchoscopy. Rigid bronchoscopy, which is often used for interventions like stent placement, foreign body removal, and LASER therapy, is assisted by BCV through the prevention of endotracheal intubation and the preservation of adequate gas exchange. Similarly, flexible bronchoscopy—often used for diagnostic procedures, bronchoalveolar lavage, and transbronchial biopsies—can be performed more safely under BCV, as it avoids the increased airway resistance and air-trapping risks of conventional mechanical ventilation [9].

BCV has also proven effective for the maintenance of oxygenation and ventilation during complex bronchoscopic interventions, such as bronchial thermoplasty and cryo-biopsy, where prolonged apnoea or hypoxemia would otherwise result [10]. BCV has been shown to reduce respiratory acidosis, reduce the need for manual ventilation, and reduce opioid requirements in anaesthesia. Its use in percutaneous tracheostomy and difficult airway management also demonstrates its versatility. By preserving spontaneous respiration and preventing endotracheal tube limitations, BCV enhances procedural safety and outcomes in bronchoscopic interventions [11].

Future Directions and Clinical Implications During Bronchoscopy The incorporation of BCV into bronchoscopy is a paradigm shift in respiratory support, with particular benefits for high-risk patients with challenging airways or those undergoing lengthy interventions. Optimization of BCV settings for individual bronchoscopic procedures and broadening its use in interventional pulmonology should be the focus of future research. With evolving technology, lighter and more conforming cuirass designs can enhance procedural ergonomics, rendering BCV an essential tool in contemporary bronchoscopic practice.

25.2.8 Biphasic Cuirass Ventilation During Emergency Rapid Sequence Induction (RSI) and Emergency Tracheal Intubation

Biphasic Cuirass Ventilation (BCV) represents a promising adjunct to rapid sequence intubation (RSI), particularly in high-risk patients who are at risk of hypoxemia or severe acidosis. Through the provision of maintained negative pressure ventilation throughout the apneic phase of RSI, BCV allows for sustained oxygenation and carbon dioxide clearance even after paralysis—transcending a basic limitation of conventional RSI. It is of particular value in hypoxemic respiratory failure, in which conventional apneic oxygenation alone might be insufficient, and in severe metabolic acidosis, in which constant ventilation is required to prevent hemodynamic collapse. A case report has also demonstrated successful BCV-facilitated intubation in a patient with unreliable pulse oximetry, suggesting the potential for broader application in emergency airway management. The technique involves preoxygenation using high-flow nasal cannula, placement of BCV in biphasic mode, and ongoing ventilation throughout laryngoscopy, theoretically optimizing first-pass success and reducing desaturation risk [12, 13].

Despite its potential, widespread application of BCV for emergent intubation is limited by factors such as device unavailability and clinician inexperience. While setup time is short (typically less than 5 minutes), it might be a deterrent in time-sensitive scenarios. BCV is also contraindicated in cardiac arrest due to interference with chest compressions and potential hindrance of emergent chest procedures. In the environment of non-arrest patients who need urgent intubation, though—particularly those with refractory hypoxemia or acidosis—BCV is a physiologically attractive option compared to traditional methods [14].

Future Direction Further research is needed to establish its benefit, but early evidence suggests BCV is a valuable strategy to contribute to enhanced safety in difficult airway scenarios.

25.2.9 BCV Uses in Total Lung Lavage in Pulmonary Alveolar Proteinosis

Biphasic Cuirass Ventilation (BCV) has been shown to be useful in optimizing the effectiveness of whole lung lavage (WLL) in pulmonary alveolar proteinosis (PAP) (Fig. 25.2). In two cases reported, BCV was utilized during WLL to provide high-frequency chest wall vibrations to augment the clearance of proteinaceous debris from alveoli. The first case was a 64-year-old man with autoimmune PAP who underwent bilateral WLL with BCV in "clearance mode" (−17 cm H_2O, 600 cycles/min) in combination with N-acetylcysteine-infused saline. This strategy yielded a 100% lavage fluid recovery rate and dramatic post-procedure clinical improvement. A 38-year-old man with severe PAP underwent WLL with BCV (300 cycles/min, −17 cm H_2O) in the second case, with 97–103% fluid recovery and pronounced radiographic and symptomatic resolution. Both reports demonstrate BCV's ability

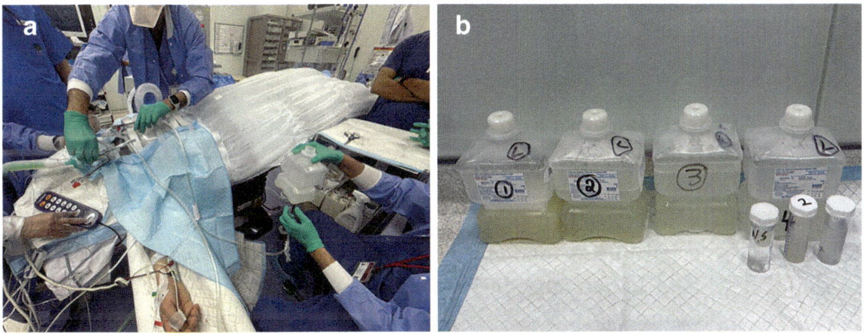

Fig. 25.2 (**a**) BCV during total Lung Wash. (**b**) Lung Saline Wash

to maximize lavage efficiency while preserving hemodynamic stability, with the potential to decrease manual percussion requirements and enhance procedural outcomes [15, 16].

Clinical Implications and Future Directions The addition of BCV to WLL provides a non-invasive, mechanized substitute for manual chest percussion, reduces residual lavage fluid, and may decrease procedure duration. Being able to sustain oxygenation and provide alveolar clearance during one-lung ventilation makes it of special utility in the setting of severe PAP. Optimal vibration parameters (pressure, frequency) are, however, undefined, and comparative research is warranted to validate BCV against conventional methods. As BCV becomes more established in WLL regimens, standardized application would be expected to improve safety and efficacy, especially in institutions without experienced physiotherapists. Research into BCV's effect on long-term PAP outcome and its synergy with adjunctive therapies such as GM-CSF should be pursued.

25.2.10 Biphasic Cuirass Ventilation in Postoperative Paediatric Cardiac Surgery: Cardiac Surgery for Congenital Heart Disease-Fontan-Fallot

Biphasic Cuirass Ventilation (BCV) has been found to be a useful modality of respiratory support in the postoperative period of paediatric cardiac surgery, especially for more complex surgeries such as Fontan and Tetralogy of Fallot (TOF) repairs. In the post-Fontan procedure, where passive pulmonary blood flow is essential, the negative pressure ventilation of BCV resembles physiological intrathoracic pressure fluctuations, maximizing preload and cardiac output without the adverse hemodynamic consequences of positive pressure ventilation [16].

In TOF patients, BCV helps to decrease right ventricular afterload and enhance pulmonary compliance in the vulnerable postoperative state. Clinical observations indicate that BCV improves oxygenation and decreases ventilator dependence with the potential for decreased risk of diaphragmatic dysfunction and shorter ICU stay. The fact that it is non-invasive also decreases the need for sedation, promoting earlier mobilization and quicker recovery in children [17].

25.2.11 Clinical Benefits and Future Considerations in Paediatrics Heart Surgery

The use of BCV in congenital heart surgery has unique benefits over traditional ventilation, especially in maintaining hemodynamic stability and favouring lung recruitment without barotrauma. In Fontan patients, the maintenance of negative intrathoracic pressure by BCV assists pulmonary circulation and prevents pleural effusion. In TOF repairs, BCV helps in the management of restrictive lung mechanics and postoperative pulmonary oedema. Initial reports emphasize its potential to facilitate extubation and decrease pulmonary complications, but larger studies are warranted to standardize the regimens. As BCV technology is refined, its incorporation into paediatric cardiac care pathways could enhance outcomes in high-risk patients, providing a bridge to recovery with less invasive support. Future studies should aim to optimize pressure and timing of initiation to derive maximum benefit in this specialized group of patients [18].

25.2.12 Intraoperative Usage of Biphasic Cuirass Ventilation with Neuromuscular Disorders

Biphasic Cuirass Ventilation (BCV) is a novel, promising option for intraoperative ventilation in neuromuscular disorder (NMD) patients with restrictive lung disease and compromised cough mechanics. Traditional positive pressure ventilation can exacerbate respiratory muscle weakness and lead to postoperative complications in such patients. BCV, on the other hand, is a more physiological form of ventilation with negative intrathoracic pressure, thus preserving diaphragmatic function and avoiding atelectasis. Studies have demonstrated its efficacy in providing adequate gas exchange during surgery with minimal requirement for invasive airway intervention. This is particularly beneficial in NMD patients undergoing surgeries such as scoliosis correction or gastrostomy tube placement, in whom long-term mechanical ventilation carries significant risks [19].

Clinical Implications and Practical Benefits: The use of BCV in NMD patients in the surgical process bypasses several obstacles, including avoidance of endotracheal intubation and preservation of spontaneous breathing. By supporting ventilation without sedation or paralysis, BCV reduces the risk of postoperative respiratory failure and enables early extubation. Its non-invasive nature also renders it suitable for patients with bulbar weakness or difficult airways. Case reports describe good experiences in Duchenne muscular dystrophy and spinal muscular atrophy patients with improvement in oxygenation and reduction in pulmonary complications. Close monitoring of chest wall compliance and CO_2 clearance is, however, obligatory as severe muscle weakness can limit the effectiveness of negative pressure ventilation. While standardized protocols must be established by additional studies, BCV represents a very valuable instrument for optimizing the perioperative care of NMD patients [20].

25.3 Conclusion

Biphasic Cuirass Ventilation (BCV) is a major development in artificial ventilation that provides a non-invasive, physiologically compatible alternative to conventional positive pressure ventilation. BCV minimizes complications of ventilator-associated lung injury, airway trauma, and ICU stay by avoiding the necessity of endotracheal intubation and sedation. The fact that BCV supports spontaneous respiration and yet assists with a controlled support makes it a very useful tool in anaesthesia, particularly for non-ENT surgery where airway manipulation is not desired.

BCV versatility is not limited to the operating room, as it has been shown to be effective in critical care, emergency medicine, paediatric anaesthesia, and even in complex situations such as radiotherapy and mass casualty resuscitation. Its application in COVID-19 management also highlights its versatility in sustaining oxygenation without the need for invasive mechanical ventilation. BCV also allows for improved preservation of respiratory muscles and cardiac function, which makes it a great choice for long-term ventilation and weaning.

As clinical experience increases, BCV will become an essential tool in anaesthesiology and intensive care, especially in patients with challenging airways, neuromuscular disease, or during procedures where conventional ventilation is not feasible. Research in the future should aim to standardize BCV techniques, broaden its indications, and streamline its application in contemporary anaesthetic practice. With its inherent benefits, BCV represents an exciting innovation that closes the gap between invasive and non-invasive ventilation, improving patient safety and outcomes in various medical specialties.

References

1. Bodhey A, Bodhey M, Shallik NA, Al Nadhari M, Griess HF, Al Ani O, Sainuddin S, Thomas KP, ElHanfi O, Jose S, Nair A. Biphasic cuirass ventilation for airway surgeries: a comprehensive review. Cureus. 2024;16(12):e75477. https://doi.org/10.7759/cureus.75477.
2. Isaac N, Mane A, Ehlers M. Letter to the editor: biphasic cuirass model. Paediatr Anaesth. 2023;33(4):288–95. https://doi.org/10.1111/pan.13923.
3. Clinkscales W, Spence M, Gleysteen J, Hayes N, Izaguirre E, Wakefield D, Schwartz D, Rhea I, Risquez C, Sharma AM. Novel use of biphasic cuirass ventilation during definitive radiation therapy: a technical report. Pract Radiat Oncol. 2021;11(3):e276–81. https://doi.org/10.1016/j.prro.2020.08.003.
4. Gur I, Bar-Yishay E, Ben-Abraham I. Biphasic extrathoracic cuirass ventilation to resuscitate victims of nerve agent exposure. Am J Emerg Med. 2005;23(4):488–91. https://doi.org/10.1016/j.ajem.2004.10.004.
5. Zitek T, Berkeley RP, Hodnick R, Davis K, Dadon N, Slattery DE. A novel technique to intubate patients without reliable pulse oximetry. Am J Emerg Med. 2018;36(12):2305–7. https://doi.org/10.1016/j.ajem.2018.07.038.
6. Borges JA, Esquinas AM. Biphasic cuirass ventilation in the escalation of non-invasive ventilation in COVID-19: case report and review. Monaldi Arch Chest Dis. 2023;93(1):2510. https://doi.org/10.4081/monaldi.2023.2510.
7. Broomhead CJ, Dilkes MG, Monks PS. Use of the Hayek oscillator in a case of failed fibreoptic intubation. Br J Anaesth. 1995;74(6):720–1. https://doi.org/10.1093/bja/74.6.720.
8. Zitek T, Berkeley RP, Hodnick R, Davis K, Dadon N, Slattery DE. A novel technique to intubate patients without reliable pulse oximetry. Am J Emerg Med. 2018;36(11):2131.e1–2. https://doi.org/10.1016/j.ajem.2018.07.038.
9. Hideaki Mori H, Shono A, Hirade R, et al. Biphasic cuirass ventilation during anesthesia for tracheobronchial stent insertion or removal by a rigid bronchoscope: a case report. A A Pract. 2018;10(8):198–200.

10. Natalini G, Cavaliere S, Seramonti V, et al. Negative pressure ventilation vs external high-frequency oscillation during rigid bronchoscopy. A controlled randomized trial. Chest. 2000;118(1):18–23.
11. Natalini G, Cavaliere S, Vitacca M, Amicucci G, et al. Negative pressure ventilation vs. spontaneous assisted ventilation during rigid bronchoscopy: a controlled randomised trial. Acta Anaesthesiol Scand. 1998;42(9):1063–9.
12. Bandyopadhyay A, Kumar P, Jafra A, Thakur H, Yaddanapudi LN, Jain K. Peri-intubation hypoxia after delayed versus rapid sequence intubation in critically injured patients on arrival to trauma triage: a randomized controlled trial. Anesth Analg. 2023;136(5):913–9.
13. Imitazione P, Annunziata A, Lanza M, Fiorentino G. Combined high flow nasal cannula and negative pressure ventilation as a novel respiratory approach in a patient with acute respiratory failure and limb-girdle muscular dystrophy. Acta Myol. 2021;40:101–4.
14. Shime N, Toida C, Itoi T, Hashimoto S. Continuous negative extrathoracic pressure in children after congenital heart surgery. Crit Care Resusc. 2006;8(4):297–301.
15. Nakamura K, Omura S, Kajiura K, Ishigaki M. Removal of lung lavage fluid during whole-lung lavage using biphasic cuirass ventilation chest percussion in a patient with autoimmune pulmonary alveolar proteinosis. Lung India. 2019;36:540–2.
16. Kato S, Kasamatsu N, Matsuda S, Sugimoto S, Yano T, Ogasawara T. Whole-lung lavage in pulmonary alveolar proteinosis supported by biphasic cuirass ventilation. AJRS. 2015;4(2):185–8.
17. Shekerdemian LS, Schulze-Neick I, Redington AN, et al. Negative pressure ventilation as haemodynamic rescue following surgery for congenital heart disease. Intensive Care Med. 2003;29(11):1869–72.
18. Alapati D, Agha H, Gowda S, et al. Biphasic cuirass ventilation in pediatric patients after cardiac surgery: a case series. Pediatr Crit Care Med. 2016;17(8):e354–9.
19. Bach JR, Gonçalves MR, Hamdani I, et al. Extubation of patients with neuromuscular weakness: a new management paradigm. Chest. 2010;137(5):1033–9.
20. Toussaint M, Chatwin M, Soudon P. Advances in respiratory physiotherapy management of neuromuscular disease. Breathe. 2016;12(4):318–28.

Postoperative Application of Biphasic Cuirass Ventilation

26

Yusuf Kahya

26.1 Introduction

Postoperative pulmonary complications are among the most common causes of morbidity following major surgical procedures and have a significant negative impact on patient outcomes. These complications include atelectasis, pneumonia, acute respiratory distress syndrome, and prolonged oxygen dependency. In patients undergoing thoracic and cardiac surgery, intraoperative lung manipulation, the effects of anaesthetic agents, and reduced respiratory effort due to inadequate postoperative analgesia contribute to decreased pulmonary capacity and an increased risk of pulmonary complications. It has been reported that approximately 5–10% of all surgical patients and 9–40% of those undergoing abdominal surgery develop at least one postoperative pulmonary complication [1–4]. This risk is particularly pronounced in patients undergoing extensive resections such as pneumonectomy, in whom morbidity rates have been reported to range from 10% to 45% [5]. Similarly, pulmonary complications have been observed in 40–90% of patients following cardiac surgery [6].

Postoperative pulmonary complications may arise as a consequence of both the surgical procedure itself and the effects of general anaesthesia. The pathophysiological alterations that occur during anaesthesia can persist in the postoperative period, thereby increasing the risk of developing such complications.

Particularly after upper abdominal and thoracic surgeries, the induction of anaesthesia may lead to a reduction in lung gas volumes, resulting in the development of atelectasis in the lower lobes. Atelectasis typically occurs in parenchymal regions adjacent to the diaphragm and may involve approximately 10% of the total lung volume. This pathophysiological condition may persist for up to 2 days following major surgical procedures [7–10]. Atelectasis is one of the principal causes of

Y. Kahya (✉)
Ankara University School of Medicine, Department of Thoracic Surgery, Ankara, Türkiye

O. Alibrahim et al. (eds.), *Biphasic Cuirass Noninvasive Ventilation*, Noninvasive Ventilation. The Essentials, https://doi.org/10.1007/978-3-032-20933-7_26

postoperative hypoxaemia and increases the risk of pneumonia in approximately 3–6% of patients undergoing cardiac surgery or lung resection [11, 12]. Similarly, hypoxaemia adversely affects the recovery process in 30–50% of patients following abdominal surgery. In approximately 8–10% of these cases, endotracheal intubation and mechanical ventilation become necessary, leading to prolonged stays in the intensive care unit and hospital and resulting in a significant increase in mortality rates [13].

In the postoperative period, dysfunction of the diaphragm and other respiratory muscles may occur. This condition typically manifests within the first few hours after surgery and may persist for several weeks. Respiratory muscle dysfunction can lead to impaired gas exchange, hypoxaemia, and ventilation–perfusion mismatch, thereby significantly increasing the risk of acute respiratory failure and the need for mechanical ventilatory support [14].

The reported incidence of acute respiratory failure is approximately 12% after thoracic surgery and 11% following cardiac surgery [15, 16]. Moreover, in 1–2% of patients undergoing cardiopulmonary bypass or one-lung ventilation, severe conditions such as acute lung injury or acute respiratory distress syndrome may develop, both of which are associated with high mortality rates [11, 12].

Positive pressure-based non-invasive ventilation (NIV) techniques—Continuous Positive Airway Pressure (CPAP) and Bilevel Positive Airway Pressure (BPAP)—have brought about a major paradigm shift in postoperative respiratory support over the past two decades and have become a cornerstone of clinical practice. Numerous studies have demonstrated that the application of CPAP or BPAP can reduce the incidence of atelectasis and improve oxygenation parameters [13, 17–19].

Mechanical ventilation administered through an endotracheal tube may adversely affect recovery by causing additional morbidities such as barotrauma-induced lung injury and nosocomial pneumonia. Clinical studies have demonstrated that the use of NIV in cases of acute respiratory failure significantly reduces the rates of endotracheal intubation, the incidence of nosocomial infections, and the length of stay in the intensive care unit and hospital, as well as overall morbidity and mortality [20–22].

NIV can be safely applied in patients who are cooperative, conscious, and able to maintain intact airway protection reflexes. When implemented by an experienced team following careful patient selection, it may help reduce respiratory complications and reintubation rates [23–25]. However, in a meta-analysis by Torres et al., positive pressure NIV was not found to have a statistically significant effect on reintubation rates, hospital length of stay, or mortality. Although NIV represents a physiologically rational approach, its clinical efficacy may remain limited depending on factors such as cardiopulmonary reserve, surgical history, and the timing of its application [26].

Biphasic Cuirass Ventilation (BCV) is an innovative NIV technique that mechanically reproduces thoracic wall movements via a specially designed cuirass applied externally to the chest, thereby generating inspiratory and expiratory cycles that closely mimic normal respiratory physiology. The principal advantage of BCV over conventional positive pressure ventilation techniques lies in its ability to achieve alveolar distension without increasing intrathoracic pressure, thus preserving cardiac preload and venous return [27]. At the same time, BCV functions as a negative pressure ventilation system capable of providing effective ventilation without the need for airway access. Owing to these characteristics, BCV may be considered for use in surgical procedures where airway management without endotracheal intubation is desired, such as airway surgery [27].

26.2 Physiopathological Basis

Positive pressure ventilation facilitates alveolar inflation during inspiration by delivering pressurised air to the lungs. However, this process increases intrathoracic pressure and consequently reduces venous return. In patients with limited cardiac reserve, these physiological alterations may compromise haemodynamic stability. In contrast, BCV generates a negative pressure cycle that closely mimics natural breathing. During inspiration, BCV expands the thoracic cage and depresses the diaphragm, thereby lowering intrathoracic pressure; during expiration, the device applies positive pressure to facilitate passive exhalation.

This biphasic mechanism enhances alveolar ventilation and optimises gas exchange without increasing intrathoracic pressure [28]. Experimental studies have demonstrated that BCV provides a more homogeneous distribution of lung volumes and reduces dynamic hyperinflation compared to positive pressure ventilation [29]. The increase in preload generated by the negative intrathoracic pressure supports cardiac output and leads to a significant reduction in NT-proBNP levels [28]. The cardiopulmonary effects of BCV are particularly pronounced in patients with pulmonary hypertension or restrictive lung disease.

In conclusion, unlike positive pressure ventilation systems, BCV preserves the physiological inspiratory and expiratory cycles, providing a more balanced haemodynamic profile across both pulmonary and cardiac systems. This characteristic offers a significant advantage in thoracic surgical patients, particularly in the postoperative period when the maintenance of cardiac output is critical.

26.2.1 Postoperative Application of BCV

Historically, BCV evolved from the negative pressure ventilation systems developed during the poliomyelitis epidemics of the 1920s, commonly known as the "iron lung" [30]. Today, these primitive and cumbersome devices have been replaced by advanced, microprocessor-controlled systems that are portable, user-friendly, and capable of operating with patient-specific parameters. Modern BCV units are equipped with sensor-based technology that detects thoracic wall movements and responds in synchrony with the patient's respiratory cycle, allowing real-time modulation of pressure between inspiratory and expiratory phases. In addition, these systems are equipped with advanced functions designed to facilitate secretion drainage and enhance airway clearance.

Thus, BCV has evolved from being merely a tool for respiratory support into a versatile, physiologic, and user-friendly ventilation platform that also contributes to pulmonary rehabilitation and non-invasive secretion management. Cuirass ventilatory devices can control both inspiration and expiration to varying degrees, depending on the selected mode of operation. There are five primary operational modes of cuirass ventilation: continuous negative pressure, controlled biphasic (also referred to as intermittent mandatory ventilation), non-invasive synchronised BCV, high-frequency oscillation, and cardiac synchronisation. The device's high-frequency oscillation mode—capable of generating up to 1200 oscillations per minute—facilitates secretion clearance, improves oxygenation, and reduces carbon dioxide levels, effectively serving as a substitute for conventional chest physiotherapy. In addition, the cardiac-synchronised mode employs electrocardiographic signals to align the ventilatory cycle with the cardiac cycle, a function known as electrocardiography-triggered BCV [31].

The use of BCV in the postoperative period represents an important alternative in situations where conventional NIV techniques are inadequate in terms of physiological effectiveness or patient tolerance. BCV is typically indicated in three main clinical scenarios. The first of these is postoperative hypoxemic respiratory failure. In this patient group, BCV has the potential to improve oxygenation by enhancing alveolar ventilation while simultaneously preventing the haemodynamic disturbances that may result from positive pressure ventilation. Following thoracic surgical procedures—such as those in which lung expansion is restricted and diaphragmatic motion is reduced due to postoperative pain—BCV can be used to support diaphragmatic movement and optimise gas exchange. Owing to these physiological advantages, the application of BCV in the management of postoperative hypoxemic respiratory failure provides superior patient comfort and greater cardiopulmonary stability compared with conventional NIV (Fig. 26.1).

The second indication group comprises patients who are intolerant to mask use or possess structural limitations in their facial anatomy. In the context of positive pressure NIV, issues such as pressure sores at the mask contact points, air leaks, and skin lesions can significantly diminish patient comfort and adversely impact adherence to treatment. For this patient demographic, BCV presents a notable advantage by providing effective ventilatory support without requiring a mask, thereby closely mimicking the physiological breathing pattern.

The third indication includes conditions characterised by secretion retention and mucociliary dysfunction. In the postoperative period following thoracotomy, pain-induced suppression of the cough reflex and the subsequent accumulation of airway secretions can hinder the maintenance of airway patency. The biphasic pressure waves generated by BCV facilitate secretion mobilisation, enhance mucus drainage, and contribute to maintaining airway clearances (Figs. 26.2 and 26.3).

The effectiveness of BCV depends on the patient's clinical condition, respiratory cooperation, and the comprehensive management of adjunctive therapies. In this context, the patient's level of consciousness and ability to cooperate are of

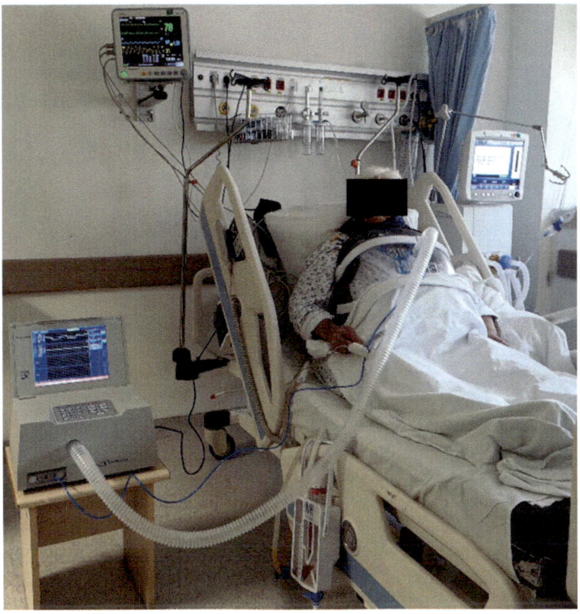

Fig. 26.1 A 78-year-old female patient underwent video-assisted thoracoscopic right lower lobectomy with systematic mediastinal lymph node dissection for squamous cell carcinoma of the lung. On postoperative day 2, she developed acute hypercapnic respiratory failure (arterial blood gas analysis: pH = 7.49, PaO_2 = 52 mmHg, $PaCO_2$ = 51.5 mmHg, SpO_2 = 87%). BCV therapy was initiated in the thoracic surgery intensive care unit using the Hayek RTX device (United Hayek Medical). The treatment was performed in control mode with the following pressure parameters: negative pressure = −21 cmH_2O, positive pressure = +7 cmH_2O, and an inspiratory-to-expiratory (I:E) ratio 1:1. The patient was continuously monitored under close haemodynamic and respiratory observation, and supplemental oxygen at 2 L/min was administered via nasal cannula. (Source: Department of Thoracic Surgery Archives, Ankara University School of Medicine)

paramount importance, as BCV demonstrates its highest efficacy in patients who can maintain spontaneous respiratory effort and synchronise with the device. Moreover, adequate pain control is a critical determinant of therapeutic success, since post-thoracotomy pain can limit respiratory effort and disrupt patient–device synchronisation. Therefore, the use of thoracic epidural or regional analgesia techniques (such as paravertebral block or erector spinae plane block) not only reduces pain but also enhances patient compliance with BCV. Furthermore, secretion control is of critical importance in preventing respiratory complications during the postoperative period. When BCV is combined with chest physiotherapy, it promotes mucociliary clearance, reduces the risk of secretion retention, and helps maintain airway patency. The coordinated management of all these elements strengthens the feasibility of BCV as a safe and effective respiratory support modality in the postoperative setting.

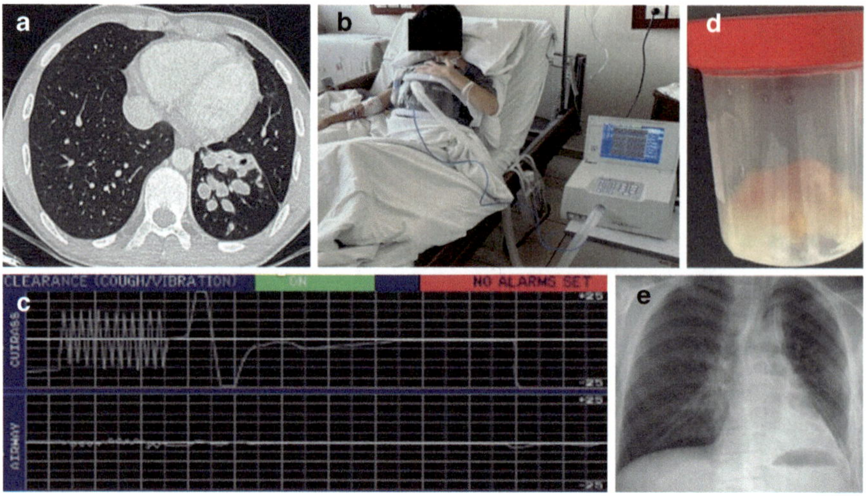

Fig. 26.2 A 13-year-old male patient underwent a left lower lobectomy via a muscle-sparing mini-thoracotomy for acquired bronchiectasis. Preoperative thoracic computed tomography (parenchymal window) demonstrated markedly dilated bronchi within the left lower lobe filled with dense secretions (**a**). In the postoperative period, BCV therapy was initiated using the Hayek RTX device (United Hayek Medical) to enhance secretion drainage and support cough effectiveness (**b**). The vibration mode of the BCV device was utilised to facilitate mucus mobilisation. In this mode, therapy was delivered at a frequency of 800 cycles per minute with a negative pressure level of −15 cmH_2O, applied in short 5-minute periods. Following the vibration phase, the cough mode was activated to promote secretion expectoration. During the cough mode, the inspiratory pressure was set at −15 cmH_2O and the expiratory pressure at +15 cmH_2O, with a frequency of 24 cycles per minute and an inspiration-to-expiration ratio of 5:1. Each cough phase lasted 2 minutes and was repeated four times during the treatment session. A total of 5 days of BCV therapy was administered (**c**). The stepwise and controlled application of BCV resulted in a reduction in secretion viscosity and facilitated mucus drainage (**d**). As demonstrated in the pre-discharge posteroanterior chest radiograph, airway patency was successfully maintained with BCV treatment (**e**). (Source: Department of Thoracic Surgery Archives, Ankara University School of Medicine)

BCV should be applied with caution in selected patient groups. In patients with thoracic wall instability (e.g., flail chest), the application of negative pressure may induce asynchronous thoracic movements and reduce ventilatory efficiency. Similarly, in patients with compromised skin integrity, burns, or open wounds, the contact surface of the cuirass may increase the risk of additional tissue injury. In cases of severe obesity or thoracic deformity, improper fitting of the cuirass may compromise the uniformity and effectiveness of ventilation. Moreover, in patients with active haemothorax or persistent air leak, negative pressure ventilation may adversely affect pleural space dynamics. Nevertheless, with proper pressure titration, appropriate cuirass selection, and individualised treatment protocols by experienced teams, these limitations can be effectively managed.

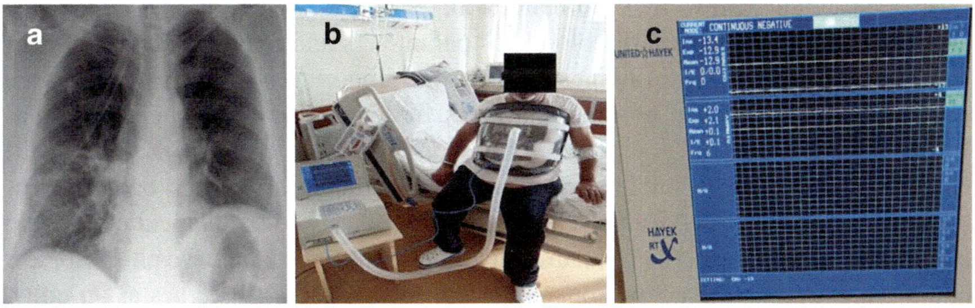

Fig. 26.3 A 64-year-old male patient had previously undergone a left upper lobectomy with mediastinal lymph node dissection for squamous cell carcinoma of the lung. Postoperatively, persistent elevation of the left hemidiaphragm, consistent with left phrenic nerve paralysis, was observed radiologically (**a**). During follow-up, a second primary lung adenocarcinoma was identified in the right lower lobe. The patient had a medical history of chronic obstructive pulmonary disease and obstructive sleep apnoea syndrome. The forced expiratory volume in one second (FEV_1) was measured at less than 50% of the predicted value. The patient, classified as high risk for surgery, underwent a right lower lobe wedge resection with mediastinal lymph node dissection for a second primary lung cancer. In the postoperative period, chest radiographs revealed findings consistent with linear atelectasis in the right haemothorax. To promote re-expansion of the atelectatic areas, BCV therapy was initiated (**b**). The continuous negative external pressure (CNEP) mode was selected for BCV treatment. This mode is particularly useful in patients predisposed to atelectasis, as it enhances alveolar recruitment, increases functional residual capacity, and improves oxygenation. An initial negative pressure of -10 cmH_2O was applied and gradually titrated up to -20 cmH_2O based on the patient's clinical response. Once adequate clinical and radiological improvement was achieved with the initial settings, the continuous negative external pressure level was reduced to -4 cmH_2O to maintain the stabilisation phase (**c**). (Source: Department of Thoracic Surgery Archives, Ankara University School of Medicine)

26.3 Evidence-Based Benefits of BCV in the Postoperative Period

Over the past decade, studies evaluating the use of BCV in the postoperative period have increased considerably. A common conclusion among these reports is that BCV provides a more physiologically balanced and clinically comfortable form of respiratory support compared with conventional positive pressure ventilation techniques.

Enhanced Recovery After Surgery (ERAS) protocols represent a modern perioperative care concept based on a multidisciplinary approach designed to reduce postoperative complications, shorten recovery time, and enhance patient satisfaction. The core philosophy of ERAS is to minimise the surgical stress response while preserving the patient's physiological reserves [32]. In thoracic surgery, an essential component of ERAS protocols includes prehabilitation and pulmonary rehabilitation programmes, within which NIV plays a pivotal role in perioperative respiratory physiotherapy [33].

In a systematic review by Chiumello et al., perioperative use of NIV was shown to significantly improve arterial blood gas parameters and reduce the rate of endotracheal intubation. These findings provided an important scientific basis for the subsequent development of modern, mask-free non-invasive systems such as BCV [34].

Considering the physiological and practical advantages of BCV over conventional NIV methods, ERAS and BCV can be viewed as two complementary modern perioperative strategies. The fundamental aim of ERAS is to preserve physiological homeostasis and accelerate postoperative recovery, and BCV emerges as an effective respiratory support modality that reinforces this goal. Accordingly, the incorporation of BCV as a routine component of thoracic surgery-specific ERAS protocols in the future may contribute substantially to reducing postoperative pulmonary complications.

Following lung resection, at least one major or minor complication has been reported to occur in approximately 21–50% of patients. The most frequently encountered complications include atelectasis, pneumonia, bronchopleural fistula, prolonged air leak, cardiac arrhythmias, and respiratory failure. Complication rates are significantly higher in patients undergoing pneumonectomy compared with those undergoing other types of lung resections, and the result has been shown to substantially increase postoperative mortality and morbidity. Among these complications, bronchopleural fistula and empyema are particularly associated with a marked rise in postoperative mortality [1, 35–39].

According to the literature, the incidence of bronchopleural fistula following pneumonectomy ranges from 1.8% to 8%, occurring either in the early or late postoperative period [40–43]. The development of postpneumonectomy bronchopleural fistula is multifactorial, and one of the predisposing factors is barotrauma. Positive pressure ventilation may induce ischaemia and necrosis at the bronchial stump, leading to dehiscence of the stapler line and, consequently, the formation of a bronchopleural fistula (Fig. 26.4).

Therefore, positive pressure ventilation should be applied with caution in patients who have undergone pneumonectomy [44].

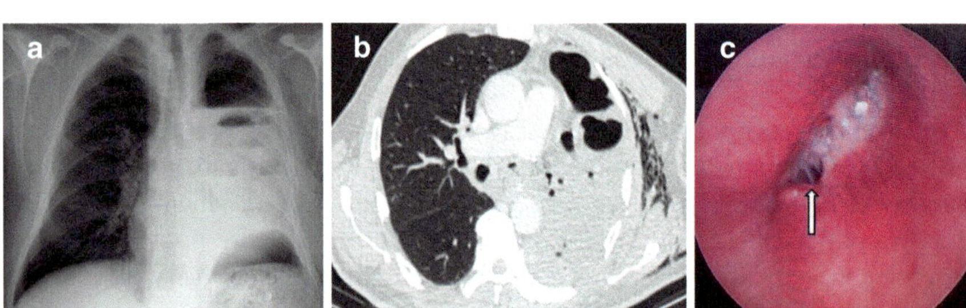

Fig. 26.4 A 56-year-old male patient underwent left pneumonectomy and systematic mediastinal lymph node dissection via a posterolateral thoracotomy for squamous cell carcinoma of the lung (**a**, **b**). The bronchoscopic image demonstrates a bronchopleural fistula located at the left main bronchial stump (**c**). (Source: Department of Thoracic Surgery Archive, Ankara University Faculty of Medicine)

BCV provides alveolar ventilation without increasing intrathoracic pressure, thereby supporting gas exchange without imposing additional mechanical stress on the bronchial stump. Consequently, it may reduce the risk of bronchopleural fistula formation and offer a safer mode of respiratory support in postpneumonectomy patients.

Following pneumonectomy, the increase in pulmonary arterial pressure and the augmented perfusion of the residual lung may lead to endothelial injury. This process results in a marked increase in capillary permeability and, particularly in cases with perioperative fluid imbalance, predisposes patients to the development of postpneumonectomy pulmonary oedema (Fig. 26.5). Postpneumonectomy pulmonary oedema occurs more frequently after right pneumonectomy and presents with a severe clinical picture resembling acute respiratory distress syndrome. Reported mortality rates exceed 50% [45–47]. Previous studies have demonstrated that BCV significantly reduces mean pulmonary arterial pressure, alleviates cardiac workload, and improves haemodynamic parameters [28]. Therefore, BCV may play a potential preventive role in the development of postpneumonectomy pulmonary oedema.

Right ventricular dysfunction (RVD) and right ventricular failure (RVF) are complications associated with increased morbidity and mortality in patients undergoing cardiac surgery [48, 49]. Current therapeutic strategies for the management of RVD and RVF are limited to reducing pulmonary vascular resistance—through optimisation of ventilation and administration of inhaled pulmonary vasodilators—maintaining adequate systemic arterial pressure to improve right ventricular myocardial perfusion and left ventricular filling pressure and using inotropic agents to

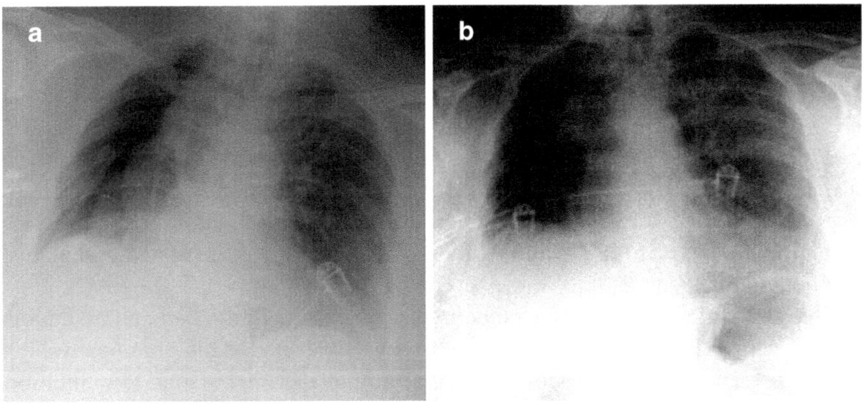

Fig. 26.5 A 62-year-old female patient underwent a complete right pneumonectomy and systematic mediastinal lymph node dissection via a posterolateral thoracotomy for lung adenocarcinoma. The following posteroanterior chest radiographs demonstrate the development of early postpneumonectomy pulmonary oedema: (**a**) the postoperative day 1 radiograph and (**b**) the postoperative day 2 radiograph, which shows diffuse pulmonary oedema in the remaining left lung. The patient died on postoperative day 2. (Source: Department of Thoracic Surgery Archive, Ankara University Faculty of Medicine)

support cardiac contractility [50–52]. However, these therapeutic strategies are often insufficient in cases of severe right ventricular failure. During positive pressure ventilation, the increase in intrathoracic pressure can elevate pulmonary vascular resistance, thereby increasing right ventricular afterload. In contrast, when oscillating negative pressure ventilation is applied using BCV, studies have reported an increase in cardiac output, improvement in oxygenation parameters, and a reduction in pulmonary arterial pressure—both in healthy volunteers and in patients who have undergone coronary artery bypass grafting [28, 53, 54].

Similarly, in their review examining the haemodynamic effects of BCV after cardiac surgery, Guarracino and Ambrosino reported that BCV enhances venous return by reducing intrathoracic pressure, significantly decreases mean pulmonary artery pressure and right atrial pressure, and increases both cardiac index and stroke volume index. These findings demonstrate that the use of BCV in the postoperative period supports cardiac output by preserving preload and optimising haemodynamic performance [55].

BCV demonstrates particularly remarkable haemodynamic effects in patients undergoing congenital heart surgery, especially in conditions characterised by elevated right heart pressures, such as Fontan circulation. The Fontan procedure is performed to improve survival in patients born with a functionally single-ventricle circulation. However, patients who have undergone Fontan-type surgery are prone to developing low cardiac output syndrome in the early postoperative period. In such cases, pharmacological support with inotropic agents may be employed; however, it should be noted that these therapies can further destabilise haemodynamics due to adverse effects such as increased pulmonary and systemic vascular resistance or tachycardia. Considering the physiologically fragile nature of the Fontan circulation, these effects may lead to significant clinical consequences. Therefore, the use of nonpharmacological strategies as alternative or adjunctive approaches to conventional therapy has gained increasing attention. The marked increase in stroke volume observed with negative pressure ventilation (NPV) represents a strong haemodynamic improvement in this patient group [56]. Shekerdemian and colleagues demonstrated that short-term use of cuirass-type negative pressure ventilation in patients with Fontan circulation increased pulmonary blood flow by 42% [56]. Moreover, this improvement continued to progress when the duration of NPV was extended, suggesting a sustained and cumulative haemodynamic benefit.

Because of the absence of a subpulmonary ventricle in the Fontan circulation, central venous pressure (CVP) tends to remain elevated. This chronically high venous pressure, combined with low cardiac output, can lead to long-term multiorgan complications—most notably affecting hepatic, renal, and gastrointestinal systems. Protein-losing enteropathy (PLE) represents a characteristic manifestation of Fontan failure and is clinically marked by peripheral oedema, ascites, pleural effusion, malabsorption, and immunoglobulin loss. Okada et al. reported a 16-year-old male patient who underwent a Fontan procedure and showed marked and rapid clinical improvement in protein-losing enteropathy and plastic bronchitis symptoms following the application of BCV. The study emphasised that BCV, through its ability to reduce central venous pressure and facilitate airway secretion clearance, provided a significant therapeutic advantage in the management of plastic bronchitis. These findings suggest that BCV may serve not only as a means of pulmonary ventilatory support but also as a potential therapeutic tool for reducing haemodynamic load in patients with Fontan physiology [57]. Toida et al. reported the use of a cuirass ventilator in continuous negative extrathoracic pressure mode in a two-year-old girl who developed lethal circulatory failure, generalised oedema, and hepatic dysfunction in the acute phase following a Fontan-type operation [58]. Following BCV therapy, improvements in hepatic function and reductions in fluid retention were observed, highlighting the potential haemodynamic benefits of this non-invasive approach in the postoperative management of complex congenital heart disease.

The haemodynamic advantages of BCV are not confined to congenital cardiac surgery but have also been documented in various other cardiac interventions. In a study by Chaturvedi et al., the application of continuous negative pressure to the thorax and upper abdomen during the early postoperative period following coronary artery bypass grafting (CABG), combined with positive pressure ventilation, resulted in significant increases in both cardiac index and stroke volume index. These findings were attributed to enhanced venous return secondary to reduced intrathoracic pressure [59].

26.4 Conclusion and Future Perspectives

Postoperative pulmonary complications remain among the most significant determinants of morbidity and mortality following major thoracic and cardiac surgery. The primary goal in preventing these complications is to preserve physiological respiratory mechanisms, optimise gas exchange, and maintain cardiopulmonary stability throughout the perioperative period. BCV represents a modern non-invasive ventilation strategy capable of achieving these objectives in a manner that closely mimics natural breathing.

By applying sequential negative and positive pressure phases externally to the thoracic wall, BCV enhances alveolar ventilation without increasing intrathoracic pressure, thereby improving gas exchange, supporting venous return and cardiac output, and eliminating discomfort associated with mask-based systems. Evidence from the literature demonstrates that BCV exerts favourable effects on multiple clinical parameters—including hypoxaemia, hypercapnia, secretion retention, and haemodynamic instability—in the postoperative management of thoracic, cardiac, and abdominal surgical patients.

In the future, the integration of BCV into ERAS protocols may yield substantial benefits by reducing postoperative respiratory complications while promoting early mobilisation and hospital discharge. Furthermore, the incorporation of advanced sensor technologies and artificial intelligence-based feedback systems into BCV units could enable the development of patient-specific ventilatory support algorithms. Through these innovations, BCV may evolve from a mere ventilation modality into a comprehensive intelligent postoperative respiratory support platform, capable of dynamically optimising physiological, haemodynamic, and digital parameters in real time.

References

1. Harpole DH Jr, DeCamp MM Jr, Daley J, Hur K, Oprian CA, Henderson WG, et al. Prognostic models of thirty-day mortality and morbidity after major pulmonary resection. J Thorac Cardiovasc Surg. 1999;117(5):969–79.
2. Wong DH, Weber EC, Schell MJ, Wong AB, Anderson CT, Barker SJ. Factors associated with postoperative pulmonary complications in patients with severe chronic obstructive pulmonary disease. Anesth Analg. 1995;80(2):276–84.
3. Esteban A, Frutos-Vivar F, Ferguson ND, Arabi Y, Apezteguía C, González M, et al. Noninvasive positive-pressure ventilation for respiratory failure after extubation. N Engl J Med. 2004;350(24):2452–60.
4. Antonelli M, Conti G, Rocco M, Bufi M, De Blasi RA, Vivino G, et al. A comparison of noninvasive positive-pressure ventilation and conventional mechanical ventilation in patients with acute respiratory failure. N Engl J Med. 1998;339(7):429–35.
5. Grapatsas K, Menghesha H, Dörr F, Baldes N, Schuler M, Stuschke M, et al. Pneumonectomy for primary lung tumors and pulmonary metastases: a comprehensive study of postoperative morbidity, early mortality, and preoperative clinical prognostic factors. Curr Oncol. 2023;30(11):9458–74.
6. Pinilla JC, Oleniuk FH, Tan L, Rebeyka I, Tanna N, Wilkinson A, et al. Use of a nasal continuous positive airway pressure mask in the treatment of postoperative atelectasis in aortocoronary bypass surgery. Crit Care Med. 1990;18(8):836–40.
7. Chawla G, Drummond GB. Fentanyl decreases end-expiratory lung volume in patients anaesthetized with sevoflurane. Br J Anaesth. 2008;100(3):411–4.
8. Hedenstierna G, Edmark L. The effects of anesthesia and muscle paralysis on the respiratory system. Intensive Care Med. 2005;31(10):1327–35.
9. Magnusson L, Spahn DR. New concepts of atelectasis during general anaesthesia. Br J Anaesth. 2003;91(1):61–72.
10. Eichenberger A, Proietti S, Wicky S, Frascarolo P, Suter M, Spahn DR, et al. Morbid obesity and postoperative pulmonary atelectasis: an underestimated problem. Anesth Analg. 2002;95(6):1788–92, table of contents.
11. Wynne R, Botti M. Postoperative pulmonary dysfunction in adults after cardiac surgery with cardiopulmonary bypass: clinical significance and implications for practice. Am J Crit Care. 2004;13(5):384–93.
12. Stéphan F, Boucheseiche S, Hollande J, Flahault A, Cheffi A, Bazelly B, et al. Pulmonary complications following lung resection: a comprehensive analysis of incidence and possible risk factors. Chest. 2000;118(5):1263–70.
13. Squadrone V, Coha M, Cerutti E, Schellino MM, Biolino P, Occella P, et al. Continuous positive airway pressure for treatment of postoperative hypoxemia: a randomized controlled trial. JAMA. 2005;293(5):589–95.
14. Ferreyra GSV, Ranieri VM. Acute respiratory failure after abdominal surgery. Year of intensive care and emergency medicine. Berlin: Springer; 2005. p. 10–8.
15. Lefebvre A, Lorut C, Alifano M, Dermine H, Roche N, Gauzit R, et al. Noninvasive ventilation for acute respiratory failure after lung resection: an observational study. Intensive Care Med. 2009;35(4):663–70.
16. Hein OV, Birnbaum J, Wernecke KD, Konertz W, Jain U, Spies C. Three-year survival after four major post-cardiac operative complications. Crit Care Med. 2006;34(11):2729–37.
17. Lindner KH, Lotz P, Ahnefeld FW. Continuous positive airway pressure effect on functional residual capacity, vital capacity and its subdivisions. Chest. 1987;92(1):66–70.

18. Stock MC, Downs JB, Gauer PK, Alster JM, Imrey PB. Prevention of postoperative pulmonary complications with CPAP, incentive spirometry, and conservative therapy. Chest. 1985;87(2):151–7.
19. Kindgen-Milles D, Müller E, Buhl R, Böhner H, Ritter D, Sandmann W, et al. Nasal-continuous positive airway pressure reduces pulmonary morbidity and length of hospital stay following thoracoabdominal aortic surgery. Chest. 2005;128(2):821–8.
20. Pelosi P, Jaber S. Noninvasive respiratory support in the perioperative period. Curr Opin Anaesthesiol. 2010;23(2):233–8.
21. Keller H, Freynet A, Puyraveau M, Falcoz PE. KINE PREOP pilot study: prehabilitation in fast-track thoracic surgery protocol. Rev Mal Respir. 2023;40(1):3–16.
22. Auriant I, Jallot A, Hervé P, Cerrina J, Le Roy Ladurie F, Fournier JL, et al. Noninvasive ventilation reduces mortality in acute respiratory failure following lung resection. Am J Respir Crit Care Med. 2001;164(7):1231–5.
23. Jaber S, Michelet P, Chanques G. Role of non-invasive ventilation (NIV) in the perioperative period. Best Pract Res Clin Anaesthesiol. 2010;24(2):253–65.
24. Olper L, Corbetta D, Cabrini L, Landoni G, Zangrillo A. Effects of non-invasive ventilation on reintubation rate: a systematic review and meta-analysis of randomised studies of patients undergoing cardiothoracic surgery. Crit Care Resusc. 2013;15(3):220–7.
25. Einav S, Lakbar I, Leone M. Non-invasive respiratory support for management of the perioperative patient: a narrative review. Adv Ther. 2021;38(4):1746–56.
26. Torres MF, Porfirio GJ, Carvalho AP, Riera R. Non-invasive positive pressure ventilation for prevention of complications after pulmonary resection in lung cancer patients. Cochrane Database Syst Rev. 2015;9:Cd010355.
27. Bodhey A, Bodhey M, Shallik NA, Al Nadhari M, Griess HF, Al Ani O, et al. Biphasic cuirass ventilation for airway surgeries: a comprehensive review. Cureus. 2024;16(12):e75477.
28. Sato Y, Saeki N, Asakura T, Aoshiba K, Kotani T. Effects of extrathoracic mechanical ventilation on pulmonary hypertension secondary to lung disease. J Anesth. 2016;30(4):663–70.
29. Grasso F, Engelberts D, Helm E, Frndova H, Jarvis S, Talakoub O, et al. Negative-pressure ventilation: better oxygenation and less lung injury. Am J Respir Crit Care Med. 2008;177(4):412–8.
30. Gorham J. A medical triumph: the iron lung. Respir Ther. 1979;9(1):71–3.
31. Linton DM. Cuirass ventilation: a review and update. Crit Care Resusc. 2005;7(1):22–8.
32. Batchelor TJP, Rasburn NJ, Abdelnour-Berchtold E, Brunelli A, Cerfolio RJ, Gonzalez M, et al. Guidelines for enhanced recovery after lung surgery: recommendations of the Enhanced Recovery After Surgery (ERAS®) Society and the European Society of Thoracic Surgeons (ESTS). Eur J Cardiothorac Surg. 2019;55(1):91–115.
33. Köhnlein T, Schönheit-Kenn U, Winterkamp S, Welte T, Kenn K. Noninvasive ventilation in pulmonary rehabilitation of COPD patients. Respir Med. 2009;103(9):1329–36.
34. Chiumello D, Chevallard G, Gregoretti C. Non-invasive ventilation in postoperative patients: a systematic review. Intensive Care Med. 2011;37(6):918–29.
35. Allen MS, Darling GE, Pechet TT, Mitchell JD, Herndon JE 2nd, Landreneau RJ, et al. Morbidity and mortality of major pulmonary resections in patients with early-stage lung cancer: initial results of the randomized, prospective ACOSOG Z0030 trial. Ann Thorac Surg. 2006;81(3):1013–9; discussion 9-20.
36. Deslauriers J, Ginsberg RJ, Piantadosi S, Fournier B. Prospective assessment of 30-day operative morbidity for surgical resections in lung cancer. Chest. 1994;106(6 Suppl):329s–30s.
37. Shapiro M, Swanson SJ, Wright CD, Chin C, Sheng S, Wisnivesky J, et al. Predictors of major morbidity and mortality after pneumonectomy utilizing the Society for Thoracic Surgeons General Thoracic Surgery Database. Ann Thorac Surg. 2010;90(3):927–34; discussion 34–5.
38. Duque JL, Ramos G, Castrodeza J, Cerezal J, Castanedo M, Yuste MG, et al. Early complications in surgical treatment of lung cancer: a prospective, multicenter study. Grupo Cooperativo de Carcinoma Broncogénico de la Sociedad Española de Neumología y Cirugía Torácica. Ann Thorac Surg. 1997;63(4):944–50.

39. Riviere S, Monconduit J, Zarka V, Massabie P, Boulet S, Dartevelle P, et al. Failure of noninvasive ventilation after lung surgery: a comprehensive analysis of incidence and possible risk factors. Eur J Cardiothorac Surg. 2011;39(5):769–76.
40. Sonobe M, Nakagawa M, Ichinose M, Ikegami N, Nagasawa M, Shindo T. Analysis of risk factors in bronchopleural fistula after pulmonary resection for primary lung cancer. Eur J Cardiothorac Surg. 2000;18(5):519–23.
41. Wahi R, McMurtrey MJ, DeCaro LF, Mountain CF, Ali MK, Smith TL, et al. Determinants of perioperative morbidity and mortality after pneumonectomy. Ann Thorac Surg. 1989;48(1):33–7.
42. Pool KL, Munden RF, Vaporciyan A, O'Sullivan PJ. Radiographic imaging features of thoracic complications after pneumonectomy in oncologic patients. Eur J Radiol. 2012;81(1):165–72.
43. Alexiou C, Beggs D, Rogers ML, Beggs L, Asopa S, Salama FD. Pneumonectomy for non-small cell lung cancer: predictors of operative mortality and survival. Eur J Cardiothorac Surg. 2001;20(3):476–80.
44. Wali A, Billè A. Complications of thoracic surgery: post-pneumonectomy bronchopleural fistula. Shanghai Chest. 2020;5
45. Algar FJ, Alvarez A, Salvatierra A, Baamonde C, Aranda JL, López-Pujol FJ. Predicting pulmonary complications after pneumonectomy for lung cancer. Eur J Cardiothorac Surg. 2003;23(2):201–8.
46. Slinger PD. Perioperative fluid management for thoracic surgery: the puzzle of postpneumonectomy pulmonary edema. J Cardiothorac Vasc Anesth. 1995;9(4):442–51.
47. Bauer P. Postpneumonectomy pulmonary oedema revisited. Eur Respir J. 2000;15(4):629–30.
48. Edward J, Banchs J, Parker H, Cornwell W. Right ventricular function across the spectrum of health and disease. Heart. 2023;109(5):349–55.
49. Haddad F, Couture P, Tousignant C, Denault AY. The right ventricle in cardiac surgery, a perioperative perspective: II. Pathophysiology, clinical importance, and management. Anesth Analg. 2009;108(2):422–33.
50. Vlahakes GJ. Right ventricular failure following cardiac surgery. Coron Artery Dis. 2005;16(1):27–30.
51. Itagaki S, Hosseinian L, Varghese R. Right ventricular failure after cardiac surgery: management strategies. Semin Thorac Cardiovasc Surg. 2012;24(3):188–94.
52. Kaul TK, Fields BL. Postoperative acute refractory right ventricular failure: incidence, pathogenesis, management and prognosis. Cardiovasc Surg. 2000;8(1):1–9.
53. McBride WT, Ranaldi G, Dougherty MJ, Siciliano T, Trethowan B, Elliott P, et al. The hemodynamic and respiratory effects of continuous negative and control-mode cuirass ventilation in recently extubated cardiac surgery patients: part 2. J Cardiothorac Vasc Anesth. 2012;26(5):873–7.
54. McBride WT, Ranaldi G, Dougherty MJ, Siciliano T, Trethowan B, Elliott P, et al. The hemodynamic and respiratory effects of cuirass ventilation in healthy volunteers: part 1. J Cardiothorac Vasc Anesth. 2012;26(5):868–72.
55. Guarracino F, Ambrosino N. Non invasive ventilation in cardio-surgical patients. Minerva Anestesiol. 2011;77(7):734–41.
56. Shekerdemian LS, Bush A, Shore DF, Lincoln C, Redington AN. Cardiopulmonary interactions after Fontan operations: augmentation of cardiac output using negative pressure ventilation. Circulation. 1997;96(11):3934–42.
57. Okada S, Muneuchi J, Nagatomo Y, Nonaka K, Iida C, Shirouzu H, et al. Successful treatment of protein-losing enteropathy and plastic bronchitis by biphasic cuirass ventilation in a patient with failing fontan circulation. Int Heart J. 2018;59(4):873–6.
58. Toida C, Shime N, Itoi T, Yamagishi M. Recovery from Fontan circulation failure by application of continuous negative extrathoracic pressure. J Anesth. 2007;21(2):282–4.
59. Chaturvedi RK, Zidulka AA, Goldberg P, deVarennes B, Iqbal S, Rahme E, et al. Use of negative extrathoracic pressure to improve hemodynamics after cardiac surgery. Ann Thorac Surg. 2008;85(4):1355–60.

Part V

Neonatology and Pediatric Section

Pediatric Acute Respiratory Failure

27

Kuniyuki Okada and Yutaka Ueda

27.1 Respiratory Support for Pediatric Acute Respiratory Insufficiency

In recent years, with the progress of non-invasive ventilation (NIV), many cases of acute respiratory failure even in children are using masks and other interfaces for non-invasive positive pressure ventilation [1]. Early intervention with NIV for respiratory distress is useful. Biphasic cuirass ventilation (BCV), in particular, is easy to install and is highly useful; hence, we use it in many cases. Table 27.1 [2] shows the benefits of BCV in children.

Because children have a smaller airway diameter and more airway secretions than adults, their airway resistance is high, which makes them prone to airway stenosis and obstruction. Furthermore, their respiratory muscles are weak, and most of the respiration is dependent on the diaphragm, causing respiratory muscle fatigue and making them prone to respiratory arrest. In addition, due to the small size of the thoracic cavity in children, positive pressure ventilation may increase the intrathoracic pressure, causing a decrease in venous return resulting in decreased cardiac output and eventually circulatory failure. As it is difficult for them to maintain a restful state due to high anxiety, cooperation in treatment is also difficult. BCV is a respiratory management technique suitable for children that can solve these problems. In this section, we will review our data and explain the use of BCV in inpatient and outpatient care for pediatric acute respiratory insufficiency, as well as the precautions to be taken when performing BCV.

K. Okada (✉) · Y. Ueda
OKADA Kodomonomori Clinic, Department of Pediatrics, Saitama Medical University and Graduate School of Saitama Medical University, Saitama, Japan
e-mail: y_ueda@saitama-med.ac.jp

O. Alibrahim et al. (eds.), *Biphasic Cuirass Noninvasive Ventilation*, Noninvasive Ventilation. The Essentials, https://doi.org/10.1007/978-3-032-20933-7_27

Table 27.1 Benefits of BCV in children

1. Simple and easy to set on or off
2. Support the patient's breath physiologically
3. Increase patient's tidal volume (improve oxygenation)
4. Impair venous circulation (decrease central venous pressure, increase cardiac output and urine output)
5. The effect of sputum excretion and resumption of the respiratory tract by Secretion Clearance mode
6. No ventilator-related complications with BCV (e.g., barotrauma, volutrauma, pneumothorax, and ventilator-associated pneumonia)
7. Each area of the lung is expanded uniformly
8. Maintain the quality of life (eat, feed, and speak)
9. In most children with respiratory failure, BCV results in rapid improvement in respiratory status

27.2 Definition of Pediatric Acute Respiratory Insufficiency

There is no clear definition to date for pediatric acute respiratory insufficiency, and it is important to check the symptoms of respiratory distress over time as shown in Table 27.2 to evaluate the respiratory status [2]. We use the Modified Pulmonary Index Score (MPIS) to objectively evaluate respiratory conditions. MPIS (Table 27.3) is an index of respiratory disorders related to intensive care unit (ICU) admission as proposed by Carrol et al. and is evaluated based on six categories: respiratory rate, heart rate, use of accessory muscles of respiration, expiratory and inspiratory time, degree of wheezing, and SpO_2 [3]. Because there is little room for bias from the evaluators, we use it as an objective indicator, and, in our institution, inpatient treatment is often required if the patient's score reaches 10 points or more [4]. Since children have little reserve for respiratory stress, the condition progresses faster than in adults, and may lead to cardiac arrest due to respiratory failure; therefore, it is necessary to judge and respond to the disease state quickly.

27.3 Indications for BCV in Pediatric Acute Respiratory Insufficiency

For the treatment of pediatric acute respiratory insufficiency, in addition to symptomatic treatments, such as inhalation therapy, oxygen therapy, and drug therapy, high-flow nasal cannulas, non-invasive positive pressure ventilation (NPPV) through masks, and conventional mechanical ventilation (CMV) with tracheal intubation are also used. Figure 27.1 demonstrates a flowchart of treatment selection according to severity, with the role of BCV shown for each severity. BCV is a simple and physiological respiratory assist technique that is particularly effective for infants who have a soft thorax and depend on the diaphragm for most of their respiratory movements. There is also a wide variety of diseases and conditions to which it can be applied. However, since BCV is a respiratory management method that is

Table 27.2 Symptoms of respiratory distress

1. Respiratory
Wheezing
Groaning
Nasal alar breathing
Tachypnea
Retraction
Orthopnea
Cyanosis
2. Cardiovascular
Tachycardia
Paradoxical pulse
Arrhythmia
Peripheral coldness
Decreased urine output
3. Neurological
Agitate
Restless
Disturbance of consciousness
Loss of sleep
Atonia
4. Digestive
Loss of appetite
Vomiting
5. Systemic
Fever
Hypothermia

performed under spontaneous breathing with an extracorporeal device, it is contraindicated in cases where the patency of the airway is uncertain or spontaneous breathing cannot be established [5–7]. In addition, sufficient consideration should be given to its use in cases with reduced consciousness, uncooperative cases, and cases with unstable general conditions such as disseminated intravascular coagulation (DIC).

On the other hand, BCV can be performed even in physically handicapped children (persons) with severe thorax deformity and scoliosis by wearing a cuirass on the side or back. In cases with thorax deformity and scoliosis, airway stenosis occurs when the curved spine presses the airway, making it difficult to discharge airway secretions, and treatment is often troublesome with repeated airway infections such as atelectasis and pneumonia [8–10]. In such cases, treatment with BCV is very useful and we often experience a rapid improvement in their respiratory status. We believe that acute respiratory distress in children (persons) with physical disabilities is a condition where the use of BCV should be recommended.

In addition, for severe acute respiratory insufficiency requiring tracheal intubation, CMV and BCV in combination often increase the tidal volume compared to when CMV is used alone, which can lead to a rapid improvement of the

Table 27.3 The Modified Pulmonary Index Score (MPIS) (Carrol [3])

	Score			
Category	0	1	2	3
Oxygen saturation, %	>95	93–95	90–92	<90
Accessory muscle use	None	Mild	Moderate	Severe
Inhalation-exhalation ratio	2:1	1:1	1:2	1:3
Wheezing	None	End expiratory	Inspiratory and expiratory wheeze, good aeration	Inspiratory and expiratory wheeze, decreased aeration
Heart rate/min <3 years old ≧3 years old	<120 <100	120–140 100–120	141–160 121–140	>160 >140
Respiratory rate/min <6 years old ≧6 years old	≦30 ≦20	31–45 21–35	46–60 36–50	>60 >50

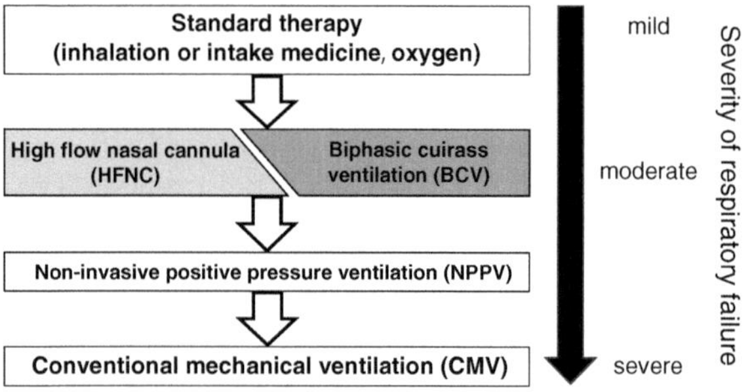

Fig. 27.1 Flowchart of respiratory therapy for acute respiratory failure in children. Standard therapy (inhalation or intake medicine, oxygen) is performed for mild respiratory failure. HFNC or BCV was performed for moderate respiratory failure, which is selected depending on each hospital or physician. If respiratory conditions get worse, it is necessary to quickly switch to NPPV or CMV

respiratory condition. Furthermore, in combination therapy, transpulmonary pressure is counterbalanced, suggesting the possibility of reducing barotrauma [11].

Since BCV improves respiratory distress soon after the start of treatment, it has been shown that hospitalization can be avoided by using it for treatment of acute exacerbation of bronchial asthma and bronchitis/bronchiolitis at outpatient clinics. Hence, the use of BCV is considered effective not only in hospitalization but also in outpatient medical care.

27.4 Effects of BCV

In BCV respiratory management, continuous negative mode is as effective as CPAP, where a pressure in continuous negative mode of –10cmH_2O is equivalent to 3–4 cmH_2O of CPAP [12, 13]. We performed a retrospective observational study of three groups: CMV, NPPV, and BCV (Continuous Negative Mode: −10 cmH_2O worn all day) for pediatric acute respiratory distress (N = 52) requiring management with mechanical ventilation. In this study, the PCO_2, respiratory rate, and SpO_2 improved significantly 24 hours after the start of treatment from before treatment with BCV, and was as effective as CMV and NPPV (Fig. 27.2a–c) [14]. In addition, compared with CMV, the time on a ventilator was significantly shorter and the hospitalization period was shortened with BCV (Fig. 27.2d, e). Minato et al. examined 70 cases of acute respiratory insufficiency in children (21 of which were RS virus infections) classified as severe (13 cases) or moderate (57 cases) using MPIS, before and after BCV (continuous negative mode: −10 cmH_2O for 1–2 hours in combination with the secretion clearance mode; four cycles per day) intervention [15]. They found that the median value of MPIS in severe cases decreased from 13 points to 9 points the following day, while the median value of moderate cases decreased from 8 points to 6 points. They also analyzed the MPIS evaluation categories and found that "accessory muscle use," "heart rate," "respiratory rate," and "degree of wheezing" significantly improved in the severe group after treatment with BCV, indicating that BCV may reduce respiratory effort. Hartman et al. reported a single-center study comparing standard treatment and BCV for acute bronchiolitis in children under 1 year of age (N = 33), and showed that a reduction in the amount of oxygen used within 1 hour was seen in a greater number of patients treated with BCV [16]. Nunez et al. reported that the therapeutic efficacy of BCV in 118 cases of pediatric acute respiratory distress (86.4% with viral bronchiolitis) was 68.6%, with a significant improvement in the SpO_2/FiO_2 ratio 1 hour after the start of treatment [17]. We also use BCV in outpatient settings in children with mild to moderate acute respiratory insufficiency. In the general pediatric outpatient clinic, continuous negative mode was used in 1384 cases and secretion clearance mode in 58,650 cases over a 15-year period (Fig. 27.3a, b), and the degree of improvement was measured based on MPIS before and after a single treatment. Continuous negative mode significantly improved MPIS from 8.5 to 6.5 points after an average of 48 minutes of use, and secretion clearance mode significantly improved MPIS from 4.8 to 3.4 points. Daily BCV treatment prevented hospitalization even in severe cases (MPIS ≥11 points, N = 9), though they required an average clinic visit of 5.0 days. For RSV bronchiolitis, continuous negative mode significantly improved MPIS from 10.1 to 7.1 after an average of 20 minutes of treatment. In particular, MPIS score significantly improved in heart rate, respiratory rate, and wheezing.

Here, we introduce the data on the effects of BCV. We measured the change in airway resistance using the forced oscillation technique (FOT) before and after BCV treatment. FOT was performed in patients with an acute exacerbation of bronchial asthma before and after continuous negative mode, and R5-R20 which indicates peripheral airway resistance decreased (Table 27.4a, b). Similarly, FOT

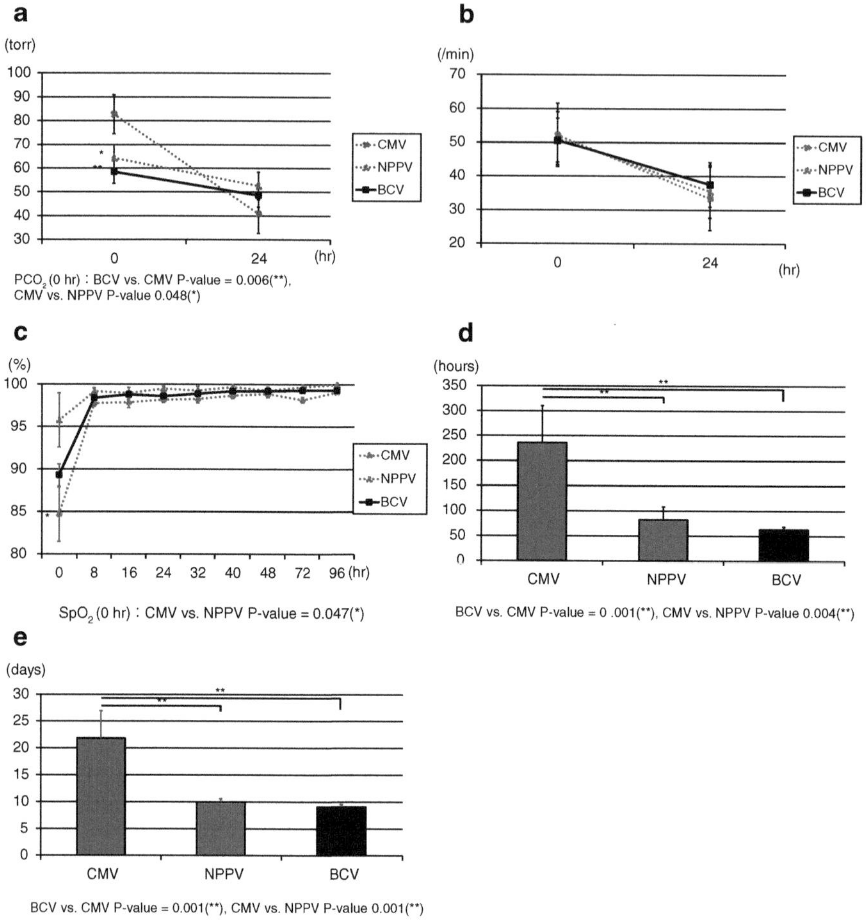

Fig. 27.2 The effect of each respiratory therapy. We performed a retrospective observational study of three groups: CMV, NPPV, and BCV (Continuous Negative mode: −10 cmH2O worn all day) for pediatric acute respiratory distress ($N = 52$) requiring management with mechanical ventilation. (**a**–**c**) The PCO_2, respiratory rate, and SpO_2 improved significantly 24 hours after the start of treatment from before treatment with BCV, and was as effective as CMV and NPPV. (**d**, **e**) Compared with CMV, the time on a ventilator was significantly shorter and the hospitalization period was shortened with BCV

measurements before and after secretion clearance mode showed a decrease in R5-R20, and subsequent bronchodilator inhalation further decreased R5-R20 (Table 27.4c). From this, one can see that BCV alone has bronchodilator and airway clearance effects, but it is more effective when used in combination with a bronchodilator.

Next, we measured the tidal volume before and after BCV treatment in cases where BCV was used in combination with a ventilator under tracheal intubation. In two patients in whom the continuous negative mode was used, tidal volume

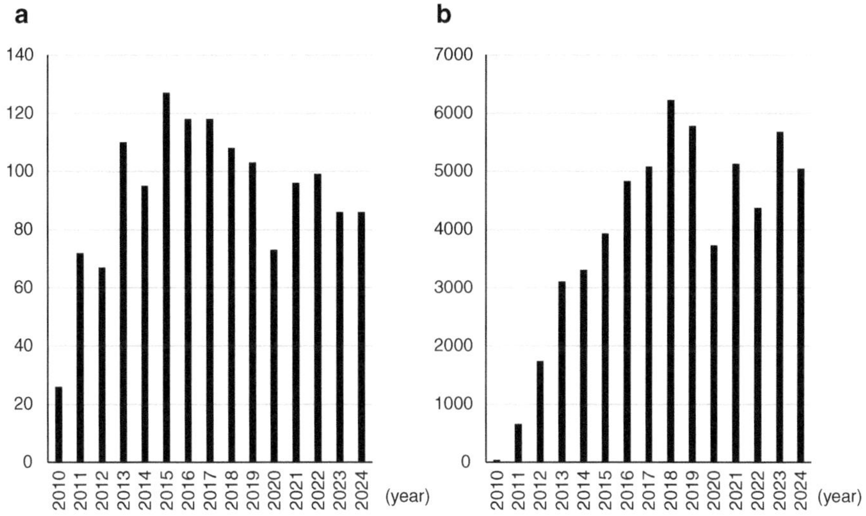

Fig. 27.3 The frequency of BCV use for outpatient. We use BCV in outpatient settings in children in the general pediatric outpatient clinic. (**a**) shows the frequency of continuous negative mode, (**b**) shows the frequency of section clearance mode over a 15-year period

Table 27.4 The change of airway resistance by BCV (Continuous Negative mode)

		R5	R20	R5-R20	X5	Fres	ALX
		(a) 7 years girl with severe exacerbation of asthma					
Ave.	Pre BCV	13.87	9.08	4.79	−6.61	26.15	67.54
	Post BCV	13.46	9.86	3.60	−5.61	27.01	58.46
		(b) 9 years boy with moderate exacerbation of asthma					
Ave.	Pre BCV	8.74	5.22	3.52	−6.29	21.83	52.73
	Post BCV	4.85	4.21	0.64	−7.35	18.10	51.83
(c) 5 years girl with mild exacerbation of asthma							
Ave	Pre BCV	6.86	4.91	1.95	−2.33	17.10	15.55
	Post BCV	6.37	4.60	1.77	−2.76	17.23	18.41
	Post bronchodilator	5.43	3.96	1.47	−2.02	14.23	11.47

increased significantly 15 minutes after BCV, from 7.3 mL/kg to 9.2 mL/kg (Fig. 27.4a) and from 7.2 mL/kg to 7.7 mL/kg (Fig. 27.4b). Although the mean airway pressure did not change in the patients in whom the secretion clearance mode was used, tidal volume improved from 1.5 mL/kg to 4.6 mL/kg (Fig. 27.4c). These results show that BCV dilates airways and decreases airway resistance by increasing negative pressure in the thorax. Furthermore, BCV induced a reduction in respiratory effort and an increase in tidal volume. In addition, clearance of airway secretions decreased airway resistance increasing tidal volume. Thus, although continuous negative mode and secretion clearance mode are effective on their own, a synergistic effect can be expected when used together.

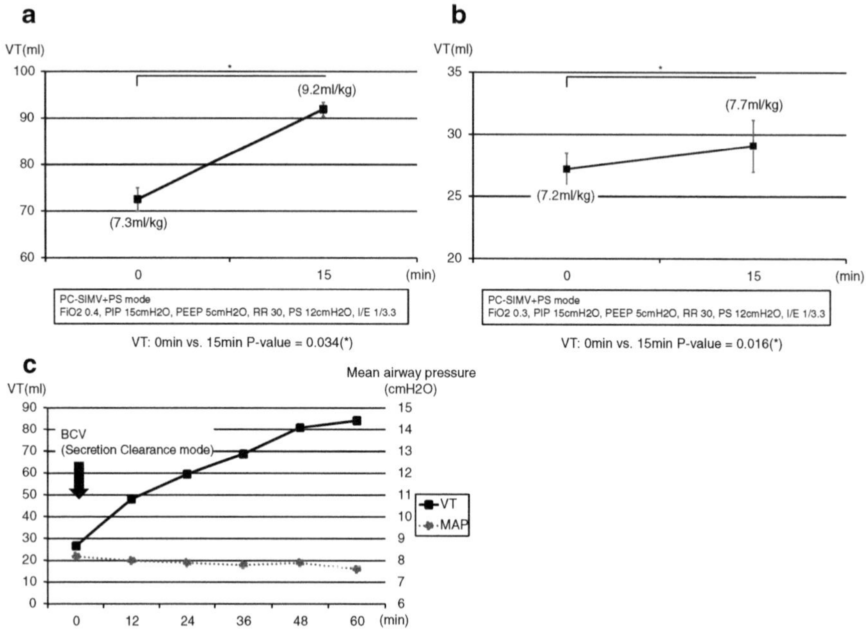

Fig. 27.4 The change of tidal volume which was treated by CMV with BCV. We measured the tidal volume before and after BCV treatment in cases where BCV was used in combination with a ventilator under tracheal intubation. (**a**, **b**) When BCV (continuous negative mode) was used in combination with a ventilator under tracheal intubation, tidal volume increased significantly 15 minutes after BCV, from 7.3 mL/kg to 9.2 mL/kg (**a**) and from 7.2 mL/kg to 7.7 mL/kg (**b**). (**c**) When BCV (secretion clearance mode) was used in combination with a ventilator under tracheal intubation, tidal volume increased from 1.5 mL/kg to 4.6 mL/kg in spite of the mean airway pressure

27.5 How to Use BCV

Installation instructions (attachment procedure: Fig. 27.5)

Since the cuirass, which is the interface of BCV, is attached to the trunk, the rejection in patients is not stronger than with other NPPVs. However, there are many children who are afraid of wearing a cuirass, especially for the first time. It can be worn smoothly by attaching the cuirass to the back or by having a parent hold the child while BCV is being performed, the patient and parents can feel safe. The cuirass is available in 11 different sizes; sizes 0–4 are often used in children.

In respiratory management by BCV, it is important to securely apply the cuirass to the body. Typically, the cuirass is secured tightly to the body and gaps are filled with towels. However, if the adhesion is too strong, it may cause skin damage, and if the adhesion is too weak, not only will the effect be insufficient due to air leakage, but the body may be cooled resulting in hypothermia. Therefore, it is necessary to

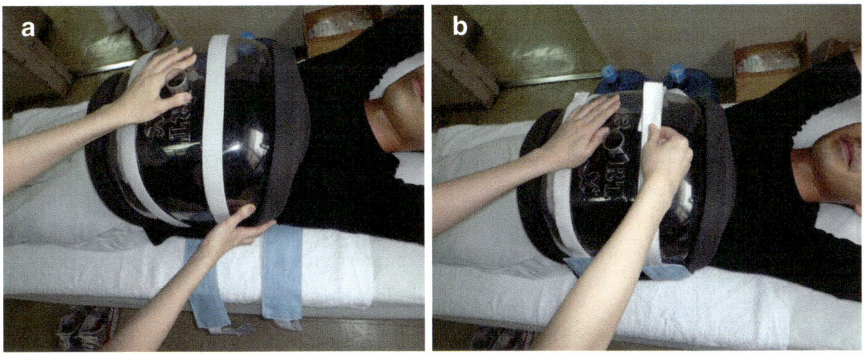

The cuirass is placed over the diaphragm. Wrap the cuirass and body with the bands.

Fig. 27.5 Steps to wear a cuirass

check whether the set value corresponds to the pressure inside the cuirass at the beginning of treatment.

Once BCV is initiated, vital signs (temperature, respiratory rate, and heart rate) should be monitored by an SpO_2 and ECG monitor. In severe cases, oxygen and carbon dioxide partial pressures, bicarbonate levels, and electrolytes should be checked over time with blood gas analysis to confirm improvement.

27.5.1 Method of Treatment

There are five modes of ventilation of BCV in the extracorporeal ventilator RTX® (United Hayek Industries, London, United Kingdom). The two main modes used for acute respiratory distress in children are Continuous Negative mode and Secretion Clearance mode, but for older children and adults, a triggered mode that detects the patient's inspiration to provide respiratory support may be used. The continuous negative mode can reduce airway resistance and increase tidal volume by expanding the thorax kept under constant negative pressure in the cuirass, which, in turn, increases the range of motion of the diaphragm. The secretion clearance mode vibrates the chest wall by alternating positive and negative pressures in the cuirass, and then promotes sputum excretion by instantly turning the pressure positive (cough) in the cuirass. This promotes clearance of the airway and oxygenation by a high-frequency oscillation (HFO) effect.

The continuous negative mode is performed when the patient has a relatively high degree of respiratory impairment. We use a negative pressure of -10 cmH_2O for all patients regardless of body size or age, and have found it to be sufficiently effective. In most cases, the respiratory condition improves within 30 minutes to 1 hour, but, in some cases, respiratory insufficiency may persist for several hours. Nebulized bronchodilator inhalation is used in almost all cases, both in- and

Table 27.5 The settings of secretion clearance mode

Parameters	Setting
Vibration mode	
Frequency vibration	600 (cpm)
Inspiratory pressure	−10 (cmH_2O)
Time	2 (min)
Cough mode	
Frequency cough	20–50 (cpm)
Inspiratory pressure	−10 (cmH_2O)
Expiratory pressure	+5 (cmH_2O)
I:E ratio	5.0:1.0
Time	1 (min)
Repeat count (for whole cycle)	4 (cycles)

outpatients, and the mode is switched to Secretion Clearance mode during inhalation. The settings we use are shown in Table 27.5.

The following are described separately in terms of in- and outpatient treatment.

27.5.1.1 BCV Treatment During Hospitalization

Patients who are admitted to the hospital have severe respiratory impairment, which inevitably leads to the use of continuous negative mode in many cases. Unlike CMV, sedatives and muscle relaxants are almost never used, but mild sedatives can be used in younger children if they express more anxiety and show resistance to wearing a cuirass. During inpatient treatment, inhalation therapy with a nebulizer every 6–8 hours is often performed in combination with the secretion clearance mode. The aforementioned MPIS is very useful in assessing respiratory status, and we evaluate and check the respiratory status every few hours. BCV is a physiological ventilatory management method that has been shown to be very effective in the treatment of acute bronchiolitis caused by RS virus. However, if there is no improvement within a short period of time (1–2 hours), the patient should immediately be converted to positive pressure ventilation such as tracheal intubation or NPPV [18, 19]. During long hours of BCV treatment, the skin in contact with the cuirass should be observed several times a day to avoid skin damage and the occurrence of ulcers. If the degree of respiratory distress is mild, "secretion clearance mode" can be used in combination with nebulizer inhalation to achieve the same effect as pulmonary physiotherapy.

Even in cases where CMV is performed because of severe respiratory impairment, BCV can often improve the respiratory condition, especially in cases where the tidal volume is low due to atelectasis. In such cases, although the main purpose is to reduce airway resistance by using the continuous negative mode, we have experienced that frequent use of Secretion Clearance mode (every 1–3 hours) improves tidal volume in a short time by promoting reopening of the airway [20]. However, although extremely rare, secretion clearance mode has been reported to cause obstruction of the central airway by peripheral airway secretions, so the patient's breathing should be checked regularly.

27.5.1.2 BCV Treatment in Outpatient Clinics

Respiratory failure in the outpatient clinic is often milder than in the inpatient hospital, and treatment mainly consists of the Secretion Clearance mode combined with nebulized bronchodilator inhalation. After the completion of BCV, the patient should be examined again, and, if respiration has not sufficiently improved, for example if wheezing remains, the same treatment should be repeated.

In the outpatient clinic, if respiratory distress is moderate with an MPIS of more than 10, continuous negative mode is usually performed for about 20 minutes, followed by secretion clearance mode. The duration of treatment may be extended depending on the severity of the patient's condition and the improvement in breathing. Admission can often be avoided when BCV treatment is performed in the morning and evening.

27.5.2 Treatment Site

When children with acute respiratory insufficiency require ventilation management with inpatient care, they are usually managed in an ICU or a hospital bed capable of providing a similar nursing system. BCV essentially requires the same settings, but it can be managed in a general ward if the only symptom is mild effortful breathing and are not accompanied by hypercapnia or severe hypoxemia. In such a case, a system that can monitor SpO_2 and pulse rate is desirable.

27.5.3 Circuit Structure and Staff Education

The circuit configuration of RTX®, a ventilator that can provide BCV, consists of a cuirass, a cuirass strap, a wide bore tube, and a pressure sensor tube, and does not require an exhalation valve (photo).

The specific procedure is as follows: (1) Select a cuirass size that suits the patient's physique. (2) Secure the cuirass with the cuirass strap. (3) Connect the wide bore tube and the pressure sensor tube. (4) Apply a negative pressure of −10 cmH_2O in continuous negative mode to confirm the fitting of the cuirass (re-fix the cuirass strap if it is loose). (5) Select the mode to be used and start.

The knowledge and experience required for staff education include the following: (1) how to attach the cuirass and cuirass straps, (2) the types of cuirass and adjustment of its fitting, (3) how to assemble the BCV equipment, (4) how to operate and troubleshoot the BCV equipment, (5) general maintenance and cleaning methods, (6) how to detect and manage complications, (7) evaluation and treatment of the response after the implementation of the BCV, (8) actual personal experience of the BCV, and (9) understanding of the pathophysiology of respiratory failure and having the necessary anatomical and physiological knowledge. In particular, it is important for medical personnel to experience wearing a cuirass and ventilation with BCV in order for them to understand how comfortable the patients would feel when using it during activities of daily living (such as mouth washing, drinking water, changing positions, and getting out from the bed).

27.5.4 Troubleshooting and Safety Management

The frequent problems are skin damage and hypothermia. Skin damage occurs when the cuirass strap is fastened to ensure that it is fitted securely, or when the cuirass seal is damaged, and the cuirass and skin come in direct contact.

To deal with areas where there is a gap between the body and the cuirass is difficult; hence, a towel placed in a plastic bag is inserted. The towel fills the large gap, and the covering plastic bag inflates by negative pressure to fill any small gaps. In this way, it is not necessary to excessively tighten the cuirass strap, and this makes it possible to reduce skin damage. In addition, wearing the cuirass with clothes on or applying a wound dressing (such as DuoActive®; ConvaTec Japan, Tokyo, Japan; or AirWall®; KYOWA LIMITED, Osaka, Japan) to the area of skin in contact with the cuirass can reduce direct irritation of the skin and prevent skin damage. Since skin damage may occur despite these precautions, when the cuirass is worn continuously, it is necessary to remove the cuirass and check for skin damage, as appropriate. Hypothermia is caused by poor fitting of the cuirass, which causes air to be drawn into the cuirass from the outside, creating a situation akin to that of the patient being exposed to strong winds. The cuirass should be fitted as described above.

27.6 Summary

BCV is a simple physiological respiratory support method that is particularly effective for acute respiratory distress in children. Since there is no interface on the face and treatment can be performed under a conscious state, oral intake and conversation are possible even during treatment, which is especially useful for children. In Japan, BCV can be covered by insurance. Depending on the mode of use, an additional fee can be charged for artificial respiration management or secretion clearance mode as support of promoting sputum excretion. However, BCV is performed under spontaneous breathing with uncertain airway control, so if it is not effective in a short period of time (1–2 hours); it is necessary to quickly switch to tracheal intubation.

References

1. Kneyber MCJ, de Luca D, Calderini E, Jarreau PH, Javouhey E, Lopez-Herce J, Hammer J, Macrae D, Markhorst DG, Medina A, Pons-Odena M, Racca F, Wolf G, Biban P, Brierley J, Rimensberger PC. Recommendations for mechanical ventilation of critically ill children from

the Paediatric Mechanical Ventilation Consensus Conference (PEMVECC). Intensive Care Med. 2017;43(12):1764–80.
2. Okada K, Ueda Y. Extra-thoracic biphasic cuirass ventilation [article in Japanese]. Jinkoukokyuu. 2010;27(1):23–9.
3. Carroll CL, Sekaran AK, Lerer TJ, Schramm CM. A modified pulmonary index score with predictive value for pediatric asthma exacerbations. Ann Allergy Asthma Immunol. 2005;94:355–9.
4. Koga T, Tokuyama K, Itano A, Morita E, Ueda Y, Katsunuma T. Usefulness of modified Pulmonary Index Score (mPIS) as a quantitative tool for the evaluation of severe acute exacerbation in asthmatic children. Allergol Int. 2015;64(2):139–44.
5. Goldstein RS, Stradling JR. An artifact induced by negative pressure ventilation. Chest. 1992;101(2):563–5.
6. Levy RD, Bradley TD, Newman SL, Macklem PT, Martin JG. Negative pressure ventilation. Effects on ventilation during sleep in normal subjects. Chest. 1989;95(1):95–9.
7. Hartmann H, Jawad MH, Noyes J, Samuels MP, Southall DP. Negative extrathoracic pressure ventilation in central hypoventilation syndrome. Arch Dis Child. 1994;70(5):418–23.
8. Kato K, Sato N, Takeda S, Yamamoto T, Munakata R, Tsurumi M, Suzuki D, Yagi K, Tanaka K, Mizuno K. Marked improvement of extensive atelectasis by unilateral application of the RTX respirator in elderly patients. Intern Med. 2009;48(16):1419–23.
9. Toyoshima M, Maeoka Y, Kawahara H, Maegaki Y, Ohno K. Pulmonary atelectasis in patients with neurological or muscular disease; gravity-related lung compression by the heart and intra-abdominal organs on persistent supine position [Article in Japanese]. No To Hattatsu. 2006;38(6):419–24.
10. Chari S, King J, Rajesh PB, Stuart-Smith K. Resolution of left lower lobe collapse postesophagectomy using the MediventRTX respirator, a novel noninvasive respiratory support system. J Cardiothorac Vasc Anesth. 2004;18(4):482–5.
11. Vincenzi U. A new mode of mechanical ventilation: positive + negative synchronized ventilation. Multidiscip Respir Med. 2021;16:788.
12. Kaneko K, Kinnno Y, Shigeta M, Nakayama K, Shimizu K, Yamaguchi O, Usuda Y, Okutsu Y. The tidal volume, arterial blood gas and functional residual capacity changes during negative extra-thoracic pressure ventilation and positive airway pressure ventilation [article in Japanese]. Masui. 1990;38(3):372–5.
13. Borelli M, Benini A, Denkewitz T, Acciaro C, Foti G, Pesenti A. Effects of continuous negative extrathoracic pressure versus positive end-expiratory pressure in acute lung injury patients. Crit Care Med. 1998;26(6):1025–31.
14. Ueda Y, Okada K. The effect of biphasic cuirass ventilation for acute respiratory failure. 10th international congress of pediatric pulmonology, 2011, Vienna, Austria.
15. Toshinori M. Clinical investigation of the efficacy and safety of biphasic cuirass ventilation in children hospitalized with respiratory distress [article in Japanese]. Nihon shoni kokyuuki gakkaishi. 2017;28(2):175–87.
16. Hartmann H, Noyes JP, Wright T, Wheatley R, Spencer A, Boon A, et al. Continuous negative extrathoracic pressure ventilationin infants with bronchiolitis. Eur Respir J. 1994;7(Suppl 18):379.
17. Nunez CA, Hassinger AB. Predictors of negative pressure ventilation response in pediatric acute respiratory failure. Respir Care. 2020;65(1):91–8.
18. Yañez LJ, Yunge M, Emilfork M, Lapadula M, Alcántara A, Fernández C, Lozano J, Contreras M, Conto L, Arevalo C, Gayan A, Hernández F, Pedraza M, Feddersen M, Bejares M, Morales M, Mallea F, Glasinovic M, Cavad G. A prospective, randomized, controlled trial of non-invasive ventilation in pediatric acute respiratory failure. Pediatr Crit Care Med. 2008;9(5):484–9.
19. Piastra M, De Luca D, Marzano L, Stival E, Genovese O, Pietrini D, Conti G. The number of failing organs predicts non-invasive ventilation failure in children with ALI/ARDS. Intensive Care Med. 2011;37(9):1510–6.
20. Chatburn RL. High-frequency assisted airway clearance. Respir Care. 2007;52(9):1224–37.

28 Biphasic Cuirass Ventilation in Patients with Congenital Myotonic Dystrophy

Hari Gourabathini, Mohammad Sallam, Vanessa Marthia, and Omar Alibrahim

28.1 Introduction

Congenital myotonic dystrophy [CMD] is a neuromuscular disorder involving multi-systems with the most severe symptom of respiratory muscle weakness. Weakness of inspiratory and expiratory muscles leads to severe respiratory complications including respiratory insufficiency and aspiration pneumonia. These complications are a common cause of mortality for these infants with a mortality rate of up to 40%. Often it can be difficult to ventilate these patients and with prolonged intubation, there is an increased risk of fatality of up to 100% [1, 2]. Patients with CMD often present in the neonatal period with severe respiratory symptoms due to weakened respiratory muscles; however, these symptoms improve as patients grow [3]. These infants often have a high risk of morbidity and mortality especially with prolonged invasive ventilation [4].

The use of negative pressure ventilation [NPV] using biphasic cuirass without engaging the face or airway is a safe, effective, and an alternative strategy that supports respiratory effort without the many associated invasive mechanical ventilation

H. Gourabathini (✉)
Beacon Children's Hospital, South Bend, IN, USA
e-mail: hgourabathini@beaconhealthsystem.org

M. Sallam
Mercy One Des Moines Medical Center, Des Moines, Iowa, USA
e-mail: mohammad.sallam@mercyone.org

V. Marthia
University at Buffalo, Buffalo, NY, USA
e-mail: vmarthia@upa.chob.edu

O. Alibrahim
Pediatric Critical Care Medicine, Duke University Hospital, Durham, NC, USA
e-mail: omar.alibrahim@duke.edu

O. Alibrahim et al. (eds.), *Biphasic Cuirass Noninvasive Ventilation*, Noninvasive Ventilation. The Essentials, https://doi.org/10.1007/978-3-032-20933-7_28

risks and long-term sedation complications in these profoundly weak patients [5]. Current NPV devices deliver negative extra-thoracic pressure to the chest wall through a plastic shell wrapped with foam as a protective barrier. These devices can provide continuous negative pressure to the chest which is comparable to continuous positive airway pressure [CPAP]. There is also a control mode to deliver biphasic pressure and secretion clearance mode where the apparatus applies rapidly alternating positive and negative pressures to the chest wall which is comparable to other chest physiotherapy and cough assist devices [6]. These devices may avoid/limit prolonged intubations, improve respiratory failure, inspiratory muscle strength, and can be a beneficial tool to bridge these individuals beyond infancy when they are at greatest risk for mortality [7–9].

28.2 Congenital Myotonic Dystrophy [CMD]

28.2.1 Etiology

Congenital Myotonic Dystrophy was first recognized and described by Vanier in 1960 [10]. Myotonic dystrophy is caused from 2 loci DM1 and DM2. DM1 is associated with CTG trinucleotide expansion on chromosome 19q13.3, and DM2 is associated with CCTG tetranucleotide expansion at 3q21 [11, 12]. These genes disrupt the coding for myotonic dystrophy protein kinase and zinc finger 9 protein. However, the pathogenesis is mostly related to accumulation of mutant mRNA in the cell's nuclei [6, 12]. Like any trinucleotide expansion repeat diseases, a larger number of repeats are associated with the severity of the disease [13, 14]. DM1 is associated with more severe clinical phenotype and manifests at an early age. The onset at earlier age in subsequent generations is due to further amplification of the CTG repeats carried by the parent during gametogenesis. This manifestation is known as Genetic anticipation. Genetic anticipation leads to congenital myotonic dystrophy [15]. The age of onset and severity of phenotype are closely correlated to the number of CTG repeats [16]. Compared to general population with 5–30 CTG repeats, patients with CMD have 50–1000 repeats [17].

28.2.2 Epidemiology

Incidence is described in the past as 1 in 3350–16,500 live births [15]. Congenital myotonic dystrophy is a rare genetic disorder affecting 2.1/100000 in Canada [4]. A mother with a previous CMD child has 20–41% increased risk for following pregnancy [3]. Pediatric mortality rates range 17–41% [3, 4]. Myotonic dystrophy is the most prevalent adult muscular dystrophy among the people of European ancestry with a minimum prevalence of 11.84/100,000 [14].

28.2.3 Clinical Features

CMD has a characteristic biphasic course. The immobility, hypotonia, respiratory insufficiency, and feeding difficulties improve over the first few weeks of life to present in later years as adult onset myotonia, muscle atrophy, and cataracts [3]. There are two major forms: Myotonic dystrophy type 1 [DM1], also known as Steinert disease; Myotonic dystrophy type 2 [DM2], which is a milder version of DM1 [16]. CDM is more than just muscular dystrophy as the affected individuals show the involvement of several organ systems [discussed in detail below] resulting in cataracts, cardiac conduction anomalies, and insulin resistance, and also the congenital form is associated with developmental disabilities [17]. Children of ages 1 to 10 years can walk with improvement in motor function; however, progressive weakness restarts in the second decade. Myotonia [by 10 years of age], intellectual disability [50–60%], autism, attention deficit hyperactivity disorder [ADHD], psychiatric disorders, vision problems, excessive daytime sleepiness, and cardiac and endocrine complications evolve in later part of life [16].

28.2.4 Neonatal Presentation

Congenital myotonic dystrophy may be misdiagnosed during neonatal period due to variant presentation from adults. Symptoms suggestive of CMD including cataracts, muscle wasting, and myotonia are rarely seen in neonates. Mothers of these children are the affected parent. These mothers often are not diagnosed or have only mild symptoms. These individuals may have a history of still births, previous neonatal deaths, or pregnancy complicated by polyhydramnios and poor fetal movements. Polyhydramnios is due to poor swallowing from fetus [3].

Neonates present with perinatal asphyxia, hypotonia or floppiness, myopathic facial features [short anteverted philtrum of the upper lip and tent-shaped mouth], skeletal deformities like pes equinovarus, and arthrogryposis. Chest X ray may reveal elevated right side of diaphragm and slender ribs. Sudden deaths can occur in neonates due to respiratory insufficiency or cardiac conduction abnormalities like adults with myotonic dystrophy. Symptoms and signs are classified into major and additional criteria. Major criteria symptoms include hypotonia, facies myopathic, muscle atrophy, respiratory problems, and feeding problems. Additional criteria symptoms include polyhydramnios, skeletal deformities, elevated diaphragm, thin ribs, edema, hematomas, and anal sphincter insufficiency [15].

28.2.5 Musculoskeletal Involvement

Individuals with DM1 characteristically have distal muscular weakness more commonly than proximal. Proximal muscle weakness is associated with poorer prognosis. As the child grows, muscular weakness leads to scoliosis, and contractures. Bulbar weakness leads to swallow difficulties, speech, and language problems [18].

Elevated diaphragm on the right side is due to immaturity of the muscle fibers and increased resistance from liver. Respiratory insufficiency is seen in all neonates due to immaturity of the diaphragmatic and intercostal muscles, associated aspiration pneumonia, and central respiratory failure. Palatopharyngeal and facial muscle weakness results in a impaired suck reflex. When exacerbated by associated gastroparesis, this significantly increases feeding difficulties. Edema observed postnatally may be secondary to decreased fetal movements [3]. Multiple contractures occur due to muscular strength imbalance and structural changes across multiple joints such as bilateral talipes equinovarus and scoliosis [19].

28.2.6 Respiratory Involvement

Weakness of inspiratory and expiratory muscles leads to major respiratory symptoms. Aspiration pneumonia and respiratory insufficiency are the most common cause of mortality in the neonatal period [19]. Children with myotonic dystrophy may present with respiratory depression after induction of anesthesia. Sudden death secondary to cardiac conduction abnormalities with muscle relaxants and anesthetic drugs has been observed in children with congenital myotonic dystrophy [3].

A case series from Rutherford et al. revealed 100% mortality in children requiring assisted ventilation for >30 days. The respiratory complications in congenital myotonic dystrophy are secondary to pulmonary hypoplasia, fetal breathing, and decreased respiratory drive from abnormal brain [1]. Children with CDM requiring intubation for >30 days have increased morbidity, mortality, and prolonged hospitalizations [4]. Developmental delay especially in motor skills was more pronounced in the longer duration ventilation group. Mortality was increased in the longer duration ventilation group but significantly lower from the previous studies. Previous studies reported 100% mortality rate in prolonged duration ventilation group. Muscular immaturity, hypotonia, and respiratory insufficiency improve with the progression of age in congenital myotonic dystrophy, resulting in lesser dependence on assisted ventilation and decreased ventilator complications. Children with longer duration of mechanical ventilation had increased number of hospitalizations due to comorbidities from respiratory illnesses and gastric dysmotility problems. Acquired air leak syndromes and pneumonia were often seen in prolonged duration ventilation group [4]. Keller et al. reported 2 cases weaned off ventilator after 127 days and 27 days to nasal CPAP. The total ventilation days were 141 and 84 days. N CPAP and methylxanthines are effective in weaning off a ventilator in very low birth weight neonates thus describing no consistent mortality in all patients [2].

28.2.7 Sleep Instabilities

Sleep disorders more commonly manifest in childhood and adults affecting memory, cognitive processing, and physical functioning. Children present with excessive daytime sleepiness, hypoventilation, sleep apnea, sleep fragmentation, periodic limb movement disorders, and rapid eye movement sleep dysregulation. Central ventilation dysregulation is secondary to neuronal loss and gliosis in the reticular activating system and brain stem. Abnormal levels of growth hormone, cortisol, and cytokinesin in DM1 also affect the sleep regulation. Sympathetic hyperactivity leads to cardiac conduction disturbances [18].

28.2.8 Other Systems

Cataracts, cardiac conduction abnormalities, diabetes mellitus, hypogonadism, growth hormone imbalance, androgen insensitivity, testicular atrophy in males, and irregular and prolonged periods of amenorrhea in females are seen [18]. Hematomas of the labia minora, skin, and cerebral region are observed. Hematomas may be caused by trauma during delivery or and capillary leakage [3]. Ventriculomegaly is observed due to hydrocephalus and brain atrophy [18]. Gastrointestinal symptoms including fecal incontinence, irregular bowel habits, gastroesophageal reflux, choking, nausea, vomiting, and gastric motility problems may be present [18]. A range of mild, moderate, and severe cognitive deficits are observed. Cognitive deficit severity is associated with muscle weakness, size of CTG repeats, and maternal transmission. CDM patients have a mean IQ of 70 with a range of 40–80 [18].

28.3 Respiratory Failure in Congenital Myotonic Dystrophy [CMD]

Respiratory failure in Congenital Myotonic Dystrophy is a complex process that, in part, resembles respiratory failure in other muscular/neuromuscular pathologies, where respiratory muscle weakness is the key factor. Other factors that play a role in respiratory failure in patients with myotonic dystrophy include central respiratory drive dysfunction, sleep apnea, upper airway dysfunction, and decreased chest wall compliance [8, 20].

28.4 Supportive Data of Negative Pressure Ventilation Use in Congenital Myotonic Dystrophies

Despite the paucity of "direct" clinical data, the use of NPV in myotonic dystrophy is supported by "indirect evidence." NPV was successfully used to support patients with respiratory failure secondary to similar mechanisms contributing to respiratory failure in myotonic dystrophies, including muscle weakness, reduced chest wall compliance, central hypoventilation, and sleep apnea. This section is a brief discussion of the direct and indirect evidence that supports the use of NPV in Congenital Myotonic Dystrophies, and the precautions that should be taken before considering NPV in this patient's population.

28.5 Direct Evidence

A case report that was recently published by Almeda et al. described a neonate with CMD who was successfully managed with polysomnography titrated biphasic cuirass ventilation [BCV] with improvement of oxygen requirement and weight gain pattern [21].

28.6 Indirect Evidence

(a) *Respiratory Muscle Weakness and Secondary Decreased Chest Wall Compliance:*

As seen in other neuromuscular/muscular pathologies, respiratory muscle weakness is one of the key factors that plays an important role resulting in alveolar hypoventilation in CMD patients [20]. Jackson et al. reported successful use of NPV in the chronic management of different neuromuscular illnesses and chest wall pathologies [7 patients with neuromuscular pathologies, 8 patients with thoracoplasty, and 10 patients with kyphosis or scoliosis] [22]. In acute settings, NPV was reported to successfully manage acute respiratory failure in different types of neuromuscular/muscular pathologies, including poliomyelitis [23], amyotrophic lateral sclerosis [ALS], muscle dystrophies and myasthenia gravis [5, 24]. Additionally, Hino et al. reported a case of Nemaline myopathy with tension pneumothorax as a complication of Non-Invasive Positive Pressure Ventilation that was successfully managed by BCV, which highlights the potential benefit of NPV "sealing" air leaks secondary to positive pressure ventilation and suggests a favorable effect of NPV on lung mechanics [25].

(b) *Central Hypoventilation and Sleep Apnea:*

Central hypoventilation and sleep apnea are known contributing factors to the development of alveolar hypoventilation in patients with muscular dystrophy [20]. A study by Goldstein et al. demonstrated an efficacy of nocturnal NPV in the management of sleep induced hypoventilation in five patients with restrictive ventilatory impairment secondary to neuromuscular pathologies [in four patients], and thoracoplasty [in one patient] [26].

28.7 Other Considerations

28.7.1 Diaphragm Atrophy

Positive pressure ventilation [PPV], including pressure support ventilation, has been shown to have a negative effect on both diaphragm thickness and strength [27]. Goligher et al. found that this atrophy is related to worse clinical outcome in acutely ventilated patients [28]. Effects of non-invasive PPV on diaphragm strength and thickness are not well studied in chronically ventilated patients with neuromuscular and muscular pathology. This finding, however, suggests that chronic PPV might have a negative impact on the strength of "weak at baseline" muscles in this patient population. NPV effect on diaphragm thickness and strength is not yet well-studied; however, one report by Gutierezz et al. showed improvement in the maximal trans-diaphragmatic pressure after intermittent nocturnal cuirass ventilation in patients with chronic airway limitation and hypercarbia [9], a finding that suggests that NPV might have a more favorable effect on diaphragm thickness and strength when compared to PPV. This theory cannot be proven in the time being and needs to be clinically tested.

28.7.2 Ventilation Strategies Using Negative Pressure Ventilation in CMD

The benefit of NPV for the management of respiratory failure secondary to neuromuscular pathologies was described more than 100 years ago, when NPV was used in the management of respiratory failure in patients with poliomyelitis during the global pandemic of the disease [29]. As discussed previously, respiratory failure is the most common complication in neonatal period and is the largest contributor of fatalities. NPV has been shown to be a beneficial option as this patient population can be challenging to treat with other forms of non-invasive modes of ventilation as the facemasks are often difficult to fit the patient's small size and can often be cumbersome to keep on patients [30].

NPV is a good option as it is portable, avoids the undesirable effects of PPV, is easy to fit and maintain on the patient, and may be titrated in an outpatient setting [21]. Overall, the use of NPV is easy to use for providers and caretakers, has little complications, and can limit, possibly even avoid, the need for intubation and mechanical ventilation. As discussed above, it is important to note that children who require prolonged mechanical ventilation also experience greater mortality and morbidity furthermore validating the benefit for the use of NPV for these individuals.

Respiratory failure occurs in this patient population when the lungs, thoracic wall, respiratory muscles, and the central nervous system respiratory control center are unable to meet the metabolic demands of the body. Limitations of the chest/abdominal wall, respiratory muscle fatigue, and depression of the respiratory control center contribute to failure. Hypercapnic respiratory failure and respiratory insufficiency are the main causes of death due to weakness of the diaphragm and intercostal muscles [31]. NPV using BCV, when compared to positive pressure ventilation [PPV], results in greater functional residual capacity [FRC] at the same transpulmonary pressure, and results in greater oxygenation with the same residual capacity. Contrary to PPV, NPV results in more homogeneous ventilation, lung distension, less injury, and improved oxygenation [30].

BCV devices consist of a plastic shell that is strapped around the patient's chest using Velcro and soft padding which is placed as a barrier around the edge of the plastic between the patient and the shell. With tubing, the shell is then connected to the ventilator that generates negative pressure. This design allows for increased freedom with the ability for the patient to participate in their care by coughing, eating, and allowing them to use their hand with overall greater mobility [26].

Cuirass devices can control both inspiration and expiration to varying degrees based on the mode used. There are three main types of cuirass modes: continuous negative pressure, controlled biphasic, and high-frequency oscillation [7, 25, 32] (Table 28.1).

(a) *Continuous Negative Pressure [CNEP]*: In this mode, negative pressure is continuous throughout breathing cycle. CNEP is equivalent to CPAP.
(b) *Biphasic Cuirass Ventilation [BCV]*: BCV modes include controlled and synchronized settings. In the controlled mode, ventilation is delivered at a preset respiratory rate independent of the patient's spontaneous effort, functionally analogous to bi-level positive airway pressure (BiPAP). In contrast, the synchronized mode triggers cuirass-assisted breaths in response to the patient's intrinsic respiratory effort, thereby coordinating ventilatory support with spontaneous breathing.
(c) *High-Frequency Oscillations [HFO]*: In this mode, the cuirass provides oscillations [up to 1200 oscillations per minute]. This mode helps with secretions clearance.

For patients with congenital myotonic dystrophy, given its ease of use for both healthcare providers and caretakers, NPV is beneficial in both homecare and hospital settings. In the inpatient setting, NPV can be used to act as a bridge to assist patients being weaned off PPV via endotracheal tube intubation; it can be used in conjunction with other forms of NIV to avoid intubation and may be used to provide additional support prior to tracheostomy placement [33]. In a home setting, NPV can be used during acute illness to prevent rapid deterioration of the patient. It may also be used for nighttime or daytime ventilation to improve endurance, lessen muscle fatigue, and assist in carbon dioxide [CO_2] clearance which improves daytime alertness along with growth and development. In both settings, NPV is a great tool

Table 28.1 Types of Biphasic Cuirass Ventilation operating modes

Operating Modes	
Continuous Negative Mode (CNEP)	Increases lung volume by creating continuous negative chamber pressure while the patient is breathing spontaneously
Control Mode	Provides full control over the patient's respiration, being able to control both the inspiratory and expiratory phases of the breathing cycle through changes in frequency: I/E ratio, inspiratory, and expiratory chamber pressures
Secretion Clearance Mode	Used as a chest physiotherapy tool and to enhance the clearance of secretions from the lungs. *Vibration Mode* [240–1200 cpm I/E 1:1], which enhances the loosening of secretions. *Cough Mode* [06–60 cpm and high I/E ratio up to 6:1] which creates a cough-like effect to assist in eliminating secretions

to assist with airway secretions and can be offered as a form of chest physiotherapy [5].

During intubation with PPV, NPV may be used in conjunction by lessening support required from a conventional ventilator causing less barotrauma and may lead to less intubated days. As the biphasic extra-thoracic pressure is applied, the requirements for pressure support are reduced assisting in improvement in oxygenation and cardiac output. Spontaneously generated tidal volumes are increased with enhanced CO2 clearance and reduce oxygen requirements. In patients who are difficult to wean from a ventilator to extubation due to inspiratory muscle weakness where pulmonary compliance and airway resistance are relatively normal, NPV would be a reasonable tool to use to facilitate a successful extubation [9, 34].

Due to the generalized hypotonia and muscle weakness associated with CMD, it is often difficult for patients to clear mucous and airway secretions especially during times of respiratory illness. This is common in the pediatric population. Weakness of the respiratory muscles affects the ability to cough and initiate deep breaths, resulting in atelectasis, chronic lung infections, chronic bronchitis, and chronic bronchiectasis. BCV assists with airway mucus clearance using the "secretion clearance mode." During this mode, there is a vibration phase where shear forces are generated, and secretion viscosity is reduced. During the cough phase, sustained inflation [negative pressure] is alternated with positive pressure which in turn compresses the thorax, producing a forced exhalation maneuver [34]. There is improvement in coughing and managing secretions while preserving muscle function which reduces the burden of the disease and resultant hospitalizations.

The relatively low cost especially when compared to the cost of hospitalizations, availability, and overall ease of use may make NPV a beneficial tool for homecare use. The device can provide daily chest physiotherapy treatments with increased treatments during time of illness. In the setting of acute on chronic respiratory failure, this treatment may be applied to restore ventilation in the home setting that may be comparable to traditional intubation with PPV [34]. Operating these devices requires minimal experience or technical skill to allow non-medically trained individuals to employ outside of a hospital setting [35].

Use of BCV may be used in the homecare setting for either daytime or nighttime application. If the devices are applied routinely, reduced muscle fatigue and improved endurance are seen. In addition, there in improvement in hypercarbia resulting in more alertness which assists in growth and development [36].

Children with CMD often have normal lung parenchyma, so the elastic recoil of the lung and airway resistance are normal. However, their muscular pressure is reduced resulting in decreased maximal airflow and lower lung volumes. The application of BPV alters chest wall mechanics and reduces a patient's work of breathing by stabilizing the chest wall and preventing inward collapse during inspiration [30].

28.8 Cautions/Contraindications

The use of NPV in patients with neuromuscular/muscular pathologies has its advantages. However, it is not without risks. Negative Pressure Ventilation is known to decrease upper airway caliber 16 [29]. The use of NPV, therefore, should be taken with caution in patients with bulbar dysfunction, pharyngeal muscles hypotonia, upper airway obstruction, and obstructive sleep apnea.

NPV may not be used in instances where there is an abnormal shape of the thorax including severe obesity and kyphoscoliosis as the cuirass device requires a tight seal over the chest wall. Absolute contraindications for the use of NPV include any open lesions on the chest or abdomen, and trauma to the thorax including rib fractures as the device may possibly make these worse. NPV should not be used in recent surgeries to chest or abdomen as it could cause further trauma to surgical sites [30].

28.9 Conclusion

Congenital Myotonic Dystrophy is a rare genetic disorder which often can be fatal especially during the neonatal/infancy period due to the profound effect on the respiratory system for these individuals. Deaths and complications are often a result of prolonged intubation. In these individuals many of these severe symptoms can improve at the age of 1 year. Negative pressure ventilation, via biphasic cuirass devices, may be an excellent option to decrease intubation rates, aid weakened respiratory muscles in ventilation, and provide chest physiotherapy. These devices may be used both in the hospital and outpatient settings due to their ease of use and offer few complications associated with their use.

References

1. Rutherford M, Heckmatt J, Dubowitz V. Congenital myotonic dystrophy: respiratory function at birth determines survival. Arch Dis Child. 1989;64(2):191–5.
2. Keller C, Reynolds A, Lee B, Garcia-Prats J. Congenital myotonic dystrophy requiring prolonged endotracheal and noninvasive assisted ventilation: not a uniformly fatal condition. Pediatrics. 1998;101(4):704–5.
3. Hageman A, Gabreels F, Liem K, Renkawek K, Boon J. Congenital myotonic dystrophy; a report on thirteen cases and a review of the literature. J Neurol Sci. 1993;115(1):95–101.
4. Campbell C, Levin S, Siu VM, Venance S, Jacob P. Congenital myotonic dystrophy: Canadian population-based surveillance study. J Pediatr. 2013;163(1):120–5.e3.
5. Corrado A, Gorini M, De Paola E, editors. Alternative techniques for managing acute neuromuscular respiratory failure. Seminars in neurology. Thieme Medical Publishers, Inc; 1995.
6. Timchenko LT. Myotonic dystrophy: the role of RNA CUG triplet repeats. Am J Hum Genet. 1999;64(2):360–4.
7. Dos Santos RA, Habre W, Albu G. Novel ventilation techniques in children. Pediatr Anesth. 2022;32(2):286–94.

8. Rimmer KP, Golar SD, Lee M, Whitelaw WA. Myotonia of the respiratory muscles in myotonic dystrophy. Am Rev Respir Dis. 1993;148:1018.
9. Gutiérrez M, Beroíza T, Contreras G, DiAz O, Cruz E, Moreno R, et al. Weekly cuirass ventilation improves blood gases and inspiratory muscle strength in patients with chronic air-flow limitation and hypercarbia. Am Rev Respir Dis. 1988;138(3):617–23.
10. Vanier T. Dystrophia myotonica in childhood. Br Med J. 1960;2(5208):1284.
11. Liquori CL, Ricker K, Moseley ML, Jacobsen JF, Kress W, Naylor SL, et al. Myotonic dystrophy type 2 caused by a CCTG expansion in intron 1 of ZNF9. Science. 2001;293(5531):864.
12. Tapscott SJ, Thornton CA. Reconstructing myotonic dystrophy. Science. 2001;293(5531):816–7.
13. Hahn C, Salajegheh MK. Myotonic disorders: a review article. Iran J Neurol. 2016;15(1):46.
14. Turner C, Hilton-Jones D. Myotonic dystrophy: diagnosis, management and new therapies. Curr Opin Neurol. 2014;27(5):599–606.
15. Wesstrom G, Bensch J, Schollin J. Congenital myotonic dystrophy: incidence, clinical aspects and early prognosis. Acta Paediatr. 1986;75(5):849–54.
16. Harley HG, Rundle SA, Reardon W, Myring J, Crow S, Harper P, et al. Unstable DNA sequence in myotonic dystrophy. Lancet. 1992;339(8802):1125–8.
17. Guida M, Marger RS, Papp AC, Snyder PJ, Sedra MS, Kissel JT, et al. A molecular protocol for diagnosing myotonic dystrophy. Clin Chem. 1995;41(1):69–72.
18. Ho G, Cardamone M, Farrar M. Congenital and childhood myotonic dystrophy: current aspects of disease and future directions. World J Clin Pediatr. 2015;4(4):66.
19. Roig M, Balliu P-R, Navarro C, Brugera R, Losada M. Presentation, clinical course, and outcome of the congenital form of myotonic dystrophy. Pediatr Neurol. 1994;11(3):208.
20. Hawkins A, Hawkins CL, Razak KA, Khoo TK, Tran K, Jackson R. Respiratory dysfunction in myotonic dystrophy type 1: a systematic review. Neuromuscul Disord. 2019;29(3):198–212.
21. Almeda M, Puranik S, Felker M, Daftary A. Biphasic cuirass ventilation in a patient with congenital myotonic dystrophy. In: A51 pediatric critical care including interventional bronchoscopy. American Thoracic Society; 2020. p. A1928-A.
22. Jackson M, Kinnear W, King M, Hockley S, Shneerson J. The effects of five years of nocturnal cuirass-assisted ventilation in chest wall disease. Eur Respir J. 1993;6(5):630–5.
23. Libby DM, Briscoe WA, Boyce B, Smith JP. Acute respiratory failure in scoliosis or kyphosis: prolonged survival and treatment. Am J Med. 1982;73(4):532–8.
24. Braun S, Sufit R, Giovannoni R, O'Connor M, Peters H. Intermittent negative pressure ventilation in the treatment of respiratory failure in progressive neuromuscular disease. Neurology. 1987;37(12):1874.
25. Hino H, Suzuki Y, Ishii E, Fukuda M. Biphasic cuirass ventilation for treatment of an air leak after pneumothorax in a patient with nemaline myopathy: a case report. J Anesth. 2016;30:1087–90.
26. Goldstein R, Molotiu N, Skrastins R, Long S, De Rosie J, Contreras M, et al. Reversal of sleep-induced hypoventilation and chronic respiratory failure by nocturnal negative pressure ventilation in patients with restrictive ventilatory impairment. Am Rev Respir Dis. 1987;135(5):1049–55.
27. Hudson MB, Smuder AJ, Nelson WB, Bruells CS, Levine S, Powers SK. Both high level pressure support ventilation and controlled mechanical ventilation induce diaphragm dysfunction and atrophy. Crit Care Med. 2012;40(4):1254.
28. Goligher EC, Dres M, Fan E, Rubenfeld GD, Scales DC, Herridge MS, et al. Mechanical ventilation–induced diaphragm atrophy strongly impacts clinical outcomes. Am J Respir Crit Care Med. 2018;197(2):204–13.
29. Woollam C. The development of appartus for intermittent negative pressure respiration. Anaesthesia. 1976;31(4):537–47.
30. Alexiou S, Piccione J, editors. Neuromuscular disorders and chronic ventilation. Seminars in fetal and neonatal medicine. Elsevier; 2017.
31. Rao F, Garuti G, Vitacca M, Banfi P, Racca F, Cutrera R, Pavone M, Pedemonte M, Schisano M, Pedroni S, Casiraghi J, Vianello A, Sansone VA, Group, U. R. Management of respiratory

complications and rehabilitation in individuals with muscular dystrophies: 1st consensus conference report from UILDM - Italian Muscular Dystrophy Association [Milan, January 25-26, 2019]. Acta Myol. 2021;40(1):8–42.
32. Linton D. Cuirass ventilation: a review and update. Crit Care Resusc. 2005;7(1):22.
33. Deep A, De Munter C, Desai A. Negative pressure ventilation in pediatric critical care setting. Indian J Pediatrics. 2007;74:483–8.
34. Nunez CA, Hassinger AB. Predictors of negative pressure ventilation response in pediatric acute respiratory failure. Respir Care. 2020;65(1):91–8.
35. Chidinma O, Rashud S, Goswami R, Treece J, Shipley L, Souza R, O'Neill L, Simberloff T, Baumrucker S. Cuirass ventulation: an alternative home-based modality for chronic respiratory failure. Home Heath Care Manage Pract. 2019;32(1):40–4.
36. Annunziata A, Coppola A, Polistina GE, Imitazione P, Simioli F, Lanza M, et al. Daytime alternatives for non-invasive mechanical ventilation in neuromuscular disorders. Acta Myologica. 2021;40(1):51.

Biphasic Cuirass Non-Invasive Ventilation: Neuromuscular/Restrictive Pulmonary Disorders

29

Mohammad Sallam, Maya Rauth, James Baxter, and Omar Alibrahim

29.1 Pathophysiology of Respiratory Impairment in Neuromuscular Disorders

Neuromuscular disorders are common causes of respiratory failure seen in the intensive care unit, both acutely and chronically. Respiratory failure in neuromuscular disorders is generally characterized by weakness of the muscles contributing to respiration. While there are many subtypes of neuromuscular disorders, they all typically result in a common pathway of progressive weakness of the respiratory musculature and subsequent "ventilatory pump failure," with varying rates of decline, some being slow, while others more rapid [1, 2].

As the respiratory muscles get weaker over time, the tidal volume they can inspire proportionally decreases. This reduction in inhaled tidal volume contributes to the creation of atelectasis and microatelectasis, which results in worsening lung

M. Sallam (✉)
Pediatric Critical Care Department, MercyOne Medical Center, Des Moines, IA, USA
e-mail: mohammad.sallam@mercyone.org

M. Rauth
Pediatric Critical Care Department, Nemours Children's Health, Studer Family Children's Hospital, Pensacola, FL, USA
e-mail: maya.rauth@nemours.org

J. Baxter
Pediatric Critical Care Department, Oishei Children's Hospital, Buffalo, NY, USA
e-mail: jbaxter@upa.chob.edu

O. Alibrahim
Pediatric Critical Care Medicine, Duke University Hospital, Durham, NC, USA
e-mail: omar.alibrahim@duke.edu

O. Alibrahim et al. (eds.), *Biphasic Cuirass Noninvasive Ventilation*, Noninvasive Ventilation. The Essentials, https://doi.org/10.1007/978-3-032-20933-7_29

compliance, and eventually can create restrictive lung disease pattern. The creation of atelectasis decreases gas exchange, ventilation to perfusion mismatching and ultimately leads to hypercapnea and hypoxia. The decreased air intake creates a reduction in functional residual capacity, and puts patients with neuromuscular disorders at increased risk for respiratory failure [3].

However, neuromuscular disorders rarely effect the muscles of inspiration and expiration alone, as these patients typically have numerous aspects of their physiology working against them. Oropharyngeal and laryngeal muscles are typically impacted in neuromuscular conditions as well, resulting in airways that become hypotonic and floppy. The hypotonic nature of these airways often results in upper airway obstruction (particularly with supine position or sleeping), which can result in hypopnea and hypercapnea, and contribute to respiratory failure [4]. Patients suffering from these conditions may also lack the ability to generate an adequate cough, further reducing their ability to clear secretions and protect their airway. The inability to adequately protect their airway through coughing and secretion clearance ultimately puts these patients at a greater risk for aspiration events, and thus worsening respiratory failure [3].

Many neuromuscular diseases may also have a central component as well, which can create inadequate ventilation and oxygenation. Patients with neuromuscular disorders can often develop forms of scoliosis and kyphoscoliosis as well, which can create restrictive lung disease, and further decrease tidal volume, setting the stage for potential respiratory failure [3].

Depending on the stage of a patient's neuromuscular disorder, some may not require respiratory support at baseline (at least in the early stages of their disease). However, due to their impaired respiratory mechanics, any potential illness or insult to the respiratory system can trigger respiratory failure. Whether it is an upper respiratory infection that yields increased secretions that are ineffectively managed, a viral lower respiratory tract infection/bacterial pneumonia, or an aspiration event, these patients can quickly become ill and develop acute respiratory failure. The risk for acute decompensation due to respiratory failure only increases if there is a chronic respiratory failure component at baseline. Typically, in healthy patients (without neuromuscular disease) who develop lower respiratory tract infections or pneumonia, the body naturally compensates by increasing minute ventilation through increased respiratory rate or tidal volume to effectively address any issues with oxygenation or ventilation. However, patients with neuromuscular diseases typically will not be able to compensate by increasing their tidal volume (and may already have significantly reduced tidal volume and compliance at baseline), and therefore must increase their minute ventilation by increasing their respiratory rate. This tachypnea puts additional stress on already weak muscles, resulting in increased respiratory fatigue and worsening hypercapnea. Lack of an adequate cough, poor secretion management, and upper airway obstruction only further worsens the degree of respiratory failure, and the ultimate need for medical intervention.

29.2 Negative Pressure Ventilation

Negative Pressure Ventilation (NPV) has been utilized as a method of managing acute and chronic respiratory failure since it was first used during the poliomyelitis pandemic, more than a hundred years ago [5]. Since the invention of the iron lung, several more practical interfaces have been developed, making the use of negative pressure ventilation more manageable both in Intensive Care Unit (ICU) and home settings.

Cuirass is one of the most practical interfaces of negative pressure ventilation. The device is comprised of a lightweight, flexible chest enclosure with large, soft seals designed to fit around the chest and abdomen, forming an airtight enclosure around the chest and abdomen [6].

29.2.1 Modes of Cuirass Ventilation [7]

Similar to positive pressure ventilation, cuirass ventilation offers variable modes of respiratory support:

- Continuous Negative Pressure Mode: It is a mode where negative pressure is continuously applied around the chest with the effect of lung inflation and increasing Functional Residual Capacity (FRC). This mode of ventilation is akin to Continuous Positive Airway Pressure Ventilation (CPAP).
- Controlled Biphasic Cuirass Ventilation (BCV): It is a mandatory mechanical ventilation mode, where the cuirass provides two different preset values of pressure to assist with inhalation and exhalation. As the name implies, "controlled" BCV provides support independent from patient's respiratory effort. The patient can breathe between the device's breathing cycles, akin to Intermittent Mandatory Ventilation (IMV).
- Synchronized Biphasic Cuirass Ventilation (BCV): As in Controlled BCV, this mode provides 2 preset values of pressure. However, with the synchronized mode, the cuirass provides preset number of mandatory breaths, and senses the patient's effort to support breaths triggered by the patient akin to Synchronized Intermittent Mandatory Ventilation (SIMV).
- High-Frequency Oscillations (HFO): It is a mode where the cuirass provides two preset values of pressure in high rates (frequency as high as 1200 oscillations per minute). This mode provides secretion clearance advantage without losing the baseline negative pressure maintaining lung inflation and FRC.
- Cardiac Synchronized Negative Pressure Ventilation: It is a relatively newer mode that synchronizes with cardiac cycle, sensing the electrical activity of the heart. The mode can affect preload and afterload by changing intrathoracic pressure, and can be used to enhance cardiac output in certain cardiac pathologies.

29.2.2 Benefits of Negative Pressure Ventilation-Supportive Data

- Lung Kinetics and Ventilator-Induced Lung Injury (VILI):
  Compared to non-invasive positive pressure ventilation, negative pressure ventilation might have a favorable effect on lung kinetics, improving oxygenation and minimizing VILI. This theory comes from the fact that negative pressure ventilation is "more physiologic," as natural breathing creates negative intrapleural pressure secondary to inspiratory muscles contraction leading to pressure gradient that moves air (or other gases to the lungs). This effect was studied by Grasso et al. [8] where NPV was shown to provide better oxygenation and less lung injury (assessed by histologic scoring), compared to positive pressure ventilation in surfactant depleted rats.
- Effects on Diaphragm:
  While positive pressure ventilation was found to have a negative effect on diaphragm thickness and strength [9], NPV seems to have a more favorable effect on diaphragm strength. In a report by Gutierezz et al. [10], it was demonstrated that patients with chronic airway limitation and hypercarbia experienced an improvement in maximal transdiaphragmatic pressure following intermittent nocturnal cuirass ventilation.
- Effects on Hemodynamics:
  Current clinical data suggests a favorable effect of negative pressure ventilation on cardiac function, lung, and systemic perfusion. Clinical studies have demonstrated that NPV can enhance pulmonary perfusion in healthy children, postoperative cardiac surgery patients [11], and children with low cardiac output syndrome following Tetralogy of Fallot repair [12]. Additionally, a report by Sidenö et al. [13] demonstrated that biphasic cuirass ventilation, in conjunction with external high-frequency oscillations, can enhance cardiac function in patients who have undergone coronary artery bypass grafting.

29.3 Negative Pressure Ventilation in Neuromuscular Disorders

Patients with neuromuscular disorders may present with both acute and chronic respiratory insufficiency due to the complications and progression of their disease. The constellation of disorders is associated with gradual respiratory muscle weakness which gives way for the development of a weak cough, the inability to clear airway secretions, and alveolar hypoventilation. The disease course in these patients may be complicated by recurrent respiratory infections and aspiration; additionally, patients may experience sleep-disordered breathing. The use of non-invasive technologies is often a preferred means to chronically managing these conditions. Negative pressure ventilation (NPV) offers an alternative to the traditional non-invasive modes of positive pressure ventilation that can be used in both acute, and chronic settings. The following is a brief discussion of NPV use and potential benefits in the management of respiratory failure secondary to neuromuscular disorders.

29.3.1 Usage in Acute Settings

Patients with neuromuscular disorders have many chronic conditions associated with their disorder; in the event of acute illnesses, they often experience more severe complications compared to other patients population that result from ineffective secretion clearance, inadequate cough, dysphagia, and inadequate lung expansion [14]. Additionally, acute respiratory failure due to illnesses can often exacerbate conditions such as chronic hypoventilation, a common respiratory complication of neuromuscular pathologies [15].

The application of a negative pressure ventilation device helps mimic the natural movement of the respiratory muscles during respiration. The ventilator applies negative pressure which then forces the movement of the diaphragm downwards while the rib muscles tend to enlarge the chest thereby creating lung expansion. The mechanism results in a greater functional residual capacity with greater oxygenation and the same residual capacity, providing a more homogenous ventilation [15]. In the pediatric intensive care unit, non-invasive therapies are often initiated in the treatment of acute respiratory failure, including NPV. Negative pressure ventilation with the biphasic cuirass ventilator offers an advantage in patients with abnormal facial structures or excessive airway secretions [16]. A major advantage in the treatment of acute respiratory failure is the preservation of a patient's physiological functions such as swallowing and coughing [17]. In the case of respiratory illnesses, NPV also allows for the management of secretions utilizing the high-frequency oscillatory mode (HFO) without interruption of respiratory support in contrast to positive pressure ventilation modes which may require removal of nasal or facial masks.

Although there is a lack of large-scale studies, there is evidence supporting the use of NPV as a viable management modality for acute respiratory failure in patients with neuromuscular pathologies. Using different interfaces, NPV was reported to manage acute respiratory failure in patients with [18], ALS, muscle dystrophies, and myasthenia gravis [19, 20].

Additionally, in pediatric population, Hassinger et al. and Nunez et al. have both demonstrated the benefits of using the cuirass interface, specifically in the CNEP and BCV modes, for managing acute respiratory failure in pediatric patients with neuromuscular diseases [16, 21].

Usage of NPV in the acute setting may be limited by a patient's neurological deficits. For example, conditions associated with bulbar dysfunction or apnea may not be ideal for the initiation of NPV. Patients may also have difficulty tolerating the NPV interface or experience musculoskeletal pain. Yet, in the setting of acute respiratory failure it still may provide a viable alternative to other non-invasive positive pressure modalities that also may not be well tolerated by a patient.

29.3.2 Chronic Use

With the progression of many neuromuscular disorders, patients often experience restrictive breathing patterns, decreased lung function and develop sleep-disordered breathing—conditions such as sleep hypoventilation, obstructive sleep apnea, and central sleep apnea [22]. Sleep-disordered breathing is a major cause of morbidity and mortality in children with neuromuscular disease [23]. Patients experience disruptions in sleep architecture and ventilation because of their neuromuscular weakness. As patients with normal respiratory function enter REM sleep, the respiratory muscles become atonic and ventilation responses to hypoxia and hypercapnia become more blunted. This effect becomes more exaggerated in patients with neuromuscular disease and requires intervention. Due to the progression in neuromuscular diseases, patients often show weakness of the muscles of the upper airway contributing to increased upper airway resistance during sleep because these muscles are required to maintain patency of the airway [23]. When lung function deteriorates, total lung capacity becomes reduced due to respiratory muscle weakness which in turn leads to air trapping and increased residual volume [22]. Intervention with ventilation can stabilize vital capacity, improve gas exchange and correct sleep-disordered breathing and promotion of growth [22]. Furthermore, presence of kyphoscoliosis can restrict lung capacity further impairing ventilation [23]. Ventilation/perfusion matching is usually preserved but patients generally develop hypercapnia due to the reduced compliance of the respiratory system combined with the weakness of the respiratory muscles [24]. Non-invasive ventilation such as high-flow nasal cannula, continuous positive airway pressure, and bi-level positive airway pressure is a means of providing respiratory support for these patients, and negative pressure ventilation is an alternative option for those that may not be able to tolerate facial or nasal masks. Ventilatory support may initially only be required at nighttime due to the likelihood of these patients developing sleep-disordered breathing and hypoventilation. Respiratory support and early intervention when lung function begins to decrease can lead to improvement in quality of life for these patients.

In patients with neuromuscular disorders, several interventions are essential to improving outcomes and management of their disease course. Long-term ventilatory support may be associated with improved quality of life, reduction in number of days spent in the hospital, and improvement in psychosocial and mental function [24].

Advantages of NPV as a modality of non-invasive ventilation in the chronic management of patients with respiratory failure secondary to neuromuscular pathologies include the following:

- Secretion Mobilization: Negative pressure devices often have functions to assist with secretion clearance using the HFO mode. The cuirass interface allows for simultaneous secretion clearance and application of negative pressure, which helps to preserve lung inflation, and prevents "derecruitment" during secretion clearance and suctioning.
- Chronically ventilated patients can be supported through the cuirass without the need for a face interface (compared to the most commonly used devices of non-invasive positive pressure ventilation), which might be more tolerated in patients with claustrophobia, facial anatomical abnormalities, and facial pressure ulcers.

NPV also helps preserve physiological functions like speech, cough, swallowing, and feeding and can prevent or delay more invasive means of ventilation such as endotracheal intubation or tracheostomy [15].
- NPV might have a more favorable effect on diaphragm strength and thickness when compared to positive pressure ventilation (as discussed under general advantages of NPV).

Disadvantage of NPV interfaces includes the need for a patient to remain on their back during sleep which may be restricted by spinal curvature or obesity. NPV use should also be taken with cautions in patients with bulbar dysfunction, and upper airway obstruction as current data suggests that NPV decreased upper airway caliber [25].

References

1. Borrelli M, Terrone G, Evangelisti R, Fedele F, Corcione A, Santamaria F. Respiratory phenotypes of neuromuscular diseases: a challenging issue for pediatricians. Pediatr Neonatol. 2023;64:109.
2. Panitch HB. The pathophysiology of respiratory impairment in pediatric neuromuscular diseases. Pediatrics. 2009;123(Suppl 4):S215–S8.
3. Bach JR, Turcios NL, Wang L. Respiratory complications of pediatric neuromuscular diseases. Pediatr Clin. 2021;68(1):177–91.
4. Katz SL. Assessment of sleep-disordered breathing in pediatric neuromuscular diseases. Pediatrics. 2009;123(Supplement_4):S222–S5.
5. Woollam C. The development of appartus for intermittent negative pressure respiration. Anaesthesia. 1976;31(4):537–47.
6. Thomson A. The role of negative pressure ventilation. Arch Dis Child. 1997;77(5):454–8.
7. Linton D. Cuirass ventilation: a review and update. Crit Care Resusc. 2005;7(1):22.
8. Grasso F, Engelberts D, Helm E, Frndova H, Jarvis S, Talakoub O, et al. Negative-pressure ventilation: better oxygenation and less lung injury. Am J Respir Crit Care Med. 2008;177(4):412–8.
9. Hudson MB, Smuder AJ, Nelson WB, Bruells CS, Levine S, Powers SK. Both high level pressure support ventilation and controlled mechanical ventilation induce diaphragm dysfunction and atrophy. Crit Care Med. 2012;40(4):1254.
10. Gutiérrez M, Beroíza T, Contreras G, DiAz O, Cruz E, Moreno R, et al. Weekly cuirass ventilation improves blood gases and inspiratory muscle strength in patients with chronic air-flow limitation and hypercarbia. Am Rev Respir Dis. 1988;138(3):617–23.
11. Shekerdemian LS, Bush A, Lincoln C, Shore DF, Petros AJ, Redington AN. Cardiopulmonary interactions in healthy children and children after simple cardiac surgery: the effects of positive and negative pressure ventilation. Heart. 1997;78(6):587–93.
12. Shekerdemian LS, Bush A, Shore DF, Lincoln C, Redington AN. Cardiorespiratory responses to negative pressure ventilation after tetralogy of Fallot repair: a hemodynamic tool for patients with a low-output state. J Am Coll Cardiol. 1999;33(2):549–55.
13. Sidenö B, Vaage J. Ventilation by external high-frequency oscillations improves cardiac function after coronary artery bypass grafting. Eur J Cardiothorac Surg. 1997;11(2):248–57.
14. Mehta S. Neuromuscular disease causing acute respiratory failure. Respir Care. 2006;51(9):1016–21; discussion 21–3.

15. Annunziata A, Coppola A, Polistina GE, Imitazione P, Simioli F, Lanza M, et al. Daytime alternatives for non-invasive mechanical ventilation in neuromuscular disorders. Acta Myol. 2021;40(1):51–60.
16. Hassinger AB, Breuer RK, Nutty K, Ma C-X, Al Ibrahim OS. Negative-pressure ventilation in pediatric acute respiratory failure. Respir Care. 2017;62(12):1540–9.
17. Annunziata A, Calabrese C, Simioli F, Coppola A, Flora M, Marotta A, et al. Negative-pressure ventilation in neuromuscular diseases in the acute setting. J Clin Med. 2022;11(9).
18. Libby DM, Briscoe WA, Boyce B, Smith JP. Acute respiratory failure in scoliosis or kyphosis: prolonged survival and treatment. Am J Med. 1982;73(4):532–8.
19. Corrado A, Gorini M, De Paola E, Editors. Alternative techniques for managing acute neuromuscular respiratory failure. Seminars in neurology; 1995: © 1995 by Thieme Medical Publishers, Inc.
20. Braun S, Sufit R, Giovannoni R, O'Connor M, Peters H. Intermittent negative pressure ventilation in the treatment of respiratory failure in progressive neuromuscular disease. Neurology. 1987;37(12):1874.
21. Nunez CA, Hassinger AB. Predictors of negative pressure ventilation response in pediatric acute respiratory failure. Respir Care. 2020;65(1):91–8.
22. Borrelli M, Terrone G, Evangelisti R, Fedele F, Corcione A, Santamaria F. Respiratory phenotypes of neuromuscular diseases: a challenging issue for pediatricians. Pediatr Neonatol. 2022;64:109–18.
23. Katz SL. Assessment of sleep-disordered breathing in pediatric neuromuscular diseases. Pediatrics. 2009;123(Suppl 4):S222–5.
24. Shneerson JM, Simonds AK. Noninvasive ventilation for chest wall and neuromuscular disorders. Eur Respir J. 2002;20(2):480–7.
25. Sanna A, Veriter C, Stanescu D. Upper airway obstruction induced by negative-pressure ventilation in awake healthy subjects. J Appl Physiol. 1993;75(2):546–52.

Pediatric Postoperative Cardiac Care: Restrictive and Single-Ventricle Physiology

30

Ryan K. Breuer, Ommul Fatmi, and Omar Alibrahim

30.1 Normal Cardiopulmonary Interactions and Physiology

While an obvious oversimplification, the "box-within-a-box" metaphor serves as an adequate starting point for appreciation of the pulmonary and cardiovascular co-dependence within the thorax. Pressure manipulations within the organs, vessels, and potential spaces occupying this finite space can exert a powerful influence over their physiologic performance—which, in turn, have the potential to drive additional change. Since "everything can impact everything else" in this space, an appreciation of these relationships under normal physiologic conditions is critical to any understanding of the derangements occurring with acute pathology.

Let us begin with the fundamental relationship between venous return to the right heart and spontaneous respiration. Recall that inspiration is primarily a negative-pressure process. Contraction of the diaphragm, its downward displacement, and the outward movement of the chest wall collectively expose residual lung to a larger overall intrathoracic volume. By Boyle's Law, this necessitates a fall in intrathoracic pressure (ITP), creating a gradient for airflow into the lungs. Concurrently, a second pressure gradient—one driving venous return to the right atrium—is also expanded. Blood from the peripheral venous system, already subjected to higher pressures than caval pressures, now sees this disparity augmented by the "pull" of negative ITP. This favors additional blood return to the right heart, serving as preload for subsequent myocardial contractions. The opposite effect is seen with rising

R. K. Breuer (✉) · O. Fatmi
Department of Pediatrics, Division of Critical Care Medicine, University at Buffalo, Buffalo, NY, USA
e-mail: rbreuer@upa.chob.edu; ommul.fatmi@nemours.org

O. Alibrahim
Pediatric Critical Care Medicine, Duke University Hospital, Durham, NC, USA
e-mail: omar.alibrahim@duke.edu

O. Alibrahim et al. (eds.), *Biphasic Cuirass Noninvasive Ventilation*, Noninvasive Ventilation. The Essentials, https://doi.org/10.1007/978-3-032-20933-7_30

ITP during expiration: venous return is relatively blunted by a dissipation of the peripheral-to-central pressure gradient.

Devices such as the biphasic chest cuirass capitalize on this physiology when providing negative-pressure, mechanical ventilation (NPV). The extra-thoracic "pull" from the cuirass promotes chest wall expansion and lung recruitment, while simultaneously dropping intrapleural and right atrial pressures. As a result, airflow into the lungs and venous return to the right heart are augmented.

Contrast this with the increase in ITP that accompanies the application of positive-pressure ventilation (PPV). We now expect a detriment to right heart loading conditions—with respect to venous return/preload—via diminishment of the previously mentioned venous pressure gradient. As numerous studies have illustrated, this is precisely the case [1–4]. It also helps explain why, as we will see later in this chapter, patients recovering from right heart surgery are often extubated as soon as possible. If early liberation from PPV is not an option, the body does have intrinsic mechanisms to aid in reestablishing enough of a gradient to ensure adequate right ventricle (RV) preload and, subsequently, RV output [5–7]. Again, as we will see later in the chapter, the benefits of lower ITP in these patients, with respect to venous flow gradients, can be amplified by the addition of negative-pressure ventilation (NPV).

The RV may also experience afterload changes related to manipulations in ITP. Excessive thoracic pressures, expanding the lungs well beyond their functional residual capacity (FRC), are known to increase pulmonary vascular resistance (PVR) through small-vessel compression. This rise in PVR must be overcome by the RV before meaningful pulmonary blood flow (PBF) is established. The absence of adequate ITP, accompanied by poor lung expansion (below FRC), will similarly raise PVR (and RV afterload), now through extra-alveolar vascular means. As such, from an RV afterload perspective, there truly is an amount of intrathoracic pressure that appears to be just right where PVR is low, RV afterload is reduced, and PBF is optimized.

The left ventricle (LV) is likewise confined to the thoracic "box," and is therefore influenced by similar forces. Studies show that raising ITP can improve pulmonary venous flow, increasing left atrial filling, and, ultimately, LV end-diastolic volume [8–10]. However, excessive intrathoracic pressures can lead to direct compression of the heart and a compromised cardiac output.

The LV will also experience afterload changes in the face of ITP manipulations, not unlike its companion ventricle. Importantly, in this instance, such changes are driven largely by alterations to the LV transmural pressure. Increasing ITP (e.g., via initiation of PPV), external to the LV, will decrease this overall difference, lowering transmural pressure and—hence—LV afterload. The opposite is true when the LV is exposed to NPV. A negative intrapleural pressure will increase its transmural pressure gradient and, consequently, its afterload. Such increases may compromise cardiac output in a "struggling" ventricle with pre-existing myocardial dysfunction.

In fact, research has shown that the impact of ITP manipulation through choice of ventilatory support does not end there. PPV also promotes an egress of blood down the thoracic aorta and into the abdomen, further decreasing LV afterload [11] and establishing this modality as a hemodynamic tool in patients with LV failure [12]. This impact would not be seen in patients supported by NPV. Taken together, one can presume that NPV is "better" for the RV, while PPV is more advantageous to the LV.

The final noteworthy component of this complicated physiologic interrelation involves the interventricular septum and its potential for encroachment into the ventricular chambers. Analogous to the LV transmural gradient, the septum is subject to its own trans-septal gradient due to the relatively non-compliant pericardial sac minimizing opportunities for a pressure "pop-off." This gradient arises from the difference between the LV end-diastolic pressure and RV end-diastolic pressure (LVEDP-RVEDP). As such, the septum is displaced into one chamber or another as they undergo diastolic filling.

Normally, as the above equation implies, this would be a rightward displacement. However, sharp increases in RVEDP can diminish this gradient and favor, instead, a leftward septal displacement to the detriment of LV stroke volume and systolic blood pressure [13, 14]. This phenomenon occurs even during spontaneous respiration, with instances of deep inspiratory effort (and the subsequent augmentation of RV filling previously described) and should therefore be anticipated during trials of NPV. In true "box-within-a-box" fashion, this fall in LV stroke volume is also promoted by the higher transmural gradient accompanying negative ITP.

The preceding paragraphs have illustrated ways in which pulmonary and cardiovascular physiology are intricately linked and perpetually dynamic. For a more in-depth physiologic discussion, we refer you to the excellent review on this topic by Verhoeff and Mitchell [15].

30.2 Tetralogy of Fallot

This classic variant of cyanotic congenital heart disease is thought to be the byproduct of a relatively simple embryologic error—a displaced infundibular septum. The resulting stages of cardiac development tend to yield patients with a malalignment ventricular septal defect (VSD), overriding aorta, and right ventricular outflow tract (RVOT) obstruction. In the context of supra-physiologic volume and pressure loads on the RV, its myocardium hypertrophies to de-escalate rises in wall stress and stroke work. The impediment to normal RV emptying and the opportunity for right-to-left shunting yield the traditional cyanotic phenotype, with severity relating directly to the degree of RVOT obstruction. While this anatomic designation is actually a spectrum of disease, we will (for the purposes of discussion) focus solely on the "classic" tetralogy of Fallot (TOF) patient undergoing "complete" surgical repair at 5–6 months of age.

Typical surgical goals for these patients include alleviation of RVOT obstruction and establishment of independent (i.e., "parallel") pulmonary and systemic circulations. Once achieved, RV myocardial function should be preserved over time. Complete repairs involve a patch closure of the VSD with RVOT expansion via muscle bundle resection and/or placement of a transannular patch. Alternatively, the narrowed RVOT can be bypassed entirely by placement of a valved conduit, sending flow directly from the ventricle into the pulmonary circulation. These patients are at risk for low cardiac output syndrome, bleeding, dysrhythmias, and residual physiologic defects at a rate as high as 12% [16–19].

As our discussion shifts toward NPV as a hemodynamic tool in the postoperative setting, we will presume a successful, "complete" TOF repair without the need for an RV-PA conduit. These children can be medically challenging during their recovery and benefit from NPV support.

It is not uncommon for the RV to demonstrate both systolic and diastolic dysfunction after coming off cardiopulmonary bypass. Inotropic support and afterload reduction have been shown to support systolic function. Diastolic dysfunction, on the other hand, relies on lusitropic agents and higher end-diastolic pressures to maintain RV filling. In fact, nearly half of postoperative TOF patients experience restrictive RV physiology, with significantly elevated central venous pressures and, oftentimes, reduced cardiac output [20]. In this setting, with a tenuous, "stiff" RV exceedingly sensitive to its own loading conditions, the traditional approach has been early extubation or—at a minimum—reducing ITP as much as possible, to preserve an adequate venous gradient for right atrial return and RV filling.

From our earlier discussion of the ITP effect on RV preload and afterload, there is compelling rationale for the use of NPV in this population. Indeed, the ability to expand the venous return gradient (filling the "stiff" RV) while also maintaining lung recruitment/minimizing the pulmonary vascular resistance (PVR) effects of hypo-inflation truly suggests NPV can be a powerful hemodynamic adjunct. Several publications to date have borne this out, demonstrating improvements in stroke volume, cardiac output, oxygen delivery, and vascular resistance in patients after right heart surgery [21]. Benefits to blood pressure and urine output, as well as amelioration of metabolic acidosis, have likewise been demonstrated, even in patients with restrictive RV physiology. Importantly, these improvements persisted after cessation of NPV therapy, and the device itself was found to be safe for use despite the presence of fresh sternotomies and indwelling chest tubes [22]. Negative-pressure ventilation has also been shown to reduce central venous pressures and augment PBF, the latter by as much as 67% after only 45 minutes of therapy [23, 24]. Again, these benefits were illustrated in postoperative patients with and without restrictive ventricular physiology.

While this modality warrants additional study in the TOF cohort, existing data and physiologic principles suggest quite a favorable role for NPV in the postoperative care of these patients.

30.3 Glenn and Fontan Management

"Single-ventricle" physiology encapsulates various cardiac malformations linked by circulatory aberrations, abnormal loading conditions, and patient cyanosis. Such manifestations include tricuspid atresia, double inlet left ventricle (DILV), double outlet right ventricle (DORV), pulmonary atresia with intact ventricular septum (PA/IVS), Ebstein's anomaly, and hypoplastic left heart syndrome (HLHS). At the core of patient symptomatology is the intracardiac mixing of venous return from the pulmonary (oxygenated) and systemic (deoxygenated) systems. This "purple" blood becomes stroke volume for the body's lone, well-developed ventricle but must be divided between the pulmonary and systemic arterial trees. In most cases, this division is driven by the ratio of the vascular resistances of the two circulations. Since PVR tends to fall below its systemic counterpart over time, these competing, parallel circuits often drive a preponderance of ventricular output into the lungs.

Early surgical interventions to stabilize these circulations reduce volume/pressure loads on the functional ventricle and/or create a total body vascular tree working in series. Operational specifics vary, of course, with the various patient permutations.

When there is deemed no opportunity for a biventricular "repair," such interventions are considered palliative (given the inevitable failure of the singular, functional ventricle). For the purposes of this discussion, we will consider HLHS as the archetype of single-ventricle physiology. The first palliative stage involves creation of a common atrium (bringing all venous return into the lone functional ventricle) and a neo-aorta (bridging the proximal pulmonary artery with the native aorta). This effectively allows most of RV output to be exported systemically, albeit at the expense of a natural source of pulmonary flow. This is addressed by creation of a modified Blalock-Taussig (BT) or Sano shunt. The relative proportion of PBF to systemic blood flow (SBF) is usually determined by the ratio of pulmonary to systemic vascular resistance (PVR:SVR) [25].

Relevant aspects of staged palliation to our discussion begin with its second stage, the bidirectional cavopulmonary anastomosis (Glenn) procedure. This is typically performed at three or four months of age. Surgeons remove any previous route for PBF in lieu of anastomosing the patients' superior vena cava (SVC) to his or her right branch pulmonary artery (PArt). This connection now serves as the main source of PBF. Patients continue to exhibit "mixing" physiology, as their IVC returns venous blood to the same RV. Importantly, the influence of vascular resistance is diminished as the patient moves away from fully competing, parallel circulations. Despite this, PVR remains paramount to the efficacy of PBF. Elevations will blunt flow and, hence, oxygenation [26].

Crucially, SVC drainage into the pulmonary arterial system, and PBF, is now a *passive* process. ITP and vascular resistance now determine Glenn flow/PBF, with movement of blood into the lungs directly proportional to the transpulmonary pressure gradient (and inversely related to the resistance across that circuit). The benefit of an NPV approach to support these patients is obvious. Decreasing ITP in this fashion maintains lung expansion/recruitment while simultaneously augmenting the pressure gradient for PBF. Conversely, excessively positive ITP may prevent intrathoracic access to valuable SVC return or promote pulmonary hyper-expansion, thereby increasing PVR.

The third and final stage of the palliative process is generally the Fontan procedure. Typically performed at about 2 years of age, the Fontan diverts IVC return directly into the pulmonary vascular bed. This ensures a near-complete bypass of the heart by systemic venous blood. As intracardiac mixing is now minimized, patients should no longer appear cyanotic. Their two circulations are fully in series, and the RV becomes as "unloaded" as patient physiology will permit. Of course, PBF remains passive and is still subject to the same pressure gradient and resistance relationships. Importantly, as the entirety of systemic return now moves directly into the lungs, these relationships—should they prove detrimental to PBF—now have the potential to substantially diminish not only oxygenation, but overall systemic output [26, 27].

Unsurprisingly, a major postoperative management goal for Glenn and Fontan patients mirrors that of children with TOF and diastolic dysfunction/restrictive physiology: *minimization of positive-pressure ventilation*. Ideally, this is accomplished by early liberation from the ventilator altogether. Spontaneous respiration, insofar as lung recruitment is maintained, will tend to provide a more generous supply of venous return into the thorax and, hence, PBF and cardiac output. This has been demonstrated in children with after both bidirectional Glenn and Fontan procedures [28]. However, in children who continue to require respiratory support, there is a legitimate argument to be made for NPV. In fact, while data are limited, published results are encouraging.

Negative-pressure ventilation has been studied in cardiac patients for several decades. In the late 1990s, Shekerdermian examined its effects in mechanically ventilated patients after various cardiac interventions, including patent ductus arteriosus closure, VSD closure, and AV valve repair. Children remained intubated and were permitted to breathe spontaneously while on NPV support. The authors found improvement in cardiac index across both groups (PDA closure and postoperative), with significant increases in mixed venous saturation and proportionate decreases in arteriovenous oxygen content difference [27]. These gains were likely a result of improved preload and reduced LV afterload, benefiting oxygen delivery. That same group also studied NPV in nearly two dozen patients with Fontan physiology and noted increases in PBF by 40–50% when they were transitioned from PPV to NPV, very likely the result of better RV loading conditions and reductions in afterload [29].

NPV support has even been found to decrease PVR and "Fontan pressure" in a majority of adults with this physiology who had been referred for cardiac catheterization [30].

While the incidence is (by definition) low, there are also case reports of NPV "rescue" in patients with complicated or failing Glenn/Fontan circuits (e.g., in the setting of severe infection or plastic bronchitis) [31–35].

Much like patients with restrictive right ventricular physiology, post-Glenn and Fontan patients may benefit hemodynamically from application of NPV under certain circumstances. Further study is warranted, but existing data—coupled with the non-invasive nature of the device—make this a promising tool for ICU physicians.

References

1. Mitchell JR, Sas R, Zuege DJ, Doig CJ, Smith ER, Whitelaw WA, Tyberg JV, Belenkie I. Ventricular interaction during mechanical ventilation in closed-chest anesthetized dogs. Can J Cardiol. 2005;21(1):73–81. PMID: 15685307.
2. Mitchell JR, Whitelaw WA, Sas R, Smith ER, Tyberg JV, Belenkie I. RV filling modulates LV function by direct ventricular interaction during mechanical ventilation. Am J Physiol Heart Circ Physiol. 2005;289(2):H549–57. https://doi.org/10.1152/ajpheart.01180.2004. Epub 2005 Mar 25. PMID: 15792988.
3. Pinsky MR. Determinants of pulmonary arterial flow variation during respiration. J Appl Physiol Respir Environ Exerc Physiol. 1984;56(5):1237–45. https://doi.org/10.1152/jappl.1984.56.5.1237. PMID: 6373691.
4. Pinsky MR. Instantaneous venous return curves in an intact canine preparation. J Appl Physiol Respir Environ Exerc Physiol. 1984;56(3):765–71. https://doi.org/10.1152/jappl.1984.56.3.765. PMID: 6368503.
5. Jellinek H, Krenn H, Oczenski W, Veit F, Schwarz S, Fitzgerald RD. Influence of positive airway pressure on the pressure gradient for venous return in humans. J Appl Physiol (1985). 2000;88(3):926–32. https://doi.org/10.1152/jappl.2000.88.3.926. PMID: 10710387.
6. Takata M, Robotham JL. Effects of inspiratory diaphragmatic descent on inferior vena caval venous return. J Appl Physiol (1985). 1992;72(2):597–607. https://doi.org/10.1152/jappl.1992.72.2.597. PMID: 1559938.
7. Takata M, Wise RA, Robotham JL. Effects of abdominal pressure on venous return: abdominal vascular zone conditions. J Appl Physiol (1985). 1990;69(6):1961–72. https://doi.org/10.1152/jappl.1990.69.6.1961. PMID: 2076989.
8. Bhatia SJ, Kirshenbaum JM, Shemin RJ, Cohn LH, Collins JJ, Di Sesa VJ, Young PJ, Mudge GH Jr, Sutton MG. Time course of resolution of pulmonary hypertension and right ventricular remodeling after orthotopic cardiac transplantation. Circulation 1987;76(4):819–26. https://doi.org/10.1161/01.cir.76.4.819. PMID: 3308165.
9. Brower R, Wise RA, Hassapoyannes C, Bromberger-Barnea B, Permutt S. Effect of lung inflation on lung blood volume and pulmonary venous flow. J Appl Physiol (1985). 1985;58(3):954–63. https://doi.org/10.1152/jappl.1985.58.3.954. PMID: 3884583.
10. Jardin F. Cyclic changes in arterial pressure during mechanical ventilation. Intensive Care Med. 2004;30(6):1047–50. https://doi.org/10.1007/s00134-004-2254-0. Epub 2004 Mar 30. PMID: 15052386.
11. Luecke T, Pelosi P. Clinical review: Positive end-expiratory pressure and cardiac output. Crit Care. 2005;9(6):607–21. https://doi.org/10.1186/cc3877. Epub 2005 Oct 18. PMID: 16356246; PMCID: PMC1414045.
12. Pinsky MR. Cardiovascular issues in respiratory care. Chest. 2005;128(5 Suppl 2):592S–7S. https://doi.org/10.1378/chest.128.5_suppl_2.592S. PMID: 16306058.
13. Kingma I, Tyberg JV, Smith ER. Effects of diastolic transseptal pressure gradient on ventricular septal position and motion. Circulation. 1983;68(6):1304–14. https://doi.org/10.1161/01.cir.68.6.1304. PMID: 6640880.
14. Thompson CR, Kingma I, MacDonald RP, Belenkie I, Tyberg JV, Smith ER. Transseptal pressure gradient and diastolic ventricular septal motion in patients with mitral stenosis. Circulation. 1987;76(5):974–80. https://doi.org/10.1161/01.cir.76.5.974. PMID: 3665002.
15. Verhoeff K, Mitchell JR. Cardiopulmonary physiology: why the heart and lungs are inextricably linked. Adv Physiol Educ. 2017;41(3):348–53. https://doi.org/10.1152/advan.00190.2016. PMID: 28679570.
16. Al Habib HF, Jacobs JP, Mavroudis C, Tchervenkov CI, O'Brien SM, Mohammadi S, Jacobs ML. Contemporary patterns of management of tetralogy of Fallot: data from the Society of Thoracic Surgeons Database. Ann Thorac Surg. 2010;90(3):813–9; discussion 819–20. https://doi.org/10.1016/j.athoracsur.2010.03.110. PMID: 20732501.

17. Pigula FA, Khalil PN, Mayer JE, del Nido PJ, Jonas RA. Repair of tetralogy of Fallot in neonates and young infants. Circulation 1999;100(19 Suppl):II157–61. https://doi.org/10.1161/01.cir.100.suppl_2.ii-157. PMID: 10567296.
18. Kirsch RE, Glatz AC, Gaynor JW, Nicolson SC, Spray TL, Wernovsky G, Bird GL. Results of elective repair at 6 months or younger in 277 patients with tetralogy of Fallot: a 14-year experience at a single center. J Thorac Cardiovasc Surg. 2014;147(2):713–7. https://doi.org/10.1016/j.jtcvs.2013.03.033. Epub 2013 Apr 18. PMID: 23602127.
19. Steiner MB, Tang X, Gossett JM, Malik S, Prodhan P. Timing of complete repair of non-ductal-dependent tetralogy of Fallot and short-term postoperative outcomes, a multicenter analysis. J Thorac Cardiovasc Surg. 2014;147(4):1299–305. https://doi.org/10.1016/j.jtcvs.2013.06.019. Epub 2013 Jul 21. PMID: 23879934.
20. Karl TR, Stocker C. Tetralogy of Fallot and its variants. Pediatr Crit Care Med. 2016;17(8 Suppl 1):S330–6. https://doi.org/10.1097/PCC.0000000000000831. PMID: 27490619.
21. Shekerdemian LS, Shore DF, Lincoln C, Bush A, Redington AN. Negative-pressure ventilation improves cardiac output after right heart surgery. Circulation. 1996;94(9 Suppl):II49–55. PMID: 8901719.
22. Shekerdemian LS, Schulze-Neick I, Redington AN, Bush A, Penny DJ. Negative pressure ventilation as haemodynamic rescue following surgery for congenital heart disease. Intensive Care Med. 2000;26(1):93–6. https://doi.org/10.1007/s001340050018. PMID: 10663287.
23. Shime N, Toida C, Itoi T, Hashimoto S. Continuous negative extrathoracic pressure in children after congenital heart surgery. Crit Care Resusc. 2006;8(4):297–301. PMID: 17227265.
24. Shekerdemian LS, Bush A, Shore DF, Lincoln C, Redington AN. Cardiorespiratory responses to negative pressure ventilation after tetralogy of fallot repair: a hemodynamic tool for patients with a low-output state. J Am Coll Cardiol. 1999;33(2):549–55. https://doi.org/10.1016/s0735-1097(98)00598-1. PMID: 9973038.
25. Kritzmire SM, Cossu AE. Hypoplastic left heart syndrome [Updated 2023 Jan 15]. In: StatPearls [Internet]. Treasure Island: StatPearls Publishing; 2023 Jan-. Available from: https://www.ncbi.nlm.nih.gov/books/NBK554576/
26. Al-Eyadhy A. Mechanical ventilation strategy following Glenn and Fontan surgeries: On going challenge! J Saudi Heart Assoc. 2009;21(3):153–7. https://doi.org/10.1016/j.jsha.2009.06.005. Epub 2009 Aug 15. PMID: 23960565; PMCID: PMC3727352.
27. Shekerdemian LS, Bush A, Lincoln C, Shore DF, Petros AJ, Redington AN. Cardiopulmonary interactions in healthy children and children after simple cardiac surgery: the effects of positive and negative pressure ventilation. Heart. 1997;78(6):587–93. https://doi.org/10.1136/hrt.78.6.587. PMID: 9470877; PMCID: PMC1892328.
28. Lofland GK. The enhancement of hemodynamic performance in Fontan circulation using pain free spontaneous ventilation. Eur J Cardiothorac Surg. 2001;20(1):114–8, discussion 118–9. https://doi.org/10.1016/s1010-7940(01)00757-6. PMID: 11423283.
29. Shekerdemian LS, Bush A, Shore DF, Lincoln C, Redington AN. Cardiopulmonary interactions after Fontan operations: augmentation of cardiac output using negative pressure ventilation. Circulation. 1997;96(11):3934–42. https://doi.org/10.1161/01.cir.96.11.3934. PMID: 9403618.
30. Peng DM, Zampi JD, Smith SM, Yu S, Rottach N, Lowery R, Lim HM, Riegger LQ, Schumacher KR, Rocchini A. Acute hemodynamic effects of negative extrathoracic pressure in Fontan physiology. Pediatr Cardiol. 2019;40(8):1633–7. https://doi.org/10.1007/s00246-019-02197-x. Epub 2019 Aug 29. PMID: 31468061.
31. Toida C, Shime N, Itoi T, Yamagishi M. Recovery from Fontan circulation failure by application of continuous negative extrathoracic pressure. J Anesth. 2007;21(2):282–4. https://doi.org/10.1007/s00540-007-0497-y. Epub 2007 May 30. PMID: 17458662.
32. Pierce JM, Jenkins IA, Noyes JP, Samuels MP, Southall DP. The successful use of continuous negative extrathoracic pressure in a child with Glenn shunt and respiratory failure. Intensive Care Med. 1995;21(9):766–8. https://doi.org/10.1007/BF01704745. PMID: 8847433.
33. Deshpande SR, Kirshbom PM, Maher KO. Negative pressure ventilation as a therapy for post-operative complications in a patient with single ventricle physiology. Heart Lung Circ.

2011;20(12):763–5. https://doi.org/10.1016/j.hlc.2011.03.010. Epub 2011 Apr 14. PMID: 21493139.

34. Okada S, Muneuchi J, Nagatomo Y, Nonaka K, Iida C, Shirouzu H, Matsuoka R, Watanabe M, Joo K. Successful treatment of protein-losing enteropathy and plastic bronchitis by biphasic cuirass ventilation in a patient with failing Fontan circulation. Int Heart J. 2018;59(4):873–6. https://doi.org/10.1536/ihj.17-292. Epub 2018 May 23. PMID: 29794380.
35. Charla P, Karur GR, Yamamura K, Yoo SJ, Granton JT, Oechslin EN, Shah A, Benson LN, Honjo O, Mertens L, Alonso-Gonzalez R, Hanneman K, Wald RM. Augmentation of pulmonary blood flow and cardiac output by non-invasive external ventilation late after Fontan palliation. Heart. 2021;107(2):142–9. https://doi.org/10.1136/heartjnl-2020-316613. Epub 2020 Jul 6. PMID: 32748799; PMCID: PMC7788264.

Part VI

Long Term Applications

BCV Long Effects and Term Applications: Summary of Clinical Studies

31

Maria Papaioannou and Fotini Ampatzidou

31.1 Introduction

The biphasic cuirass ventilator is noteworthy for its capacity to apply both positive and negative pressure to the chest wall. This biphasic approach is especially helpful for patients who encounter elevated CO_2 levels because it promotes both inspiration and expiration. The biphasic cuirass ventilator provides clinicians with flexibility in customizing ventilation support to accommodate the needs of patients attributable to its multifunction capabilities, which include controlled ventilation.

This ventilator does not require a mask, in contrast to conventional positive pressure ventilation devices, which resolves concerns about mask discomfort and interface complications. It makes use of negative pressure ventilation, which promotes improved gas exchange, lung recruitment, and volume expansion [1].

With a foam backing for comfort, the device is made up of a shell that is placed over the patient's chest. To ensure that different patients can wear it comfortably and properly, it comes in a range of sizes. A straightforward hose connects the ventilator to the shell, allowing for the adjustment of respiratory rate and other parameters, like positive and negative pressure. Even with its sophisticated features, the device is easy to operate, which makes it appropriate for a variety of patients, including young children. Because it can simulate natural breathing patterns by applying negative pressure during inspiration, it is especially useful for patients with a variety of respiratory disorders, including those who may need multiple surgeries due to congenital heart defects [1].

The BCV significantly enhances cardiac function by boosting cardiac output and blood return to the chest. With just one interface and multiple functions, it makes respiratory support for patients easier by removing the need to switch between various devices for ventilation or chest wall oscillation. This combined method reduces

M. Papaioannou (✉) · F. Ampatzidou
General Hospital of Thessaloniki, 1st ICU, Thessaloniki, Greece

O. Alibrahim et al. (eds.), *Biphasic Cuirass Noninvasive Ventilation*, Noninvasive Ventilation. The Essentials, https://doi.org/10.1007/978-3-032-20933-7_31

the need for sedation and alleviates patient discomfort, especially in acute care settings where endotracheal tube discomfort may necessitate sedation [1].

Synchronizing the ventilator with the patient's spontaneous breathing reduces the risk of hospital-acquired infections in intubated patients. For patients who could benefit from non-invasive ventilation in both acute and post-acute care settings, the cuirass ventilator is a worthwhile option to take into consideration because its use has generally been linked to shorter hospital stays [1].

It has proven beneficial for several patient groups, including those with cystic fibrosis, COPD, neuromuscular diseases, and even acute respiratory distress syndrome (ARDS). Negative pressure ventilation is important for respiratory care because of its adaptability and improved care outcomes [1].

Compared to positive pressure ventilation, negative pressure ventilation—like that provided by the Hayek Biphasic Cuirass ventilator—offers several benefits. Unlike positive pressure ventilation, which may only inflate the areas of the lung that are already inflated, negative pressure ventilation ensures that all parts of the lung receive adequate ventilation by providing more homogeneous lung inflation. This method eliminates the need for potentially hazardous interventions such as lung recruitment maneuvers and is safer and more effective [1].

31.2 Long Effects

Biphasic cuirass ventilation is an alternative method for patients suffering from chronic obstructive pulmonary disease (COPD) who are characterized by carbon dioxide retention, secretion clearance, and muscle fatigue [2].

Negative pressure ventilation (NPV) was successful in lowering $PaCO_2$ and strengthening respiratory muscles in patients experiencing an acute exacerbation of COPD. NPV decreased the electrical and mechanical activity of the inspiratory muscles in patients with COPD and restrictive diseases that cause chronic respiratory failure [2].

For cough assistance and secretion clearance by High Frequency Oscillation (HFO), the cuirass can be applied while seated in a chair or on the bed. Forced vital capacity, blood gases, and inspiratory muscle strength have all improved when BCV is applied periodically, daily, or weekly [2]. Especially in patients presenting with cystic fibrosis, an inherited disease with mucociliary dysfunction, facilitating the cuirass ventilator's "secretion clearance" mode, mucus plugging is mobilized and extracted out of the airways, thus protecting patients from infections [3].

Individuals diagnosed with neuromuscular disorders, including Duchenne muscular dystrophy, myotonic dystrophy, spinal muscular atrophy, Pompe disease, and amyotrophic lateral sclerosis, exhibit an ineffective cough, impaired clearance, airway obstruction, restrictive lung disease, dysphagia and aspiration-related swallowing difficulties, recurrent respiratory infections, sleep-disordered breathing, alveolar hypoventilation, and respiratory failure. These patients requiring constant respiratory support often cannot adjust to non-invasive ventilation (NIV) due to claustrophobia, excessive airway secretions, or inability to wear a face mask. Given that they maintain physiological functions like speaking, coughing, swallowing, and feeding, biphasic cuirass ventilation might be a suitable option for them when compared to positive pressure ventilation [4].

Cuirass ventilatory devices can be a helpful tool in emergency or combat situations to quickly resuscitate patients experiencing acute respiratory distress. Caregivers wearing protective gear can quickly and easily apply the cuirass to apneic victims, and a portable respirator can initiate biphasic external cuirass-based ventilation if needed. Therefore, this ventilation technique may be useful if an adult victim of nerve agent (NA) poisoning needs immediate resuscitation respiratory support. Even with heavy protective gear on, non-medical staff without prior experience with patient ventilation could effectively operate the device and quickly initiate respiratory support. When facilitated for immediate respiratory support, this technique helps remove secretions and avoids the need for laryngoscopy [5].

Additionally, external biphasic ventilation has been used for adequate ventilation of neurosurgical patients after trauma, during general anesthesia for ear, nose, and throat (ENT) surgery (e.g., severe tracheal stenosis, microlaryngeal surgery), and failed endotracheal intubation [2].

Following coronary artery bypass grafting, biphasic cuirass ventilation with external high-frequency oscillations has also been demonstrated to enhance cardiac function. Increased intrapulmonary pressure in right ventricular failure or cardiogenic shock can be harmful to cardiac function, even though positive pressure ventilation is known to support a failing heart. A constant negative pressure can enhance oxygenation and provide the best possible alveolar ventilation. The right ventricle's afterload can be decreased and the pulmonary circulation can be improved with synchronized biphasic external cuirass ventilation. Continuous negative pressure can also be used to support the FRC [2].

Implementing cuirass ventilation could help to lessen the risks associated with invasive PPV. Weaning patients from invasive PPV not only improves quality of life but also lowers the risk of respiratory muscle atrophy, laryngeal damage, and ventilator-associated pneumonia—all of which are linked to prolonged mechanical ventilation [3].

According to published reports, negative pressure ventilation may play a significant role in treating patients who have acute respiratory failure secondary to SARS-COV-2 [6]. Given its ability to effectively support breathing, its favorable effects on cardiopulmonary hemodynamics, and its potential to reduce the risk of viral transmission to healthcare workers, NPV has been linked to a possible benefit during this pandemic. Furthermore, a combination of BCV and high-flow nasal oxygenation (HFNO) utilized in a COVID-19 pneumonia patient resulted in the successful weaning of prolonged NIV and de-escalating therapy [7].

31.3 Term Applications

In addition to chronic respiratory and neuromuscular diseases, biphasic cuirass ventilation has been used in a variety of other conditions.

In the literature are described cases of successful anesthesia wherein biphasic cuirass ventilation was used to support adequate ventilation and oxygenation during tracheobronchial stent implantation or removal procedures involving rigid bronchoscopy. It must be verified that the airway is kept open before utilizing BCV for stenting operations. Other supportive measures, such as ECMO, should be considered when the airway is almost completely blocked prior to surgery and tumor resection is planned. This would significantly increase the risk of total obstruction from bleeding and tumor debris [8].

The use of BCV during interventional bronchoscopy with a rigid bronchoscope enabled the preservation of minute ventilation during treatment and the administration of adequate anesthesia, indicating the potential clinical utility of this technique [9].

BCV enabled a patient suffering from inherited spinocerebellar degeneration to be weaned off positive pressure ventilation without oxygen administration. It was possible to successfully facilitate secretion clearance and chest physical therapy during BCV. Increased ventilation and the resolution of respiratory failure could have been caused by improved pulmonary thorax compliance and decreased atelectasis [10].

BCV can decrease the duration of time required to wean off PPV and increase the probability of success in the short and long terms by offering an additional therapeutic tool. BCV offers an alternative that does not require a trach or facial interface, allowing patients who cannot consider the loads on the cardiopulmonary system or who are neurologically incapable in the foreseeable future. This method maximizes pulmonary health and maintains clear lungs. For these patients, BCV can create new avenues for discharge and offer a way to reduce the risk of pulmonary disease-related readmission [11].

31.4 Summary of Clinical Studies

Vincenzi and colleagues [12] combined positive and negative ventilation on elderly patients suffering from severe acute respiratory failure in order to maximize their advantages while lowering their drawbacks and side effects. A novel mechanical breathing technique developed out of this research; it employs two ventilators concurrently to administer positive pressure (either non-invasively or invasively) within the airways and negative pressure externally to the thorax via a chest shell [12].

The potential for increased pulmonary recruitment, particularly in the posterior regions of the lungs that were previously challenging to recruit with positive pressure ventilation and were also having trouble determining the optimal driving pressure, is undoubtedly a significant advantage of this coordinated approach [12].

An observational study by Sato et al. [13] found that using BCV significantly improved gas exchange and cardiac function in patients with acute exacerbation of chronic respiratory failure and secondary pulmonary hypertension (PH), suggesting that this treatment modality is promising for these patients [13].

Compared to positive pressure ventilation, ex situ lung perfusion (ESLP) prior to transplantation employing negative pressure ventilation results in reduced ventilator-induced lung injury [14]. A single-arm interventional study demonstrated that this mode of ventilation enabled the preservation and evaluation of donor lungs with all grafts. Patients managed to survive up to 30 days and recovered enough to be discharged from the hospital. With no patients exhibiting primary graft dysfunction scores of grade 3 at 72 hours or needing postoperative extracorporeal membrane oxygenation, this trial further proved the safety and viability of ex situ lung perfusion [14].

Following a transplant, patients who need invasive bridging techniques still experience worse outcomes than recipients who do not. Negative pressure ventilation (NPV) offers a less invasive respiratory support strategy for a group of patients as a transition to lung transplantation. In order to ensure effective airflow into the lung, NPV alternately applies atmospheric (zero) and sub-atmospheric (negative) pressures around the abdomen and thorax [15].

Comparing Fontan subjects to controls, short-term, non-invasive external thoraco-abdominal ventilation has been linked to significantly higher CO and pulmonary blood flow (PBF) as determined by cardiovascular magnetic resonance imaging. When compared to negative pressure ventilation, biphasic ventilation increased vascular flow to a greater extent [16].

Biphasic Cuirass Ventilation has the potential to reduce central venous pressure (CVP) in the Fontan circulation and to expectorate casts as a respiratory physical therapy tool, which makes it a potentially useful treatment for plastic bronchitis (PB). Intractable dyspnea associated with plastic bronchitis (PB) was treated with BCV, which improved protein-losing enteropathy (PLE) symptoms the patient also exhibited. The patient with Fontan circulation may see an improvement in their hemodynamics as a result of BCV increasing CO, according to the non-invasive hemodynamic monitor [17].

Using BCV has been effective in ensuring sufficient ventilation and secretion clearance, leading to the resolution of atelectasis. It is simple to use, well tolerated, and does not exhibit any side effects. An additional benefit of BCV is that it can postpone the unavoidable requirement for a tracheostomy and traditional mechanical ventilation.

31.5 Conclusion

Standardizing the use of BCV is a challenging task due to the limited scope of current research on the subject, which consists of case reports and review articles. Randomized controlled trials are required to fully evaluate the benefits and drawbacks of cuirass ventilators and to expand the range of medical applications for them.

References

1. Aloan C. Non-invasive ventilation in the post-acute care setting. Continued.com - Respir Ther. 2024:218. Available at www.continued.com/respiratory-therapy
2. Linton DM. Cuirass ventilation: a review and update. Crit Care Resusc. 2005;7(1):22–8.
3. Onweni C, Rashid S, Goswami R, et al. Cuirass ventilation: an alternative home-based modality for chronic respiratory failure. Home Health Care Manag Pract. 2020;32(1):40–4.
4. Annunziata A, Calabrese C, Simioli F, Coppola A, Flora M, Marotta A, Di Spirito V, Didonna F, Cicalese M, Fiorentino G. Negative-pressure ventilation in neuromuscular diseases in the acute setting. J Clin Med. 2022;11(9):2589.
5. Gur I, Bar-Yishay E, Ben-Abraham R. Biphasic extrathoracic cuirass ventilation for resuscitation. Am J Emerg Med. 2005;23(4):488–91.
6. Sallam M. Is negative pressure ventilation a reasonable answer during COVID era? MAR Pediatr. 2023;3(4)
7. Almeida Borges J, Esquinas AM. Biphasic cuirass ventilation in the escalation of non-invasive ventilation in COVID-19: case report and review. Monaldi Arch Chest Dis. 2023;93(4).
8. Mori H, Shono A, Hirade R, Nikai T, Saito Y. Biphasic cuirass ventilation during anesthesia for tracheobronchial stent insertion or removal by a rigid bronchoscope: a case report. A A Pract. 2018;10(8):198–200.
9. Kanda H. The Clinical Usefulness of Biphasic Cuirass Ventilation in the Prevention of Hypoventilation During Interventional Bronchoscopy Using a Rigid Bronchoscope. Chest. 2012;142(4_MeetingAbstracts):866A.
10. Nishiyama K, Sakaguchi Y, Sato T, Kodaka M, Nishimura Y, Komori M. Improvement of postoperative atelectasis in response to biphasic cuirass ventilation in a patient who was receiving noninvasive positive pressure ventilation at home. J Jpn Soc Intens Care Med. 2012;19(2):247–8.
11. Mefford G. Biphasic cuirass ventilation as a tool to expedite weaning from positive pressure ventilation. Respir Ther. 2014;9(2).
12. Vincenzi U. A new mode of mechanical ventilation: positive + negative synchronized ventilation. Multidiscip Respir Med. 2021;16(1):788.
13. Sato Y, Saeki N, Asakura T, Aoshiba K, Kotani T. Effects of extrathoracic mechanical ventilation on pulmonary hypertension secondary to lung disease. J Anesth. 2016;30(4):663–70.
14. Buchko MT, Boroumand N, Cheng JC, Hirji A, Halloran K, Freed DH, et al. Clinical transplantation using negative pressure ventilation ex situ lung perfusion with extended criteria donor lungs. Nat Commun. 2020;11(1):5765.
15. Martínez MDP, Alvarez FG, Mallea JM, Shah SZ, Pham SM, El-Sayed Ahmed MM, Jacob S, Janik AB, Haddad T, Erasmus DB, Narula T. Negative pressure ventilation as a bridge to lung transplant. Oxf Med Case Rep. 2020;2020(8):omaa056.
16. Charla P, Karur GR, Yamamura K, Yoo SJ, Granton JT, Oechslin EN, Shah A, Benson LN, Honjo O, Mertens L, Alonso-Gonzalez R, Hanneman K, Wald RM. Augmentation of pulmonary blood flow and cardiac output by non-invasive external ventilation late after Fontan palliation. Heart. 2021;107(2):142–9.
17. Okada S, Muneuchi J, Nagatomo Y, Nonaka K, Iida C, Shirouzu H, Matsuoka R, Watanabe M, Joo K. Successful treatment of protein-losing enteropathy and plastic bronchitis by biphasic cuirass ventilation in a patient with failing Fontan circulation. Int Heart J. 2018;59(4):873–6.

32 Biphasic Cuirass Ventilation (BCV): Ethics, Palliative Medicine, and Quality of Life

Mehmet Gökhan Gök and Dilek Özcengiz

32.1 Introduction

Another area of use of noninvasive mechanical ventilation (NIMV) is palliative care. Since one of the main goals of palliative care is to reduce dyspnea in terminally ill patients, NIMV can be used for this purpose [1, 2]. The application standards of NIMV treatment may differ in patients receiving palliative care. The issue of when to start and when to stop respiratory support is still controversial. The respiratory status of the patients prior to palliative care, including factors like chronic respiratory disease, previous long-term oxygen use, and home ventilation devices, should be considered. Although there are no clear boundaries regarding this issue, there is literature data defining some classifications. Since palliative care is a dynamic process, scenarios may change. During the process, risks, benefits, and treatment preferences are evaluated periodically with families, patients, and the healthcare team; it should be remembered that goals may change [2, 3].

When patients and their families do not accept invasive life support such as endotracheal intubation (ETI) during the palliative care process, NIMV may be a treatment option. However, this approach may conflict with their decision to reject all life support measures. It should be emphasized that NIMV treatment is used only to reduce dyspnea. In the palliative care process, treatment options should contribute to the patient's comfort and to the goal of a comfortable end-of-life. They should not prolong the death process [4, 5].

Several issues may arise with the use of NIMV in palliative care. One significant concern is that NIMV might contradict the patient's or family's decision to refuse all life support measures. Additionally, patients might feel discomfort with the NIMV mask, be unwilling to use it, experience increased claustrophobia, or believe

M. G. Gök · D. Özcengiz (✉)
Department of Anesthesiology and Reanimation, Intensive Care Unit, Cukurova University, Adana, Turkey

O. Alibrahim et al. (eds.), *Biphasic Cuirass Noninvasive Ventilation*, Noninvasive Ventilation. The Essentials, https://doi.org/10.1007/978-3-032-20933-7_32

they are unable to communicate while using it. Biphasic cuirass ventilation (BCV) may be an option both in terms of its suitability for combination with other respiratory support options and in cases where other treatment options that provide NIMV with positive pressure are difficult to use [2–5].

32.2 Advantages of BCV in Palliative Care

BCV is a noninvasive ventilation method that can significantly help alleviate respiratory distress and enhance the quality of life for end-of-life patients. BCV's portability, lightweight design, and ease of use in a home setting make it a more accessible option for palliative care patients compared to other mechanical ventilation methods. Research indicates that BCV can increase patient comfort and reduce anxiety more effectively than other ventilation techniques in palliative care.

Studies have demonstrated that the use of BCV in palliative care can improve the quality of life and decrease suffering by alleviating respiratory distress. However, its tolerability may be limited by factors such as mask discomfort or patient anxiety. At the end-of-life stage, BCV has been reported to enhance both the quality and duration of life. Caregivers have also noted improvements in patient comfort and reductions in anxiety with the use of BCV [6, 7].

32.3 Ethical Considerations

Caregivers must carefully balance comfort and symptom management in patients receiving BCV therapy. BCV use should not merely prolong the dying process without improving the patient's symptom burden and quality of life. It is important to consider whether BCV truly improves patient comfort and dignity or merely delays the natural process of dying [6].

The use of BCV in palliative care raises several ethical issues, including the distinction between allowing patients to die with dignity and hastening death and the potential for claims of euthanasia or physician-assisted suicide. Clinicians must carefully balance the patient's wishes for comfort and quality of life with the risk of inadvertently shortening the patient's life through the use of BCV and related medications [6, 7].

Clinicians should consider the wishes of the patient and family, primarily regarding quality and dignity of life, when determining the appropriate use of BCV. A structured professional framework for support and ethical guidance is important to ensure confidence in patients, families, and caregivers when using BCV in palliative care [8]. Family members often provide the patient's daily care and best understand the patient's needs and wishes, so they should be closely involved in the decision-making process. Open communication among the patient, family, and healthcare team is essential, as families may have different perspectives or preferences regarding BCV use than the patient [9]. Families can ensure that the patient's wishes are met and that BCV use is consistent with the patient's goals of care [10, 11].

Apart from all these ethical principles, another important point during the use of BCV is the application of palliative sedation. The doctrine of double effect (DDE) is an important ethical principle in palliative sedation practices in end-of-life care. This principle is often invoked to justify actions that have both positive and negative consequences, particularly when the intention is to achieve a good outcome while accepting the possibility of a harmful side effect. The DDE is frequently cited to justify this practice, as it allows healthcare providers to relieve suffering even when there is a risk that sedation may hasten death. The ongoing debate highlights the need for careful ethical consideration and a nuanced understanding of the complexities involved in end-of-life care [12].

The personal beliefs of family caregivers can significantly impact decision-making regarding the care of their loved ones, especially in end-of-life situations. Some key ways beliefs impact decisions include the following.

Spiritual and Religious Beliefs: Caregivers who are religious or spiritual may rely on their faith to guide difficult decisions. They may consult with clergy, pray for guidance, or make choices that align with their religious values [13].

Moral and Ethical Principles: Caregivers' personal moral compasses shape their views on issues such as quality of life, life extension, and euthanasia. Dutiful beliefs that focus on duties/rules may lead to different choices than consequentialist beliefs that weigh consequences [14].

Cultural Background: Cultural norms around family obligations, gender roles, and the meaning of illness/death may influence caregiving decisions. Collectivist cultures emphasize family harmony over individual autonomy [14].

Past Experiences: Caregivers draw on their own or their families' previous experiences with illness, death, and the healthcare system. Positive and negative memories shape expectations and decisions [15].

Emotional Factors: Guilt, fear, grief, and love profoundly influence caregiving choices. Caregivers may make decisions to avoid regret or to honor their loved one's wishes, even when this is difficult [15].

As caregivers aim to act in their loved one's best interests, their personal beliefs inevitably shape their perceptions of what this means. Recognizing these influences can help caregivers make more value-oriented decisions. Open communication with healthcare providers about beliefs and values is key to collaborative decision-making. Establishing a structured professional framework for support and ethical guidance is crucial to providing confidence to patients, families, and caregivers during the use of BCV in palliative care [15, 16].

References

1. Rochwerg B, Brochard L, Elliott MW, et al. Official ERS/ATS clinical practice guidelines: noninvasive ventilation for acute respiratory failure. Eur Respir J. 2017;50(2):1602426.
2. Tripodoroa VA, Rabecc CA, Vito EL. Withdrawing noninvasive ventilation at end-of-life care: is there a right time? Curr Opin Support Palliat Care. 2019;13(4):344–50.
3. Curtis JR, Cook DJ, Sinuff T, et al. Noninvasive positive pressure ventilation in critical and palliative care settings: understanding the goals of therapy. Crit Care Med. 2007;35:932–9.
4. Davies JD. Noninvasive respiratory support at the end of life. Respir Care. 2019;64:701–11.
5. Wilson ME, Majzoub AM, Dobler CC, et al. Noninvasive ventilation in patients with do-not-intubate and comfort-measures-only orders: a systematic review and meta-analysis. Crit Care Med. 2018;46:1209–16.
6. Onweni C, Rashid S, Goswami R. Cuirass ventilation: an alternative home-based modality for chronic respiratory failure. Home Health Care Manag Pract. 2019;32(1):108482231987511.
7. Krivec U, Caggiano S. Noninvasive ventilation in palliative care and ethical dilemma. Front Pediatr. 2020;8:483.
8. Szalados JE. Discontinuation of mechanical ventilation at end-of-life: The ethical and legal boundaries of physician conduct in termination of life support. Crit Care Clin. 2007;23(2):317–37.
9. Symmons SM, Ryan K, Aoun SA. Decision-making in palliative care: patient and family caregiver concordance and discordance— systematic review and narrative synthesis. BMJ Support Palliat Care. 2023;13:374–85.
10. Wu X, Wang L, Wang N, et al. Influencing factors of decision-making for palliative care in family members of elderly people. J Nurs. 2022;29(18):12–7.
11. Oosterhout SPC, Daisy J, Amstel FKP, et al. Experiences of bereaved family caregivers with shared decision making in palliative cancer treatment: a qualitative interview study. BMC Palliat Care. 2021;20:137.
12. Faris H, Dewar B, Dyason C, et al. Goods, causes and intentions: problems with applying the doctrine of double effect to palliative sedation. BMC Med Ethics. 2021;22:141.
13. Koenig TL. Caregivers' use of spirituality in ethical decision-making. J Gerontol Soc Work. 2005;45(1–2):155–72.
14. Mitnick S, Leffler C, Hood VL, et al. Family caregivers, patients and physicians: ethical guidance to optimize relationships. J Gen Intern Med. 25(3):255–60.
15. When caregivers have to make difficult decisions for their parents. CICOA Aging and In-Home Solutions. December 20, 2019.
16. Bechthold AC, Azuero A, Puga F, et al. What is most important to family caregivers when helping patients make treatment-related decisions: findings from a National Survey. Cancers (Basel). 2023;15(19):4792.

GPSR Compliance

The European Union's (EU) General Product Safety Regulation (GPSR) is a set of rules that requires consumer products to be safe and our obligations to ensure this.

If you have any concerns about our products, you can contact us on ProductSafety@springernature.com

In case Publisher is established outside the EU, the EU authorized representative is:

Springer Nature Customer Service Center GmbH
Europaplatz 3
69115 Heidelberg, Germany

Batch number: 10726060

Printed by Printforce, the Netherlands